Foundation for Medical Communication

Foundation for Medical Communication

ESTHER CALDWELL
BARBARA R. HEGNER

RESTON PUBLISHING COMPANY, INC.
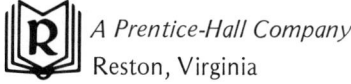
A Prentice-Hall Company
Reston, Virginia

Library of Congress Cataloging in Publication Data

Caldwell, Esther.
   Foundations of medical communication.

   Includes index.
   1. Medicine—Terminology 2. Communication in medicine. I. Hegner, Barbara R., joint author.
II. Title. [DNLM: 1. Nomenclature. 2. Communication. W15 C147r]
R123.C18   610'.1'4   77-17349
ISBN 0-87909-299-8
      0-87909-298-x(pbk.)

©1978 by Reston Publishing Company, Inc.
A Prentice-Hall Company
Reston, Virginia 22090

All rights reserved. No part of this book may be reproduced in any way, or by any means, without permission in writing from the publisher.

10 9 8 7 6 5 4 3 2 1
Printed in the United States of America

Table of Contents

Preface ix

1 The Community Health Team 1
DOCTORS AND PATIENTS 1,   NURSES AND NURSE PRACTITIONERS 4,
EMERGENCY SERVICES 6,   PHARMACISTS 6,   HOMEMAKING
SERVICES 7,   COMMUNITY HEALTH FACILITIES 7,   CLINICS AND
CLINICAL CARE 8,   LONG-TERM CARE FACILITIES 10,   HOSPITALS—
GENERAL AND SPECIAL 10,   VOLUNTARY HEALTH ASSOCIATIONS 11,
SUMMARY 14,   *PRACTICE & REVIEW* 15

2 The Hospital Health Team 17
HOSPITAL VOLUNTEERS 17,   HOSPITAL PROFESSIONALS 17,
MEDICAL SPECIALISTS 18,   NURSING STAFF 23,   SUPPORTIVE
SERVICES 24,   HOSPITAL ORGANIZATION 25,   THE PATIENT UNIT 26,
HOSPITAL DEPARTMENTS 27,   *SUMMARY* 33,   *PRACTICE &
REVIEW* 33

3 Non-oral and Symbolic Communications 35
SIGNS AND SYMBOLS 36,   LOGOS FOR HEALTH GROUPS 36,
PROFESSIONAL ORGANIZATIONS 37,   THE HOSPITAL AS WORK
ENVIRONMENT 39,   WARNING SIGNS 39,   *SUMMARY* 47,
PRACTICE & REVIEW 48

4 Combining Word Forms 51
SUMMARY 66,   *PRACTICE & REVIEW* 66

5 Common Medical Abbreviations 69
HEALTH WORKER ABBREVIATIONS 72,   HOSPITAL DEPARTMENT
ABBREVIATIONS 73,   ABBREVIATIONS FOR TESTS 75,
ABBREVIATIONS FOR COMMON HEALTH PROBLEMS 75,   THE PHYSICAL
EXAMINATION 76,   BODY PLANES AND LANDMARKS 81,   TIME AND
MEASUREMENTS 88,   ROMAN NUMERALS 89,   *SUMMARY* 93,
PRACTICE & REVIEW, 93

6 **Basic Medical Asepsis** 96
   MICROORGANISMS 96, IDENTIFICATION OF BACTERIA 101, BODY DEFENSES 104, EXTERNAL CONTROL OF MICROBES 107, NOSOCOMIAL INFECTIONS 110, *SUMMARY* 111, *PRACTICE & REVIEW* 111

7 **The Patient: Focus of Concern** 113
   PERSONAL CHARACTERISTICS 117, EXPLANATION TO PATIENT 117, PROFESSIONAL COMMUNICATIONS 118, ORDERS FOR PATIENT CARE 118, HOSPITAL ASSIGNMENTS 120, LEGAL CONSIDERATIONS 121, ETHICS 122, DISEASE 124, THE DIAGNOSIS 126, THERAPEUTIC REGIMES 126, *SUMMARY* 128, *PRACTICE & REVIEW* 128

8 **Human Development** 130
   CELLS—BASIC UNITS OF HUMAN STRUCTURE 130, EMBRYOLOGY 133, OBSTETRICS 136, *SUMMARY* 143, *PRACTICE & REVIEW* 143

9 **The Integumentary System** 146
   STRUCTURE OF THE SKIN 147, *SUMMARY* 158, *PRACTICE & REVIEW* 158

10 **The Respiratory System** 160
    CELLULAR RESPIRATION 160, THE RESPIRATORY TRACT 161, RESPIRATION 166, *SUMMARY* 172, *PRACTICE & REVIEW* 172

11 **The Musculoskeletal System** 174
    THE BONES 175, JOINTS 181, MUSCULOSKELETAL PATHOLOGY 186, *SUMMARY* 190, *PRACTICE & REVIEW* 191

12 **The Cardiovascular System** 193
    THE BODY FLUIDS 193, THE HEART 198, THE VASCULATURE 203, *SUMMARY* 209, *PRACTICE & REVIEW* 210

13 **The Endocrine System** 212
    ENDOCRINE GLANDS 212, *SUMMARY* 222, *PRACTICE & REVIEW* 222

14 **The Nervous System** 224
    NERVOUS SYSTEM DIVISIONS 228, *SUMMARY* 239, *PRACTICE & REVIEW* 240

15 **The Gastrointestinal System** 242
    THE NUTRIENTS 242, ALIMENTARY CANAL 244, ACCESSORY STRUCTURES 251, *SUMMARY* 254, *PRACTICE & REVIEW* 254

16 **The Urinary System** 257
    ENZYME SYSTEMS 258, THE KIDNEYS 260, *SUMMARY* 268, *PRACTICE & REVIEW* 268

17 The Reproductive System   271
    THE INTERNAL FEMAL ORGANS 271,   THE EXTERNAL FEMALS GENITALIA 277,   THE MALE GENITALIA 278,   VENEREAL DISEASE 279,   *SUMMARY* 282,   *PRACTICE & REVIEW* 282

18 Respiratory Care   284
    AIR POLLUTANTS 285,   PULMONARY FUNCTION TESTS 287,   MEDICAL GASES 289,   AEROSOLS 290,   CHEST PHYSICAL THERAPY 291,   *SUMMARY* 297,   *PRACTICE & REVIEW* 298

19 Radiology and Radiotherapy   300
    CHEMICAL ELEMENTS 301,   DIAGNOSTIC RADIOLOGY 302,   SAFETY PRECAUTIONS 305,   FLUOROSCOPY 309,   RADIOTHERAPY 310,   NUCLEAR MEDICINE 310,   *SUMMARY* 313,   *PRACTICE & REVIEW* 313

20 Communication with Medical Records   315
    UNOFFICIAL RECORDS 315,   OFFICIAL RECORDS 318,   PATIENT IDENTIFICATION 323,   RECORD STORAGE 327,   *SUMMARY* 329,   *PRACTICE & REVIEW* 330

    Glossary   333

Preface

The language of medicine is verbal and symbolic and seemingly filled with mystery to the uninformed. It is the purpose of this text to unshroud the mystery while laying a foundation for understanding the fascinating work in the medical and allied health disciplines.

The authors believe that words learned out of context become meaningless signs and symbols which can be memorized fleetingly but are rarely retained. So the format of this text has been designed to help you as a beginning health student to master new medical terms and modes of communication. Then with basic terms well understood, you can continue to build an "on-the-job" or functional vocabulary while pursuing your career specialty.

Medical personnel communicate vital information to each other constantly—directly through conversations, oral reports and the use of symbols, and indirectly through written reports and orders, laboratory reports and case summaries. You will find all these in use in the narratives about the sick people whose health problems are outlined here. New words and their pronunciations are always introduced on the opening page of each chapter. Study them carefully.

Foundation for Medical Communication is not intended to replace a good medical dictionary. Be sure to make one a part of your medical reference library. Remember, health personnel, such as doctors, nurses, medical assistants, dental assistants, radiologists, inhalation therapists, and others must communicate effectively in order to maintain continuity in health care. Not only will you as a health worker need to communicate with other health staff, but often your interpretive ability will also ease the anxiety and frustration of patients. Make notes in this book's margins, and ask your instructor to give you additional exercises whenever you want to learn more about a special topic.

E.C.
B.R.H.

Foundation for
Medical Communication

After studying Chapter 1
The Community Health Team
You should be able to:

* Pronounce and define each of its new medical words and phrases and use the new technical jargon.

* Name ten community health workers.

* List three long-term care facilities.

PRONOUNCE THESE TEN NEW WORDS WITH YOUR TEACHER: MEDICAL WORDS

milieu (me-lyuh′)
catastrophic (kat″as-trah-fĭk)
therapeutic regime (ther″ah-pu′tĭk)
rehabilitation (re″hah-bil″ĭ-ta′shun)
obesity (o-bes″ĭ-te)

genes (jēns)
primipara (pri-mip′ah-rah)
continuum (kon′tin-u-um)
orthopedics (or″tho-pe′diks)
obstetrics (ob″stĕ-triks)

Within the framework of any community, there is a wide range of health services. The nature of a community partly determines the types of health services that are offered and the kinds of personnel required to fulfill the need.

The people providing community health care make up a team of professional and **ancilliary** (assisting) workers. They offer their skills and services in a variety of diverse settings—to people in their homes, in clinics or centers, at their place of work or study, and in the more formal setting of the hospital.

Everyone is aware that **physicians** (medical doctors) work within hospitals but their presence is also very much in evidence within the community. The **practicing** (active and performing the normal duties) physician usually has an office in the community where he sees patients and provides treatment. People who use the doctor's service and the services of other health workers are called patients.

DOCTORS AND PATIENTS

DOCTORS AND PATIENTS 1 *

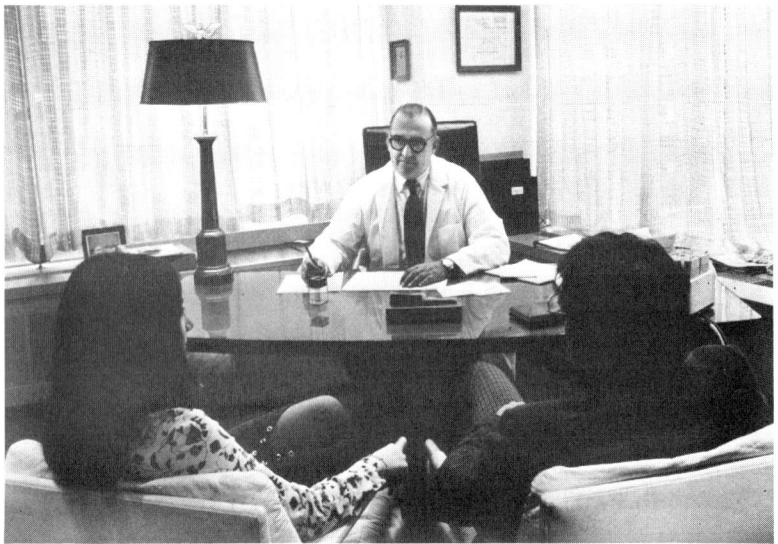

Figure 1-1: The physician sees patients in his office *(courtesy of Holland-Rantos Company, Inc.)*

Patients, then, are people who are being treated for an illness or disease. The doctor is a professional health worker who provides direct primary care to patients, assessing their ill condition and prescribing the **therapeutic regime** (treatment program). Frequently the doctor sends patients to the hospital for special care that cannot be provided in the office. He or she supervises and directs the **in-patient** (hospitalized) care during the hospital stay and continues seeing patients as **out-patients** (not hospitalized) after discharge.

While some doctors work independently, there is a trend today toward group practice. These groups vary in size, but their members frequently provide basic surgical and medical services in addition to specialty services, such as **orthopedics** (bone) and **obstetrics** (maternity).

The **surgeon** is a doctor who treats patients with unhealthy conditions that respond best to **surgery** (operations with instruments) or to certain other manual treatments. When any physician member of a group has a patient requiring an operation, he notifies the surgeon and refers that patient to that doctor for treatment.

For example, Mrs. Swanson went to see Dr. Gienofsky, her family doctor, because she was sick to her stomach and had a severe pain in her side. After examining her, Dr. Gienofsky referred her to Dr. Faulkner because he suspected that she was suffering from an inflamed appendix. After examining Mrs. Swanson, Dr. Faulkner agreed with Dr. Gienofsky's evaluation.

That afternoon Mrs. Swanson entered the hospital as an inpatient, where her appendix was **surgically** (pertaining to surgery) removed by Dr. Faulkner, the surgeon.

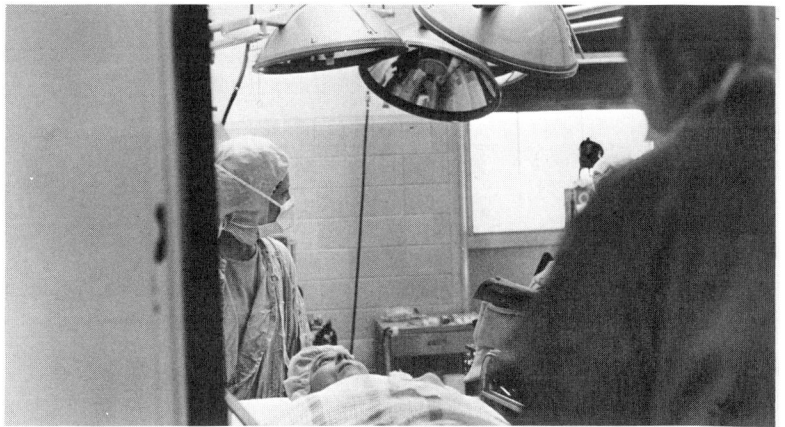

Figure 1-2: The patient's appendix was surgically removed by the surgeon *(courtesy of Northwestern Memorial Hospital, Chicago).*

The doctor does not handle all the office work himself. Other members of the office health team include nurses or **medical assistants** (persons particularly trained to assist the physician and clerical personnel).

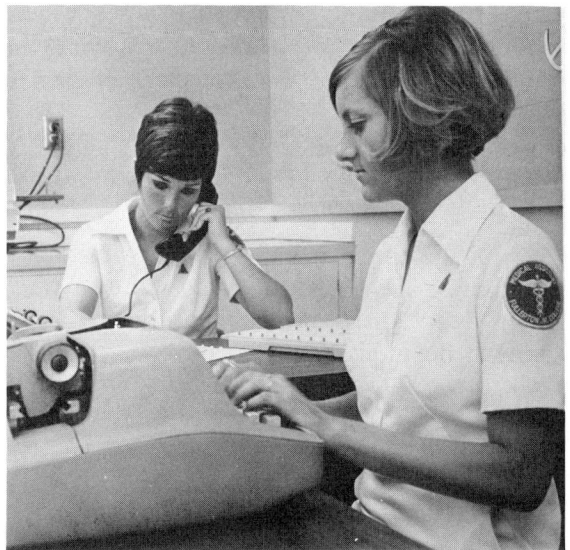

Figure 1-3: The medical assistant is specially trained to assist the physician *(courtesy of American Association of Medical Assistants, Inc.).*

In some communities, the primary care by physicians in private practice is augmented by another specially trained person called the **Physician's Assistant**. The Physician's Assistant is a relatively new member of the physician's team. He or she is a person who has been trained to assume some of the doctor's routine work, thus freeing the doctor for other duties. Physician's Assistants sometimes use the initials P.A. after their names.

Physicians also work in most of the other community health care settings that will be described later.

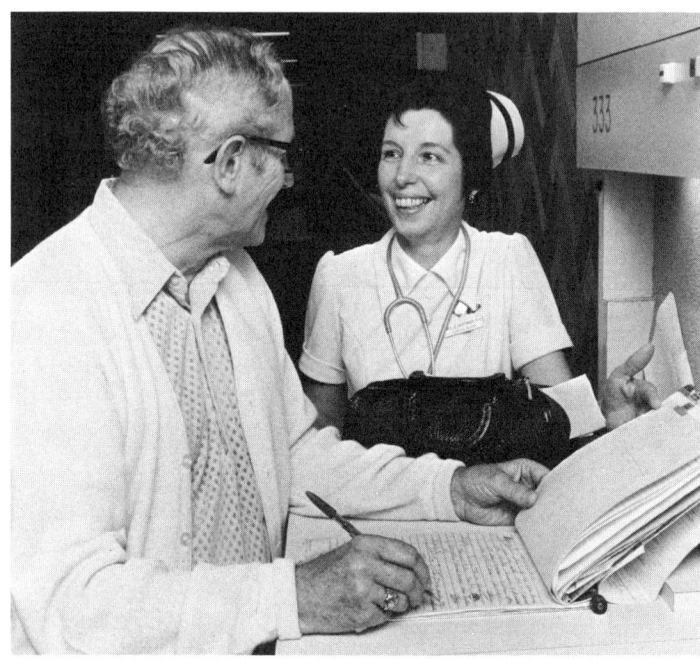

Figure 1-4: The nurse functions in a variety of community health settings

NURSES AND NURSE PRACTITIONERS

Nurses are persons who are specifically trained in caring for the sick who are receiving either medical or surgical treatment. Nurses are professional health workers. They usually work in hospitals but they are found within the community as well. Nurses function in doctors' offices, clinics, schools and industry. Their services are very diverse, ranging from direct care in a person's home to the direct nursing service offered by private nurse practitioners.

Many nurses today are adding to their educations by earning degrees at universities and colleges and by increasing their level of professional competeny with clinical training. Some of these nurses who are additionally prepared, provide nursing services to patients from their own offices in the community. They are called **nurse practitioners**.

* 4 *THE COMMUNITY HEALTH TEAM*

Private nursing practice is a fairly new trend in **primary** (direct) care. The nurse in private practice has advanced training. In addition to giving direct care, such as checking blood pressure, a nurse practitioner spends considerable time teaching health care, interpreting physicians' orders, and counseling outpatients. Patients utilizing this professional nursing service are frequently referred to as "**clients**." You will find nurses working in every community health setting.

Public health nurses provide health assistance through the operation of health clinics and in some cases, home visits. They focus their attention primarily on health matters which affect large numbers of people in the community, such as tuberculosis screening. Public health nurses are also involved in public health education, enforcement of community health laws, and the gathering of health statistics.

Visiting nurses provide direct nursing care for patients who remain in their own homes. Often a family member can provide much of the physical care for a sick person so long as a professional like the visiting nurse can come periodically to provide particular nursing services. These often include special medications.

Nurses are found in industry, offering health care for the injured and also teaching about preventative health practices.

School nurses perform a similar function for teachers, students, and their families. Nurses spend much of their time teaching regardless of the other nursing services offered.

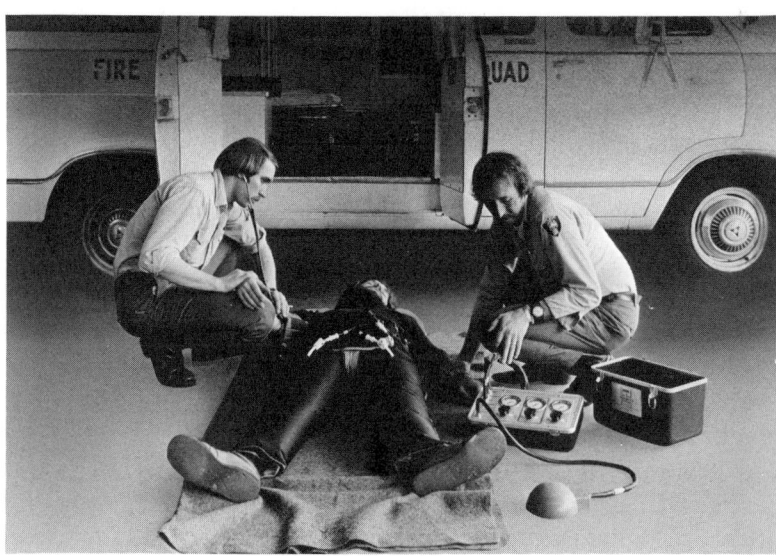

Figure 1-5: Paramedics (EMT's) are community health workers who provide emergency care *(courtesy of Jobst Institute)*.

NURSES AND NURSE PRACTITIONERS 5 *

EMERGENCY SERVICES Emergency care for citizens is provided in many communities by an important and rapidly growing branch of health personnel called **paramedics**, or emergency medical technicians. These paramedical workers are frequently assigned to work with fire departments because emergency medical techniques are often needed at fires. They also answer general accident or emergency calls, assess the injury or illness, communicate the situation to a doctor, and give immediate care as instructed.

In some communities, emergency care is offered in a special hospital department called the **Emergency Room**. Hospitals that operate emergency rooms or **accident rooms** have equipment and personnel available at all times to meet sudden, unexpected health needs.

Dentists are persons who are licensed to practice **dentistry**, the healing art concerned with the teeth and oral cavity. Dentists are professional community health workers who maintain community based offices and who are assisted in their work by dental assistants.

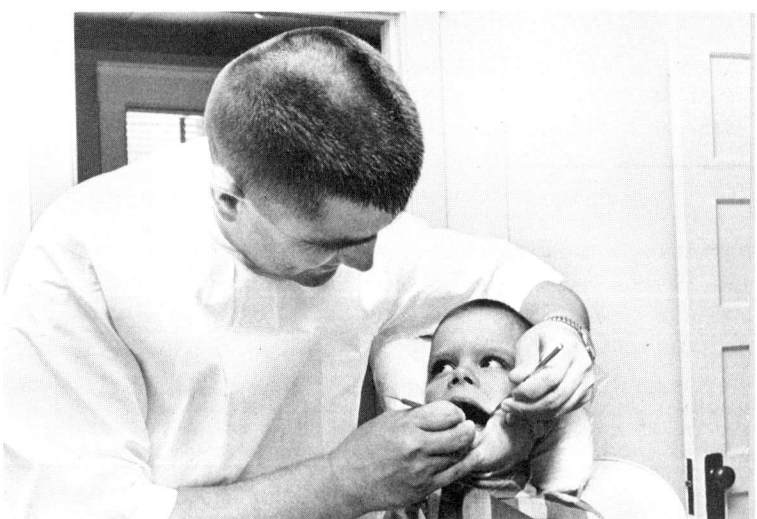

Figure 1-6: Dentistry, the healing art concerned with care of the teeth and oral cavity

PHARMACISTS **Dental Assistants** are persons specially trained to understand and facilitate the work of the dentist. The Dental Assistant helps the dentist maintain his office routines and his actual practice.

Pharmacists are also professional members of community health teams. They compound and dispense medications and drugs according to doctors' **prescriptions** (written instructions).

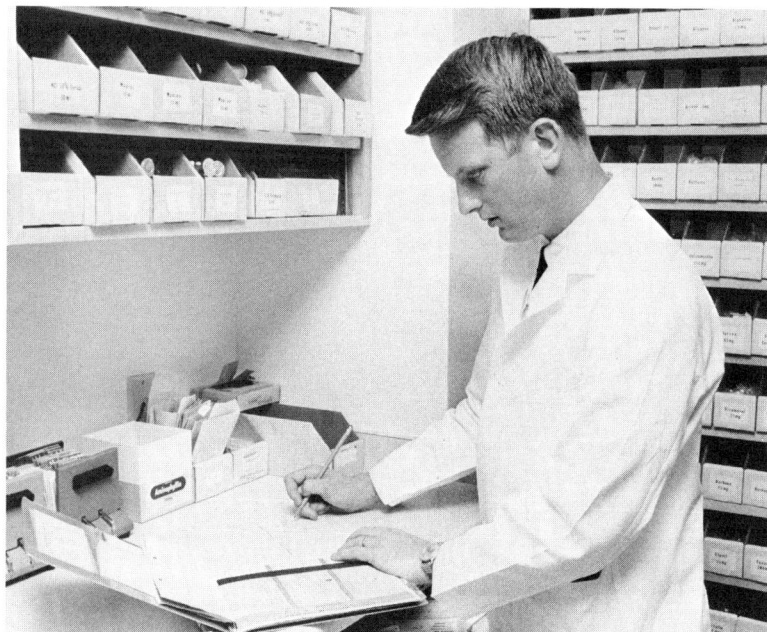

Figure 1-7: The pharmacist compounds and dispenses medicine

Many people in the community also see an expanding role for the pharmacist in teaching the correct use of the numerous non-prescription drugs which are available.

HOMEMAKING SERVICES

In some communities, **homemaking services** make it possible for sick people to remain in their own homes rather than be hospitalized. Such homemakers are responsible for maintaining a healthful **milieu** (environment). They may have purely household responsibilities or they may be one of the growing number of ancillary health workers who also have some basic nursing skills. They then provide some nursing care as well as housekeeping services.

Not all communities provide this service, but the number is growing. Homemaker services allow a **convalescent** (a person recovering) to come home from the hospital at a much earlier stage than would be otherwise possible.

COMMUNITY HEALTH FACILITIES

Many other members of the community health team are located in various community health facilities. Often community health **facilities** (agencies) offer services to patients with a wide range of needs.

Publicly supported health departments offer testing for and protection against diseases that are easily passed from one

COMMUNITY HEALTH FACILITIES 7 *

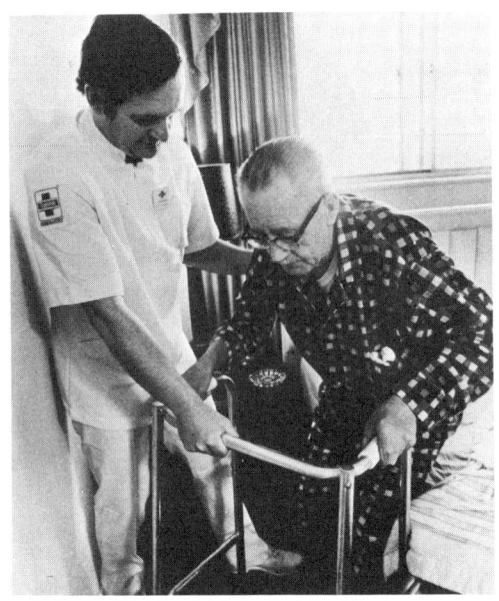

Figure 1-8: The Homemaker health care service makes it possible for a convalescent to come home earlier *(courtesy of Homemakers Home & Health Care Services, Inc.)*

CLINICS AND CLINICAL CARE person in the community to another. Many of the services provided by such a health department meet needs not met by the other agencies.

Clinics are facilities where patients are seen and treated by groups of physicians who are medical specialists. Such clinics are often part of a large hospital, or they may function as an independent agency.

Figure 1-9: Two outpatient pediatric clinics

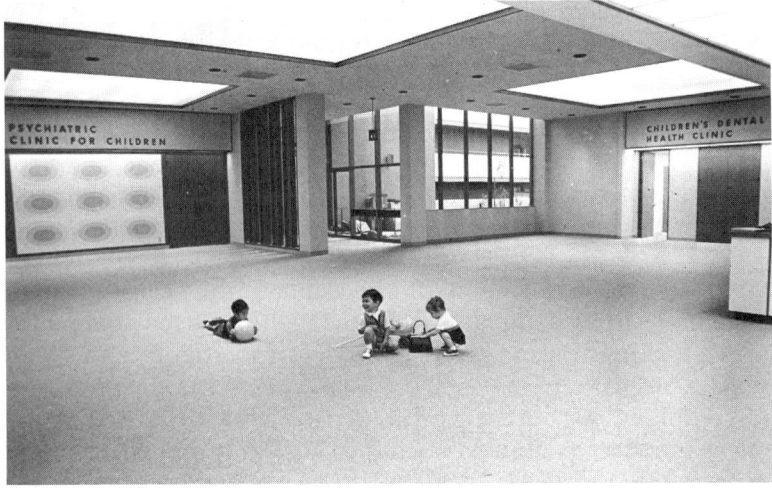

* 8 *THE COMMUNITY HEALTH TEAM*

Clinics offer concentrated special services that help patients make the transition from in-patient to out-patient and subsequently to independent status. A large general hospital may provide multiple clinical services. One such clinic might be the **rehabilitation** (restoration) clinic for **stroke** patients. A stroke patient has suffered damage to the nervous system because a blood vessel in the brain was broken or blocked.

Another clinic might be the **pulmonary** (pertaining to the lung) rehabilitation clinic. It offers help for those persons suffering from breathing problems. Still another clinic, the **arthritis** (inflammation in joints) rehabilitation clinic, is provided for those who find it difficult to carry out the normal physical activities of daily life because of painful joints.

Each of the preceding examples describes a clinic designed to help patients find ways to live more effectively with ongoing physical problems. When a severe physical burden, such as arthritis is present, the emotional life of the person is affected as well. Clinic personnel usually try to deal with all aspects of the patient's physical and emotional well-being. Sometimes a person's physical health deteriorates too because of emotional stress.

Other special clinics provide services to deal primarily with the emotional aspects of certain conditions such as **alcoholism** (drunkenness), **obesity** (overweight), compulsive smoking, and uncontrolled gambling.

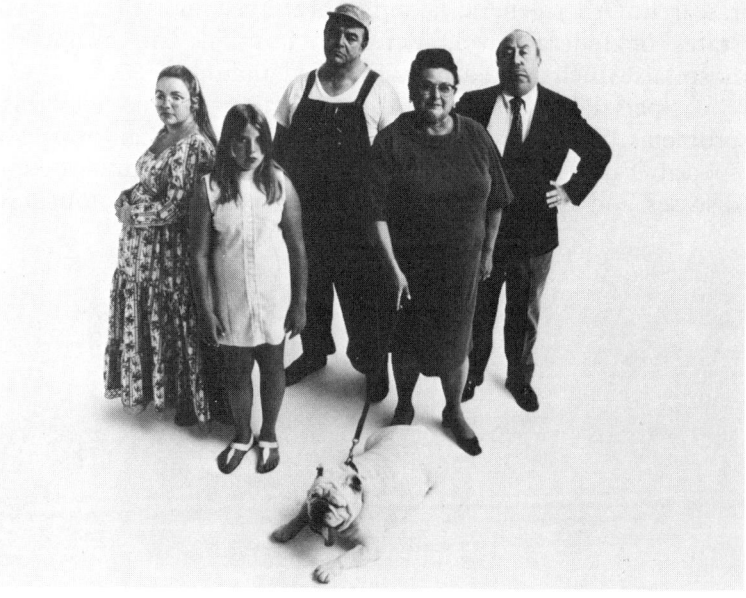

Figure 1-10: Obesity can be a health problem for people of all ages *(courtesy of Riker Laboratories, Inc.).*

LONG-TERM CARE FACILITIES

As people age, their health needs change, and sometimes they are not able to successfully cope with the stresses of aging and illness. Some of them who require total nursing care are housed and cared for in **long-term** facilities. Frequently called **nursing homes, rest homes,** and **convalescent hospitals,** these facilities try to meet all a patient's needs. Sometimes these facilities are used by older persons for short periods during times of increased stress or illness. Then, once improved, they return to their own homes. Many times, however, people spend their remaining years in such a facility.

There are many older patients who do not need the continued intensive care of the long-term health facility, of course. They continue to live in their own homes and care for themselves, selecting from the total community only the specific services that fulfill their health needs. You will meet them outside as "patients" in any one of the community facilities described.

HOSPITALS— GENERAL AND SPECIAL

Some communities have no hospital and some have several. A **general hospital** accepts patients of all ages regardless of their particular illness or need. Some general hospitals are privately operated and provide their service as a profit earning endeavor. Others are financed by citizens through charitable contributions.

The hospitals supported through public contributions are managed by groups or "boards" of trustees who return any profits to the hospital for expansion, equipment purchase, or research. Other general hospitals are tax-supported at the local, state, or federal level. Veterans' hospitals are examples of hospitals which are federally financed and operated.

Special hospitals care for patients with unique or related problems. For example, The "City of Hope" in California offers special care to patients with **catastrophic** (overwhelming) diseases and is dedicated to relieving pain and prolonging life

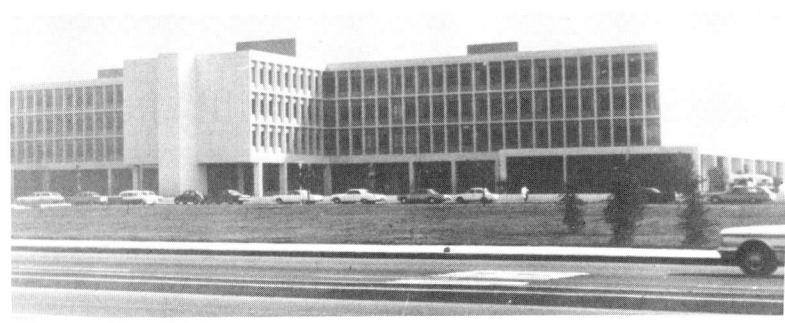

Figure 1-11: Naval Regional Medical Center, a federally supported hospital.

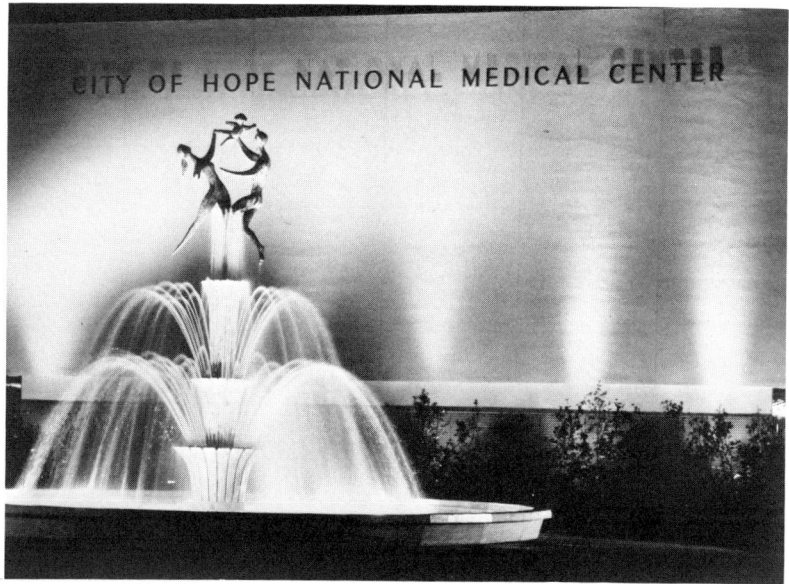

Figure 1-12: A special hospital caring for people with catastrophic diseases *(courtesy of City Hope Medical Center).*

with dignity. This hospital provides direct care to patients and carries out extensive research and education. It is recognized nationally for its excellence of service.

Doctors who are officially related to, or supportive of a particular hospital are "**on staff**" at that hospital and have the privilege of admitting their patients to the hospital for care.

Both general and special hospitals that meet certain high standards are accredited by the Joint Commission on Hospital Accreditation. Members of this Joint Commission represent the several branches of medicine including The American College of Physicians, The American College of Surgeons, The American Medical Association, and The American Hospital Association. Some hospitals provide clinical services which follow patients through the changing situations of a **potential** (possibly developing) health problem. Trained technicians and therapists man the clinics, offering their special skills to meet specific health needs.

VOLUNTARY HEALTH ASSOCIATIONS

There are local chapters of voluntary health associations, societies, or foundations located in many communities. These organizations are supported through voluntary contributions and devote themselves to educating the public about a specific health problem. Some also provide direct assistance to the patient or his family during his illness. The Heart Association Cancer Society, and Multiple Sclerosis Society are examples of voluntary service agencies which serve the community.

CASE STUDY

Esther Dorson was a 32 year-old black woman who had been married to Richard Dorson for several years. She thought she was at last pregnant and told her husband. They were both very excited, so she made an appointment with Dr. Rowlands to confirm the pregnancy.

Figure 1-13:
The older primipara is at risk for fetal abnormalities *(courtesy of City of Hope Medical Center).*

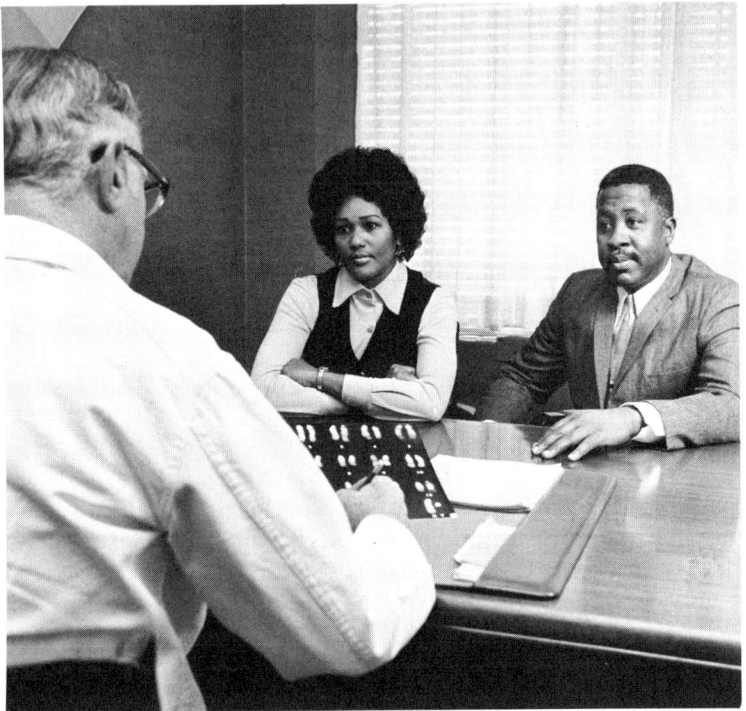

Dr. Rowlands examined Mrs. Dorson, found her to be truly pregnant, and then suggested a conference with her husband. He explained to them that he shared their joy but cautioned that two areas needed to be investigated for possible complications.

First, women of Mrs. Dorson's age who are **primipara** (pregnant for the first time), are **at risk** (more likely) to develop a dangerous condition leading to **fetal** (pertaining to the baby before birth) **abnormalities** (defects).

The second area for concern was the fact that Mrs. Dorson had a cousin with sickle cell anemia. The doctor explained that **sickle cell anemia** is a condition which harms the red blood cells. It seems to affect

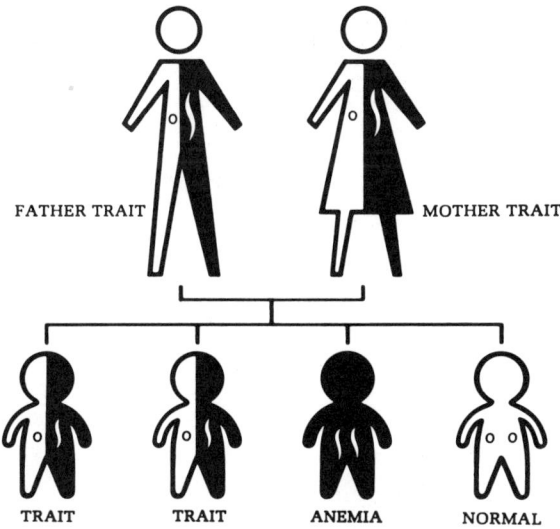

Figure 1-14: The trait for sickle cell anemia is carried in the genes of the parents *(courtesy of The National Foundation March of Dimes)*.

more black people than people of other races. Unfortunately the tendency toward sickle cell anemia is transmitted from one generation to another in the genes.

The **genes** (cell proteins), he explained, carry characteristics from one generation to the next and determine how a baby will be formed. A defective gene causes sickle cell anemia. Since Mrs. Dorson's cousin had sickle cell anemia there was a greater than ordinary likelihood that Mrs. Dorson also had that defective gene.

Dr. Rowland did say, however, that there was no cause for excess alarm. But it was always best to know what might have to be faced. Greatly disturbed, the couple agreed to see a physician in the **genetic** (pertaining to genes) counseling clinic at the medical center.

At the clinic, blood studies were made and an amniocentesis was performed. **Amniocentesis** is a technique for withdrawing a small amount of the fluid that surrounds the growing baby. It is then examined to determine if there are any problems. After encouraging genetic counseling reports, Mrs. Dorson continued to see her doctor while attending the **prenatal** (before birth) clinic at the hospital. There as an out-patient she learned special ways of

VOLUNTARY HEALTH ASSOCIATIONS 13 *

Figure 1-15: Aminocentesis being performed *(courtesy of The National Foundation March of Dimes)*.

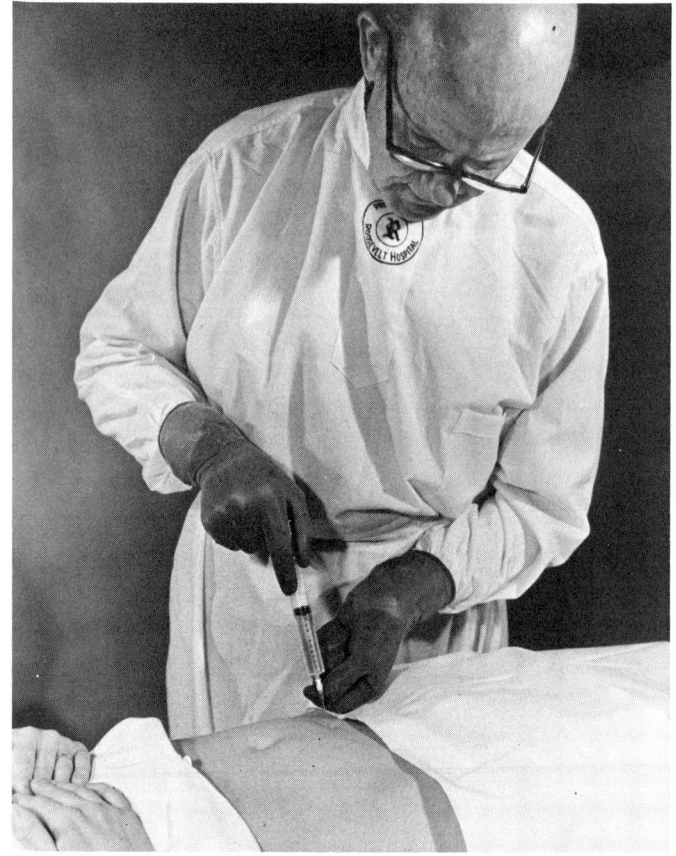

helping herself at the time of delivery. Finally, for the delivery and immediate aftercare, she was admitted as an in-patient to the **maternity** (motherhood) service of the medical center.

On June 5th, Mrs. Dorson gave birth to a healthy boy. After discharge, she and the baby returned to the hospital for services as out-patients in the **postpartum** (after delivery) and **neonatal** (newborn) clinics.

A community that offers all these related services provides a **continuum** (continuous flow) of optimum care for its citizens.

SUMMARY *The community health team is composed of a variety of professional, semi-professional, and ancillary workers. Their services are offered through privately and publicly financed facilities as well as on an independent basis. Health needs are complex, and many different health services and types of personnel are required to meet these needs.*

Explain and define the new special terms you have been using. Remember, you learned to pronounce them at the beginning of this chapter.

PRACTICE & REVIEW

1. milieu _____

2. catastrophic _____

3. therapeutic regime _____

4. rehabilitation _____

5. obesity _____

6. genes _____

7. primipara _____

8. continuum _____

9. orthopedics _____

10. obstetrics _____

Now, double-check the meaning of the terms above by studying the brief definitions given in the Glossary-Index at the back of this text.

Test yourself quickly before going on to learn other medical and professional terms. Use these short review exercises to practice for your new work in health services. Your teacher will also help by recommending various other Study Activities.

A. Match the terms at the left to the definitions at the right:

____ 1. ancillary   a. refers to baby before birth
____ 2. arthritis   b. defects
____ 3. pulmonary   c. lungs
____ 4. fetal   d. obstetrics
____ 5. maternity   e. direct
____ 6. abnormalities   f. assisting
____ 7. postpartum   g. drunkenness
____ 8. primary   h. health agencies
____ 9. alcoholism   i. overweight
____ 10. facilities   j. after delivery
                            k. inflammation of a joint

B. Complete the following statements by writing in the missing word or words:

1. The protein that transmits the characteristics of the parents to the child are the _____ .
2. The group which provides emergency care in the community are called _____ .
3. The health worker that compounds and dispenses medications is called the _____ .
4. A planned treatment program is called the _____ .
5. List below the three long-term care facilities that you learned about in this chapter:
   a _____ b _____ c _____
6. Patients who live at home but use community services are called _____ .

C. Underline the new word or words you recognize in the sentences below:

1. Patients with pulmonary conditions frequently have a cough.
2. The stroke patient has sustained damage to his brain.
3. Patients with arthritis may be out-patients at an orthopedic clinic.
4. Older primipara women are at risk for fetal genetic abnormalities.
5. Long-term primary care is provided by the physicians and nurses on staff at the convalescent hospital.

After studying Chapter 2
The Hospital Health Team
You should be able to:

* *Pronounce and define each of its new medical words and phrases and use the new technical jargon.*

* *Name and describe ten specialists in the medical field.*

* *Describe the duties of both the volunteer and the volunteen.*

PRONOUNCE THESE TEN NEW WORDS WITH YOUR TEACHER: MEDICAL WORDS

therapeutic (ther″ah-pu′tĭk)
expertise *knowledge*
pathologist (pah-thol′o-jist)
consultant (kon-sul′tant)
psychiatrist (si-ki′ah-trist)

diagnosis (di″ag-no″sis)
procedure
prognosis (prog-no′sis)
liaison (li′a-e′son)
physician (fi-zĭsh′un)

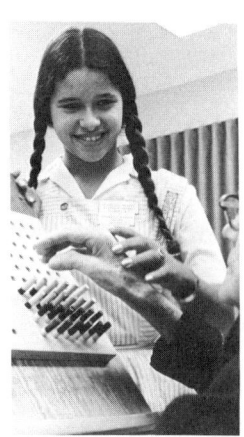

Many of the health care providers working in the community are also found within the hospital walls. Hospital health workers, like people in general, whether paid or unpaid, come in all sizes and in all ages from 16 years on up.

Volunteers are frequently called **Candy Stripers** from their gay striped uniforms. They help in various chores and duties such as transporting patients to and from treatment appointments, assisting patients as they eat, delivering mail and flowers, and generally bringing cheer and comfort to lonely, frightened persons. Their activities free more highly trained workers to concentrate on carrying out their specialized functions. The youngest volunteer worker is usually called a **volunteen** (teenage worker).   HOSPITAL VOLUNTEERS

One of the oldest hospital health workers often is an experienced doctor who has given up general private practice. But, because of some special **expertise** (expertness, knowledge) and long experience such a person often serves as a **consultant** (an   HOSPITAL PROFESSIONALS

HOSPITAL PROFESSIONALS 17 *

additional doctor whose opinion is sought) for difficult or unusual cases.

Of course, one person is always the center of attention and the focus of all activity in any health care setting. That one person is the patient. Each member of the hospital health team who comes in contact with the patient uses his special **therapeutic** (effective in treatment of disease) skills in the overall program that has been designed to help the patient get well.

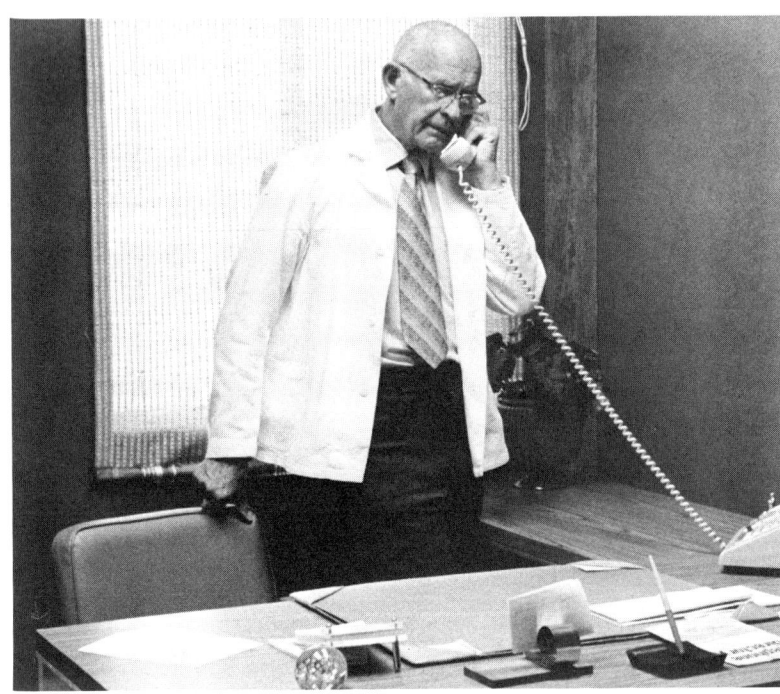

Figure 2-2: A consultant offers his special expertise in unusual cases

MEDICAL SPECIALISTS

Today, many doctors work only as specialists in one aspect of patient care. They limit treatment to patients with conditions relating to their **specialty** (special area of education). Many different specialists often have offices in the same building in a community or in the hospital itself. Look at Webster's Medical Directory in Figure 2-3 to see some of the numerous classifications of specialty medical practice.

Doctors who are **radiologists read** (interpret) and sometimes take the X-rays which help to establish the presence or absence of a disease process. Usually highly-trained technicians take these diagnostic photographs of the interior of the body

WEBSTER MEDICAL BUILDING		
Brown, S. , M.D.	Radiologist	101
Butler, L. , M.D.	Otologist	317
Caldwell, N. , M.D.	Surgeon	321
Cavanaugh, P. , M.D.	Radiologist	101
Copeland, J. , M.D.	Pathologist	104
Decker, R. , M.D.	Obstetrician/Gynecologist	211
Dunbar, S. , M.D.	Opthalmologist	302
Dyler, A. , M.D.	Dermatologist	312
Evenly, D. , M.D.	Cardiologist	301
Farham, M. , M.D.	Pediatrician	201
Haley, S. , M.D.	Endocrinologist	304
Henzelman, C. , M.D.	Internist	111
Hogan, D. , M.D.	Pediatrician	201
Kline, J. , M.D.	Pediatrician	204
Maddox, P. , M.D.	Neurologist	300
Mall, J. , M.D.	Anesthesiologist	309
Williams, B. , M.D.	Obstetrician/Gynecologist	211

Figure 2-3: Typical hospital sign listing medical staff.

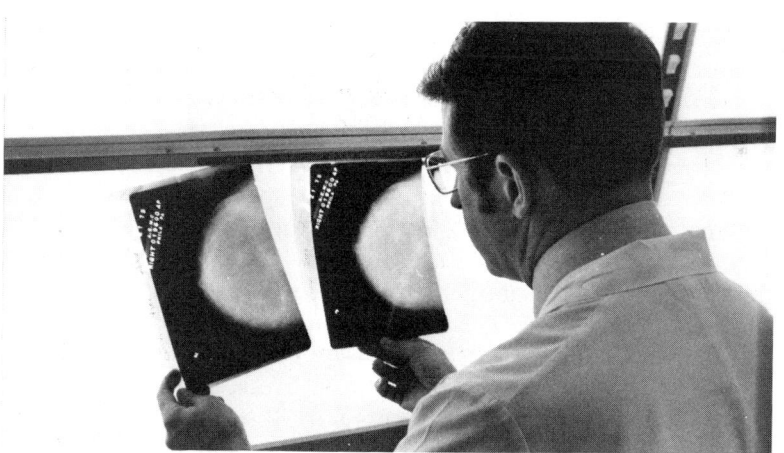

Figure 2-4: Radiologist "reads" the X-ray.

for the doctors. The **pathologist** studies and describes the disease process, aiding the **attending physician** (doctor in charge) to determine the cause of a particular illness. **Pediatricians** care for children. Some pediatricians specialize in the treatment of infants while others care for young people all the way through the teen years.

Figure 2-5: The pediatrician cares for infants and children *(courtesy of A-H Robbins Company)*.

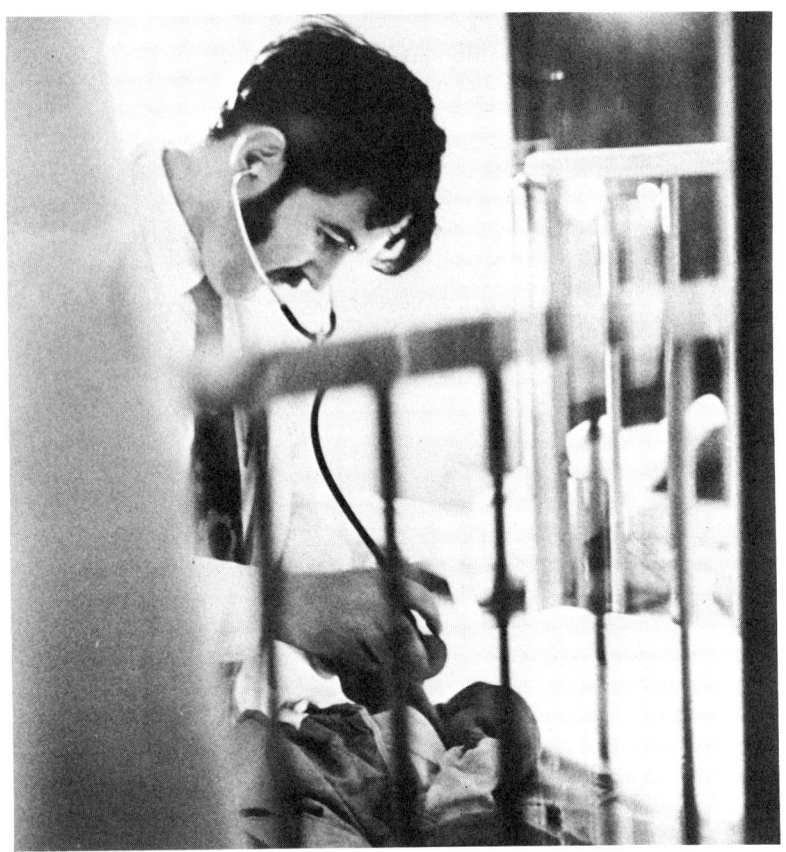

Frequently, a physician who has been trained and educated in the care of women, combines two specialities. The first is **gynecology** (the study of female reproductive problems). The second is **obstetrics** (the care of the woman during pregnancy, delivery and in the immediate after delivery period known as **postpartum** or **P.P.**). This specialist is called either a gynecologist/obstetrician or an obstetrician/gynecologist (Ob/gyn).

The **otologist** treats patients with diseases of the ear and the **opthalmologist** treats patients with diseases of the eye. The **dermatologist** specializes in skin diseases and the **cardiologist** cares for persons with heart problems. The **endocrinologist** provides care for diabetics—people whose medical problems involve the glands which produce hormones in the body. The **neurologist** specializes in that branch of medicine which diagnoses and treats abnormalities of the nervous system.

The **anesthesiologist** keeps patients comfortably unaware of pain during otherwise painful procedures such as **surgery**

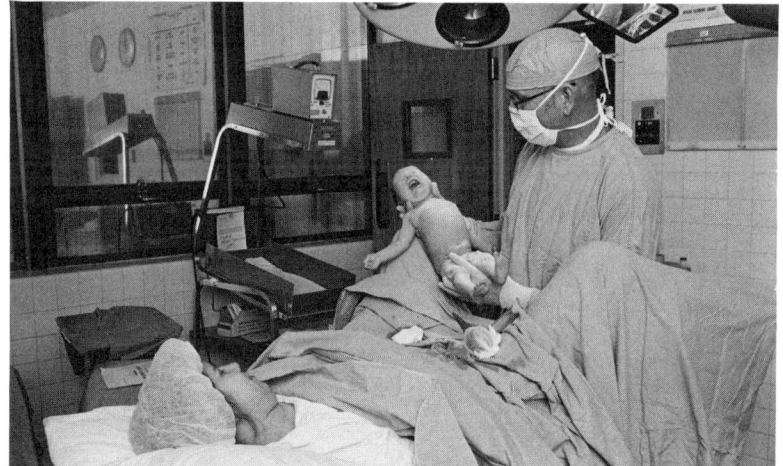

Figure 2-6:
The obstetrician cares for the woman during delivery

(operation). From a position near the patient's head, he or she carefully **monitors** (watches, observes) all the patient's **vital signs** (living signs). This doctor watches the patient's temperature, blood pressure, and respiration while he is under the partial or total **anesthesia** (techniques that reduce sensation or feeling) during surgery.

The anesthesiologist keeps the surgeon informed of the patient's overall general condition throughout the surgical procedure.

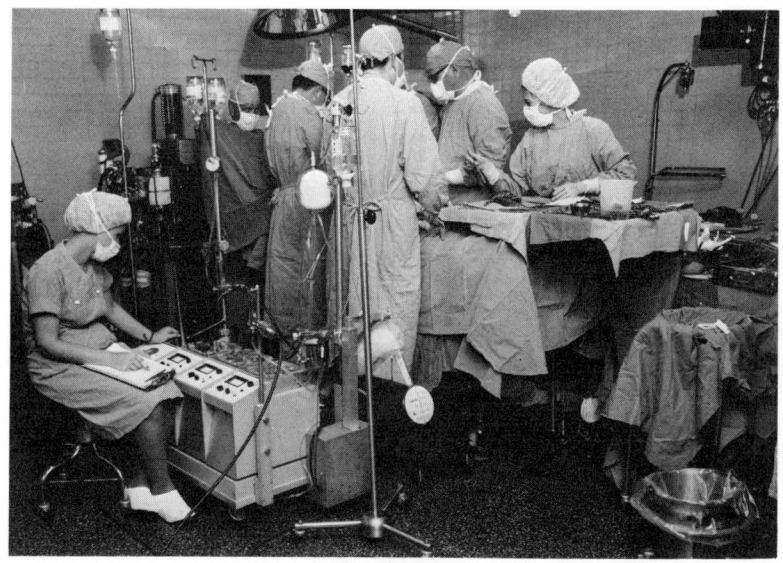

Figure 2-7:
The anesthesiologist who is just seen at the head of the operating table monitors the patient

MEDICAL SPECIALISTS 21 *

Other medical specialists include: the **psychiatrist**, who treats emotional illness; the **urologist**, who treats problems of the kidneys and urinary organs; and, the **orthopedist**, who treats persons suffering with diseases of the bones and joints. These are just a few of the highly trained physicians who are part of the hospital health team.

The attending physician determines the **diagnosis** (labels the condition), establishes a probable **etiology** (cause), and prescribes the appropriate **therapy** (treatment). Frequently, this doctor is able to indicate a **prognosis** (probable outcome) for the patient. The attending physician will call in one of the specialists for consultation when needed. These same physicians who see and treat patients in their offices in the community serve on hospital staffs and use hospital facilities as well.

In addition to those doctors already registered to practice, future doctors engaged in the learning process at various levels are also found in the hospital setting. Larger hospitals, with special **accreditation** (approval) are teaching institutions for medical students and interns.

Under the guidance and supervision of the doctors, the medical students and interns assist in the care of patients. In America **medical students** are those persons still enrolled in a medical school. **Interns** are people who have completed their medical school education and are gaining more direct, general experience in patient care by working full time in the hospital. Internships and residencies permit doctors to further increase their knowledge and capabilities in some special field of medical treatment before they begin independent practice.

The **physician of record** (attending physician) requests all the laboratory tests needed to determine the diagnosis. He also

Figure 2-8: Interns and medical students work under the guidance of professional physicians

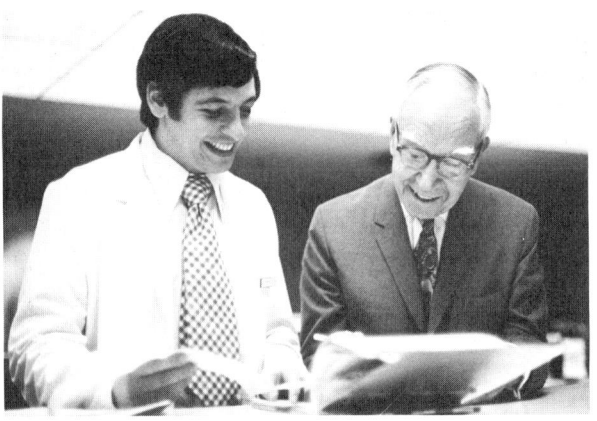

writes **orders** (directions) for the patient's care that are to be carried out by all of the health workers. The doctor's orders are part of the official legal patient records which must be cared for properly.

NURSING STAFF

Nursing care (direct physical and emotional support-activities) is provided by several categories of health care workers in the hospital. The average person thinks of a person in a white uniform as a "nurse" and is often unaware that the **nursing staff** (team of people providing care) is made up of several levels or categories of workers. These all carry out the **procedures** (series of events designed to promote a specific goal) which fulfill the doctor's orders.

The nursing staff functions under the overall supervision of a registered nurse, entitled "The Director of Nursing."

The **health assistant** is a person trained in basic care. The health assistant is sometimes called an **aide** or **orderly**. The health assistant always works under the direct supervision of either a Registered Nurse (R.N.) or a Licensed Vocational Nurse (L.V.N.).

The initials R.N. stand for Registered Nurse and indicate that this person has been professionally trained and prepared to give direct nursing care and has successfully passed a registered nursing state licensing examination. A nurse so registered coordinates the total care that she and the other health workers render to the patient. Part of an R.N.'s responsibility is overseeing the care given by L.V.N.s and health assistants. R.N.s also give direct nursing care as a member of the nursing team.

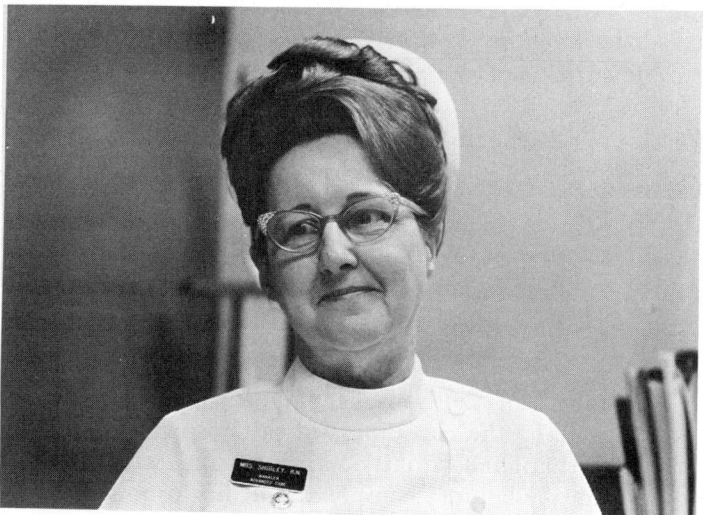

Figure 2-9: The registered nurse coordinates patient care

NURSING STAFF 23 *

The **Licensed Vocational Nurse** is usually prepared for his/her role in an educational institution with clinical practice in various hospitals and other health agencies. The length of the educational program varies from one year to eighteen months. In Texas and California, a person prepared in this way, and having successfully passed the state licensing examination is designated a Licensed Vocational Nurse and may use the initials L.V.N. after his/her name. In other states, a person with the same preparation and state board licensing is called a **Licensed Practical Nurse** and may use the initials L.P.N. after his/her name.

SUPPORTIVE SERVICES

In the hospital, ancillary workers of many kinds augment direct nursing services. **Porters** transport patients, **runners** pick up **specimens** (samples of body tissues or fluids, such as urine) from the patient units and deliver them to the proper laboratory facility, and adult **volunteers** do many of the same chores and errands as the volunteens. Hospital staffs depend heavily upon the ancillary workers to augment their direct care. The many services that the volunteers render are much appreciated by all busy hospital professionals.

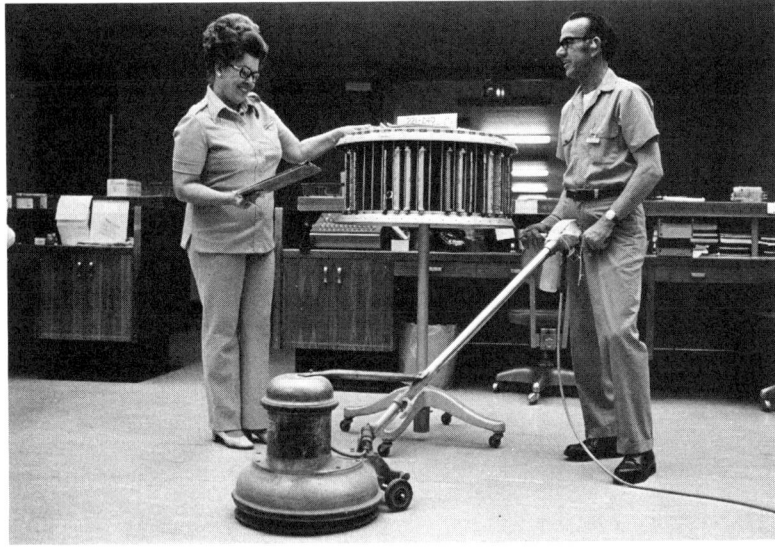

Figure 2-10: The housekeeping staff is responsible for the cleanliness of the hospital

Members of the housekeeping department are responsible for maintaining the cleanliness of the hospital. Some give direct service to patient's rooms, corridors, and service areas, while others man the laundry, supply and utility rooms.

* 24 *THE HOSPITAL HEALTH TEAM*

Operating a hospital also requires a business office and clerical personnel to handle the business affairs and records of the patient and hospital. In large hospitals, a patient representative acts as a special **liaison** (link) between the patient and the hospital staff. Many hospitals have adopted the American Hospital Association's "Patient's Bill of Rights" and see that each patient receives a copy so that he/she will know exactly what services are due to a sick person—that is, what a sick person has a right to expect.

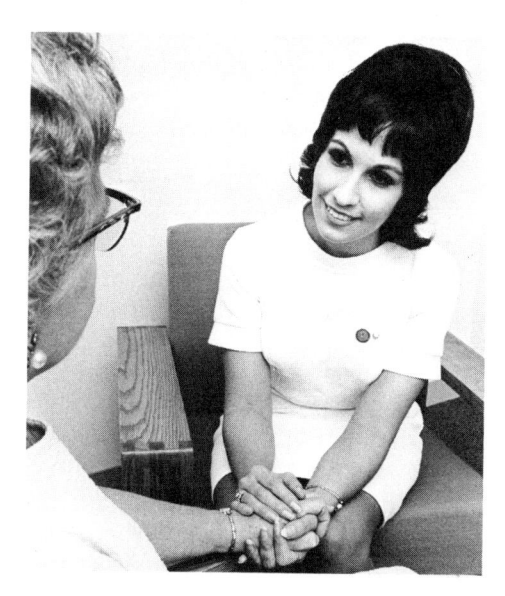

Figure 2-11: The liaison serves as a link between the patient and hospital administration

HOSPITAL ORGANIZATION

Hospitals cannot always offer all the same services. The degree of service and type of care provided depends upon the size of the facility, the base of financial support and the community need. But almost all general community hospitals provide certain basic services and are generally organized in a similar manner.

The hospital is itself a kind of community since it is made up of many different departments working as a unit. It is staffed by various people trained for specific roles in patient care or therapy.

Ordinarily hospitals are separated into adult and **pediatric** (children) divisions. Adult patients may be further divided according to their diagnosis and placed on **services** (patient care areas) according to the type of treatment they need, such as **medical** (those requiring treatment with medicines) patients or

Figure 2-12: Pediatric department

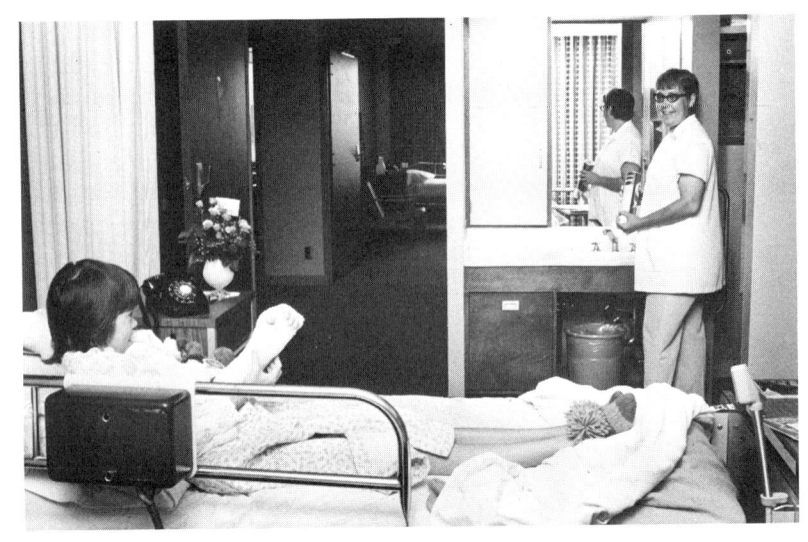

surgical (those who have had or will have an operation) patients. Patients may be further separated according to their type of surgical or medical condition. For example, two surgical patients may be placed on separate floors because one has an orthopedic problem and the other a gynecological problem, even though both require surgery.

THE PATIENT UNIT
Patients in the hospital are cared for in patient units. A **patient unit** consists of a bed, bedside stand, overbed table, usually a storage closet, chair and individual equipment such as a **bedpan** (receptacle used for bodily elimination), wash basin, and water pitcher and glass together on a tray. Patients are housed in **private rooms** (one patient unit), in **semi-private** rooms (two or three patient units), or **wards** (four or more patient units). Curtains or screens partition the semi-private room and wards, providing for patient privacy. Privacy is a basic human need and a basic patient right.

Patient units are developed near or around a nursing station where records are kept and nurses are able to monitor patients and plan for their care.

Each patient care area service usually has a medicine room where patient medications are prepared and a utility room where sterile and non-sterile supplies are kept. Many have additional rooms for special therapies. For example, on the orthopedic service, in addition to the specific patient rooms or units, there usually is a room for the application of casts and splints for broken bones.

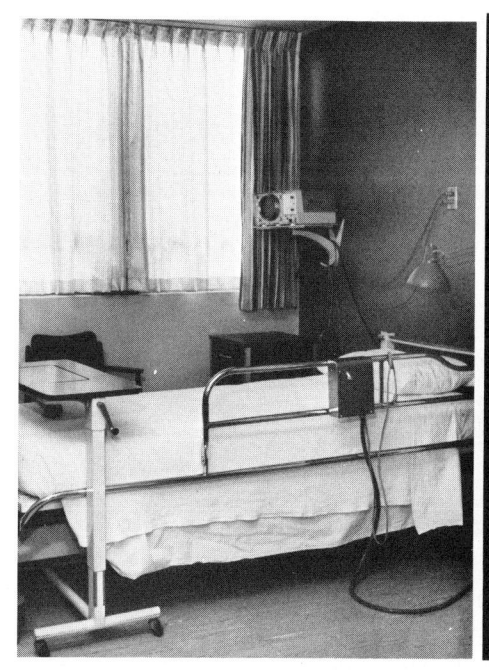

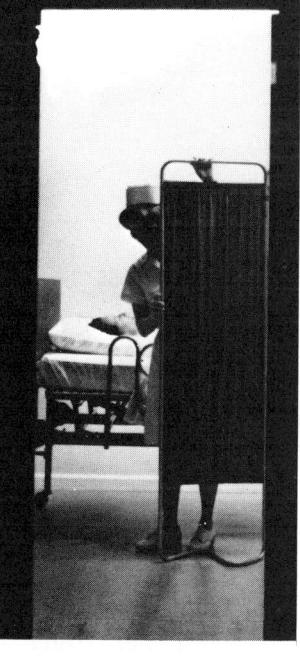

Figure 2-13: (left) Standard patient unit

Figure 2-14: (right) Screens provide privacy in a semi-private or ward accommodation *(courtesy of Eli Lilly and Company).*

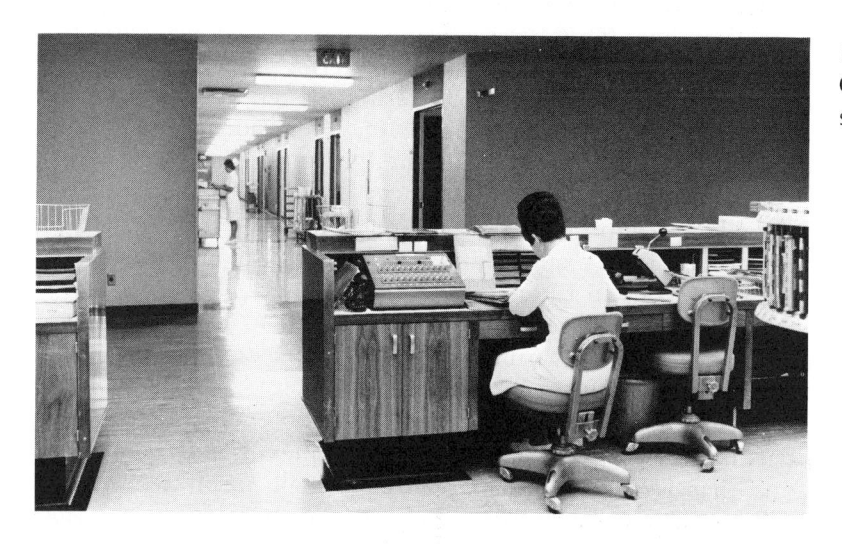

Figure 2-15: Central nursing station

Hospitals that provide care for pregnant women and for newborn babies operate an **obstetrical** (pertaining to obstetrics) unit, department, or suite. First, the new mothers are cared for in the labor room while preparing for delivery. The babies born in the **delivery room** are then cared for in the newborn **nursery**.

HOSPITAL DEPARTMENTS

Figure 2-16: (left) The labor room is part of the obstetrical department

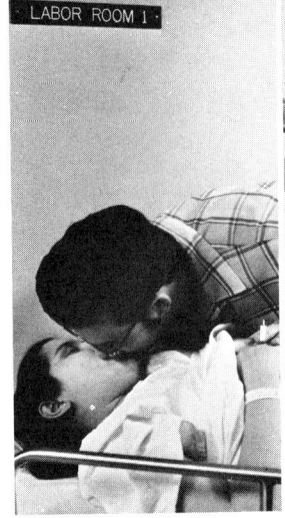

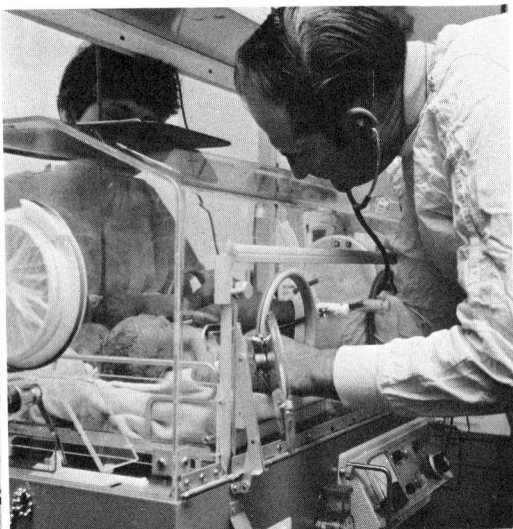

Figure 2-17: (right) The pediatrician exams the newborn in the nursery *(courtesy of The National Foundation March of Dimes).*

After delivery, the mothers are cared for in the postpartum section of the unit.

Other departments of the hospital and their specially trained staffs augment the care given in the patient unit. The **operating room (O.R.)** or surgery is staffed by people who carry out the necessary surgical procedures. The **postoperative recovery room** is adjacent to the operating room. Patients remain in the recovery area, under the close supervision of nurses and doctors, until they have recovered from the anesthesia. The **X-ray** or **Radiology Department** personnel include the radiologic technologist who takes X-rays and the radiologist who analyzes special radiologic examinations. An **upper gastrointestinal series** would be done in the radiology department. This procedure is also called a **barium swallow** since the patient is asked to swallow a solution of barium which outlines the digestive tract. X-ray films are taken to reveal any pathology.

The emergency room or accident room receives **emergency** patients who are stricken with sudden, unexpected crisis conditions that require immediate care. Not all hospitals have the facilities to operate an emergency service so you may not find this department in your hospital. Most hospitals operate one or more **laboratory departments** where patient specimens are examined and treated. Sometimes the laboratory is a very large department which carries out a wide variety of test procedures. In very large hospitals or medical centers, the laboratory department may be so active and busy that it is divided into several

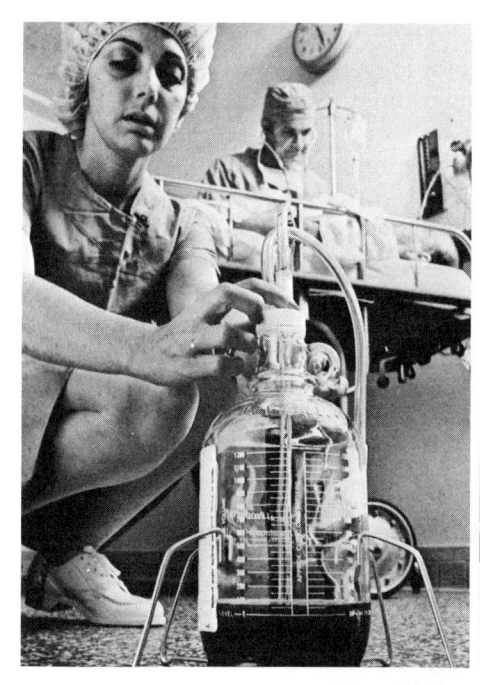

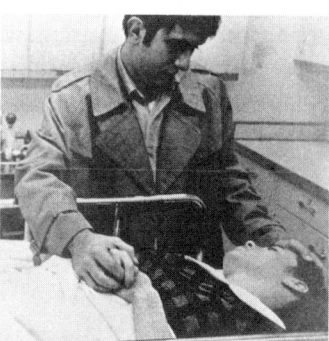

Figure 2-18: (left) Postoperative recovery room *(courtesy of Chesebrough-Pond's, Inc.)*.

Figure 2-19: (right) The ER, a busy hospital department *(courtesy of Ortho Diagnostics, Inc.)*.

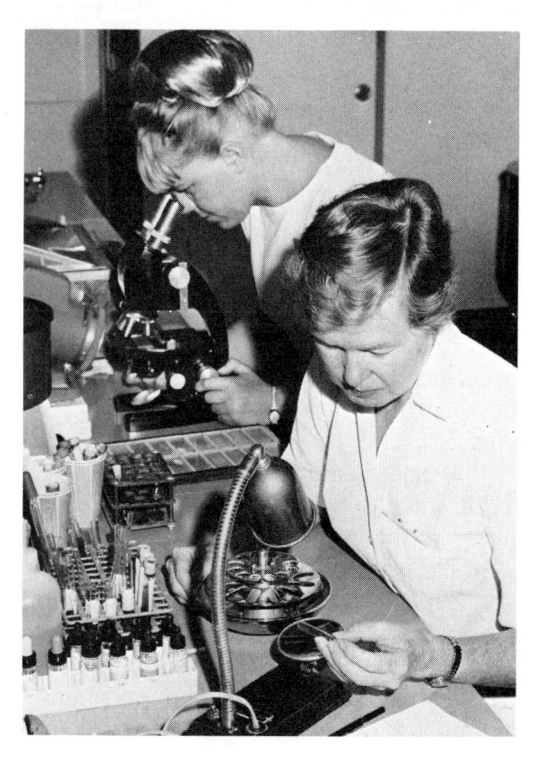

Figure 2-20: The laboratory department

HOSPITAL DEPARTMENTS 29 *

sub-laboratory departments. There may be laboratories for **hematology** (blood study), **cytology** (cell study), **parasitology** (study of parasites), or **bacteriology** (study of bacteria). In smaller hospitals the laboratory staff carry out only routine procedures. Specimens requiring more thorough or complex examinations are sent to a larger laboratory.

Every hospital has a department which keeps the service areas supplied with essential materials and equipment called the **central supply department** or Central Service. Special procedure trays and equipment are stored in this department and are sent to the patient care areas when needed. Some of this equipment is returned, cleaned, and prepared for re-use. But much of the equipment and supplies used in patient care is **disposable** (used once and then destroyed). These materials are also **dispensed** (supplied) from the central supply area.

Figure 2-21: The central supply department

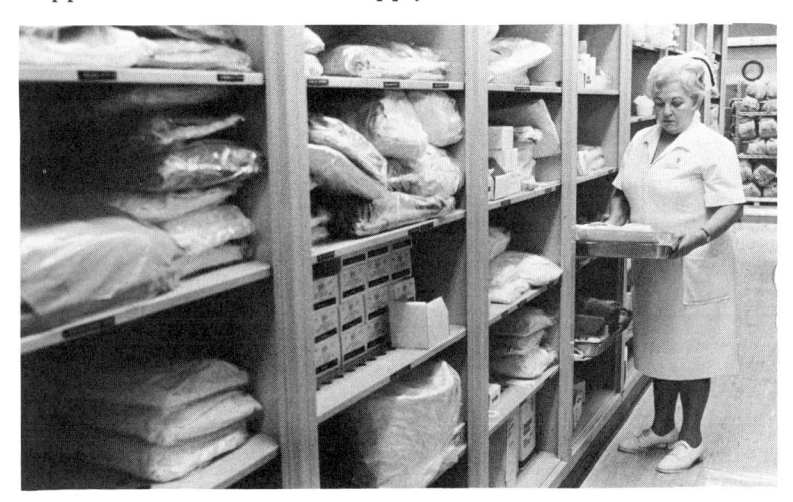

Each hospital has a dietary department to supply the nutritional needs of both patients and staff. Food is prepared to suit the special diets of persons recovering from various illnesses and injuries.

Every hospital has a pharmacy which prepares and dispenses medications. These medicines are sent to the medicine room of the individual service units where the nurses dispense them to the patients.

Larger hospitals have diverse departments depending on the type of service they offer to the community. For example, a large medical center may also have an orthopedic rehabilitation department, respiratory care department, pathology department, and nuclear medicine department.

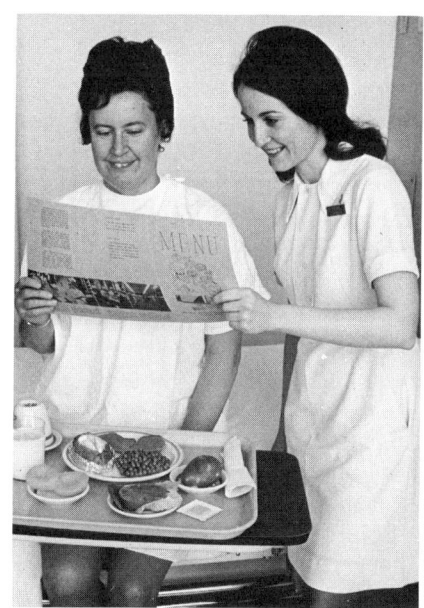

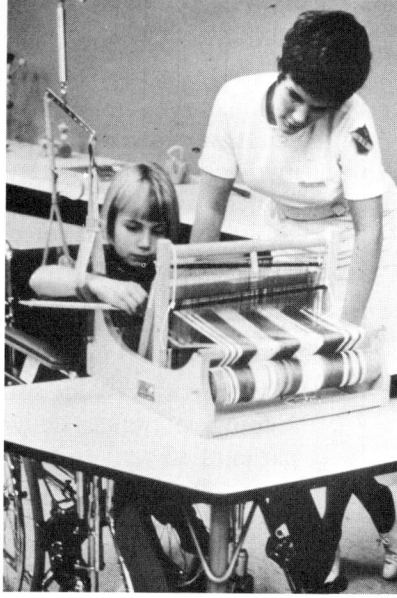

Figure 2-22: (left) The dietary department provides for the nutritional needs of patients and staff

Figure 2-23: (right) Orthopedic rehabilitation department

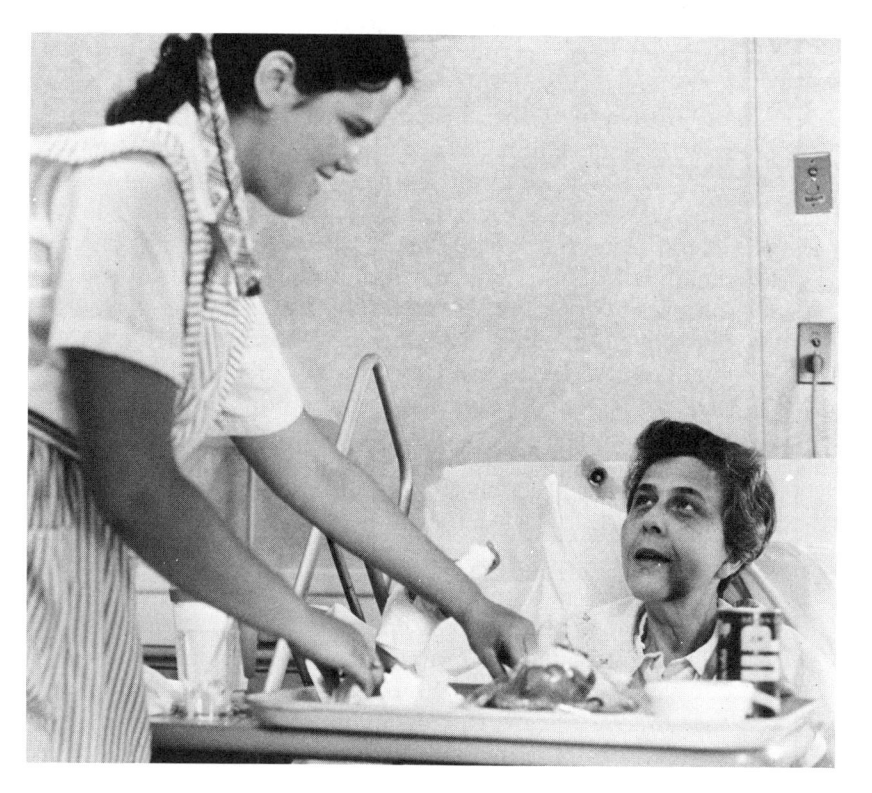

Figure 2-24: The volunteer volunteers for service.

HOSPITAL DEPARTMENTS 31 *

CASE STUDY

Penny Stevens, 17 years old and a senior in high school, hopes someday to enter the field of medicine. She is thinking of becoming a pediatrician so she can care for the children in the pediatric department. Because she realizes that a great deal of time will be involved in achieving a premedical education, in being a medical student, and intern, Penny is undecided about her final choice. She feels that becoming a volunteer may help in her decision.

Penny has been a volunteer at Webster Memorial Hospital for a year and has learned a great deal about the staff members and the departments of the hospital. Part of her time was spent on the surgical service, feeding patients, delivering mail, and transporting patients to and from other departments. One afternoon she visited five different departments in the hospital; the hematology laboratory, central supply, radiology, and emergency department. She also accompanied the surgery porter who took one of her patients to surgery.

A friendly person, Penny soon became acquainted with many hospital physicians and staff members. For example, she now knows short, graying Dr. Brown, is an internist, and that Dr. Copeland who is always in a hurry is a pathologist. She also recognizes Dr. Caldwell, the youngest woman surgeon on the staff, and Dr. Green and Dr. Hamilton who are in a group practice with several other staff doctors. The members of the group take care of each others' patients when one of them is busy elsewhere. Her favorite physician is Dr. Decker, whose practice is in gynecology/obstetrics. His patients all call him Dr. "D" and seem to appreciate the amount of time he spends talking with them. Penny thinks that she would like to have him care for her when she is married and pregnant. Her closest friend on the staff is Robert Baker, R.N.

As Penny works with the patients, she hears and learns many new terms each day. At one time, words like "prognosis, therapy, diagnosis, and etiology" seemed foreign, but now they are part of her everyday vocabulary. Like many others, Penny belongs to the ancillary staff that is an important part of the hospital health team.

Patients are people who are ill and who are being treated for disease or injury. The treatment often takes place in complex institutions called hospitals which are staffed by professional, technical, and ancillary workers of many kinds.

Each member of the hospital health team has special responsibilities designed to promote patient welfare. Hospitals are highly organized so that the staff members of each department contribute to the total team effort and the ultimate goal of optimum patient care.

SUMMARY

Explain and define the new special terms you have been using. Remember, you learned how to pronounce them at the beginning of this chapter.

PRACTICE & REVIEW

1. therapeutic _____
2. expertise _____
3. pathologist _____
4. consultant _____
5. psychiatrist _____
6. diagnosis _____
7. procedure _____
8. prognosis _____
9. liaison _____
10. physician _____

Now, double-check the meaning of the terms above by studying the brief definitions given in the Glossary-Index at the back of this text.

Test yourself quickly before going on to learn other medical and professional terms. Use these short review exercises to practice for your new work in health services. Your teacher will also help by recommending various other Study Activities.

A. Five areas of specialty in medicine are listed in the center column. To the left, write a brief definition; to the right, write the name of the physician who practices that specialty:

Study of	*Specialty*	*Specialist*
_____	Dermatology	_____
_____	Neurology	_____

HOSPITAL DEPARTMENTS 33 *

Study of	Specialty	Specialist
_____	Otology	_____
_____	Cardiology	_____
_____	Opthalmology	_____

B. Match the name of the specialist with the best description of his work by writing the appropriate letter at the left:

_____ 1. Treats disease of bones and joints
_____ 2. Treats diseases of women
_____ 3. Treats children's diseases
_____ 4. Treats diseases of the skin
_____ 5. Treats heart diseases
_____ 6. Usually treats diseases of the urinary tract
_____ 7. Treats emotional illness
_____ 8. Studies disease process and tells when disease is present
_____ 9. Takes and reads X-rays
_____ 10. Diagnoses and treats conditions of the nervous system

a. pediatrician
b. radiologist
c. obstetrician
d. otologist
e. opthalmologist
f. dermatologist
g. urologist
h. cardiologist
i. pathologist
j. anesthesiologist
k. gynecologist
l. psychiatrist
m. orthopedist
n. neurologist
o. endocrinologist

C. Complete the following statements by writing in the correct word:

1. A doctor uses his special knowledge or _____ in the care of the sick.
2. The attending physician calls in another doctor to see his patient as a _____ .
3. The physician's special area of education is his _____ .
4. A sudden, unexpected occurrence is called an _____ .
5. The _____ treats patients with ear conditions.
6. The anesthesiologist carefully observes or _____ the patient during surgery.
7. The physician names the disease when he makes a _____ .
8. The probable outcome or _____ is not always easy to predict.
9. The attending physician is also called the physician _____ .
10. Directions for the patient's care are called the _____ .

After studying Chapter 3
Non-oral and Symbolic Communications
You should be able to:

* *Identify six logos of health associations, foundations, or societies.*

* *Identify six warning signs used in hospitals.*

The three symbols that are pictured in Figure 3-1 have been adopted by the United Nations for use in traffic control. Since they are international symbols, strangers in a country can easily follow these directions even if they are unfamiliar with the language. **Symbols** are special signs. They are an emphatic way to communicate information without using many words. In some cases no words at all are used. For example, look at the sign in Figure 3-2. It takes very little imagination to realize you cannot enter and must stop. Another important highway sign which is frequently seen directs drivers to the nearest hospital. See Figure 3-3. Symbols are signs, emblems or tokens which stand for or mean something definite. A symbol may be a picture which conveys a message, or words which convey a message beyond the meaning of the actual words that are used. A symbol may also be a token, such as a flag which signifies a country or some other political community.

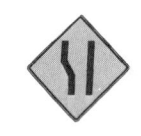

Fewer lanes ahead

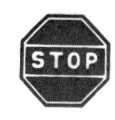

Stop sign

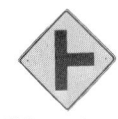

Side road

Figure 3-1:

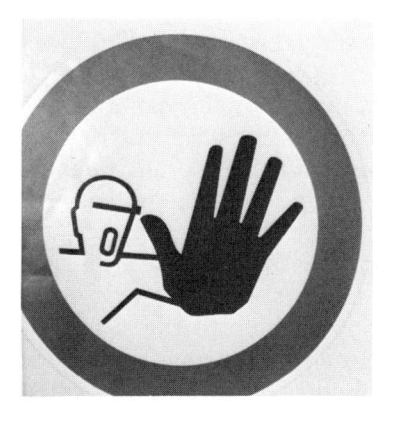

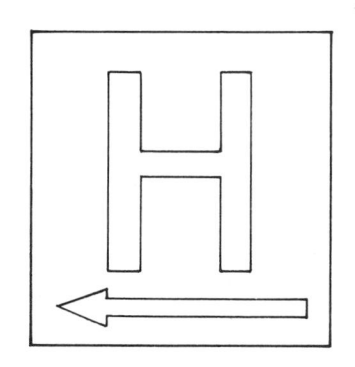

Figure 3-2: (left) "Do not enter" *(Courtesy of Bel-Arts Products).*

Figure 3-3:

HOSPITAL DEPARTMENTS 35

Figure 3-4:

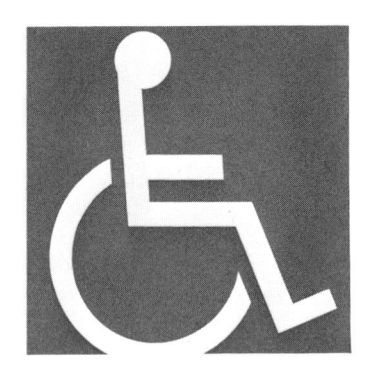

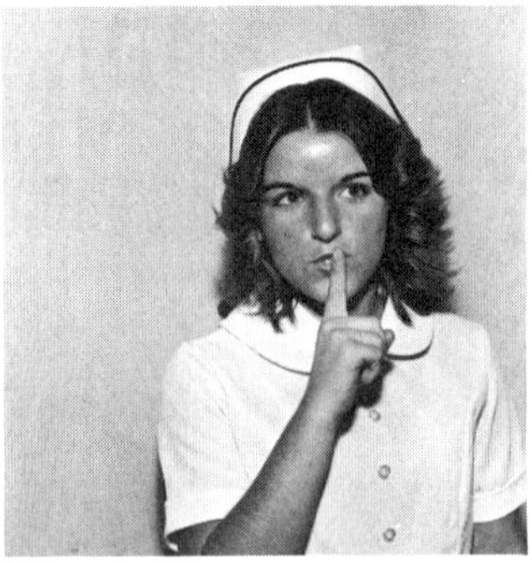

Figure 3-5:
International
symbol of access.

SIGNS AND   Look at Figure 3-4. It conveys a definite message without
SYMBOLS using any words. Similar pictures hang in hospitals all over the country and everyone who sees it understands the message "Quiet Please."

      Figure 3-5 is a pictorial representation of a mobile chair for people who cannot walk. It is also the international symbol meaning "this area is accessible to wheelchairs." It tells all who see it in a parking area or over a doorway to a public facility that space has been reserved for a person who is **handicapped** (has a limitation of physical activities). You will notice that the actual spaces under such signs are larger than usual. This is because disabled people who use wheelchairs and drive cars need more space—to maneuver wheelchairs out of cars, adjust themselves safely in them, then close the car doors, and so forth. This symbol can be seen wherever there is wheelchair accessibility to buildings. It is used to point out ramps, ground level entrances, elevators, crosswalks without curbs, public rest rooms, telephones, and drinking fountains that can be easily approached by persons in wheelchairs.

LOGOS FOR   Many health organizations use special symbols called **logos**.
HEALTH GROUPS Like a trademark, they are a token representation of a particular group. Seeing the logo reminds people of the name of that special organization and the important work it supports. Because many serious health problems cause great stress and financial strain, voluntary health associations, foundations, and societies have been organized to help. They offer financial, physical and emotional support to persons afflicted with a particular disease.

      For example, the Cancer Society is a widely recognized voluntary organization that offers direct help to the cancer patient in the form of supplies such as clean dressings (bandages). The Society also uses much of its budget to inform the general public about cancer—the ways to recognize danger signals, and how to avoid improper treatment at the hands of **quacks** (unauthorized persons).

The Cancer Society also produces many educational materials that provide health workers with up-to-date information about cancer. Whenever you see the symbol shown in Figure 3-6, you know the Cancer Society is at work. Not all voluntary health societies carry out exactly the same supportive services but they are similar in nature and center their activities around a specific health condition.

The logos of eight voluntary health agencies are pictured for you in Figures 3-7a through Figures 3-7h. Study the logos and the name of the society, association or foundation so that these symbols will have meaning for you. Then you will be able to recognize them when you meet them again.

Figure 3-6: Logo of the American Cancer Society, Inc.

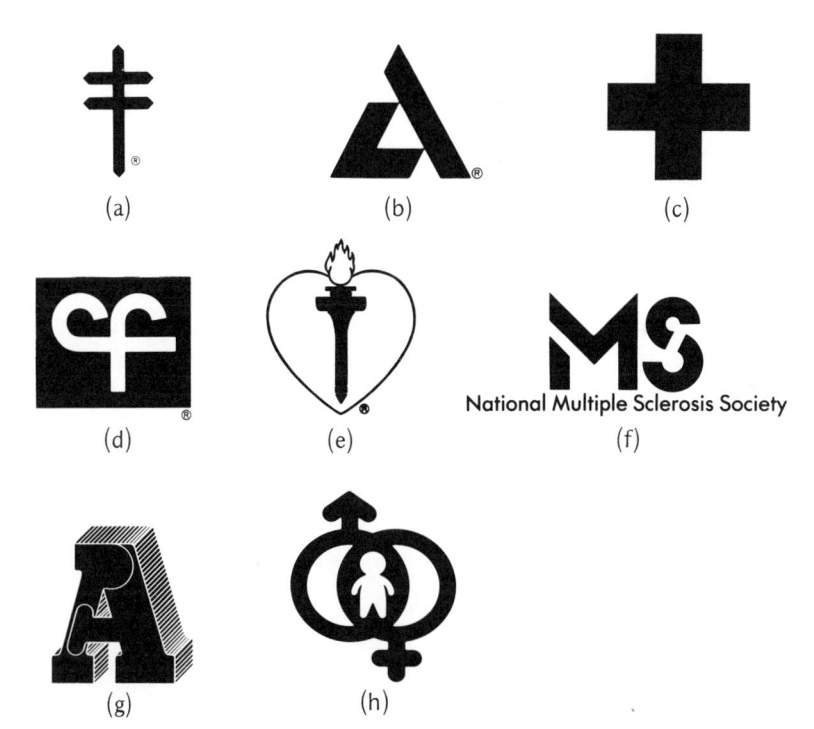

Figure 3-7: (a) Registered Trademark of the American Lung Association; (b) logo of the American Diabetes Association; (c) logo for the American National Red Cross; (d) logo for the Cystic Fibrosis Foundation; (e) logo of the American Heart Association; (f) logo of the National Multiple Sclerosis Society; (g) logo for Arthritis Foundation; (h) logo for The National Foundation March of Dimes.

PROFESSIONAL ORGANIZATIONS

Logos have been adopted by professional organizations as well as voluntary health associations. Some of the organizations of professional health personnel that have easily identifiable logos include:

PROFESSIONAL ORGANIZATIONS 37

Figure 3-8:
(a) Star of Life, EMT Symbol;
(b) logo of the American Association of Medical Assistants, Inc.;
(c) logo of the American Dental Assistants Association;
(d) logo of the American Medical Association.

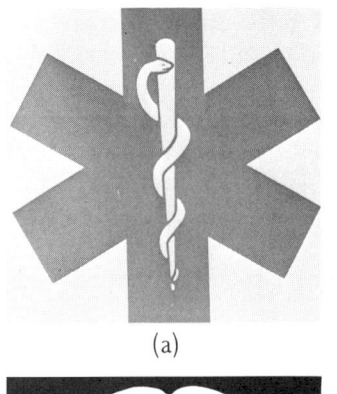

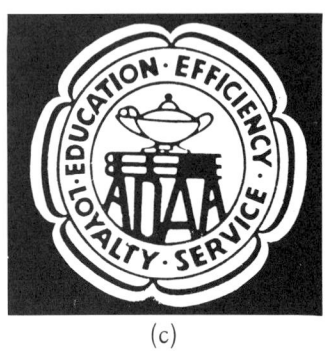

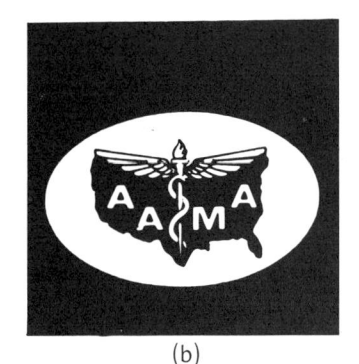

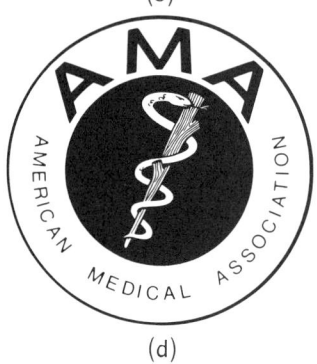

The Bowl of Hygeia has rapidly gained favor as a true international symbol of the pharmacy profession, although the Pharmaceutical Association uses another logo to represent it.

Some professional associations adapt a logo for the state association so that it is slightly different from the one used at the national level. Compare the logo of the California Podiatry Association with the logo of the American Podiatry Association.

Figure 3-9: Bowl of Hygeia, symbol for health concerns.

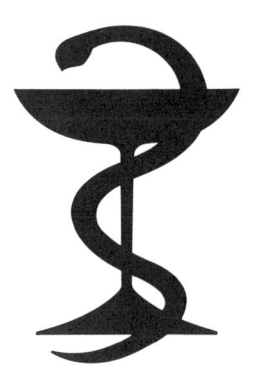

*38 NON-ORAL AND SYMBOLIC COMMUNICATIONS

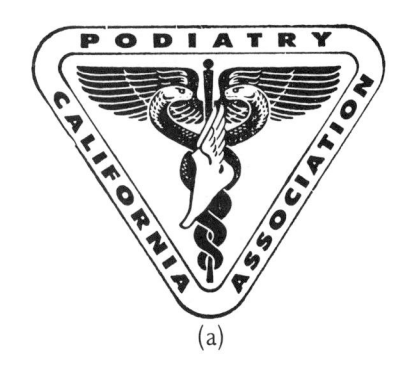

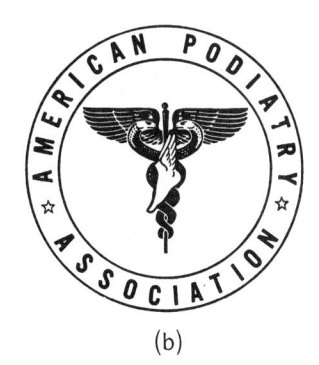

Figure 3-10:
(a) Logo for the California Podiatry Association;
(b) logo of the American Podiatry Association.

In some ways working in the hospital or some other medical situation is similar to moving into a strange country. Until you are familiar with the medical **milieu** (environment), many things will seem unusual. The hospital will seem less frightening and strange if you become familiar with the symbols that are commonly used to communicate important information and to signal important messages.

THE HOSPITAL AS WORK ENVIRONMENT

Some signs you see will guide your actions without words. Several such signs you may see include:

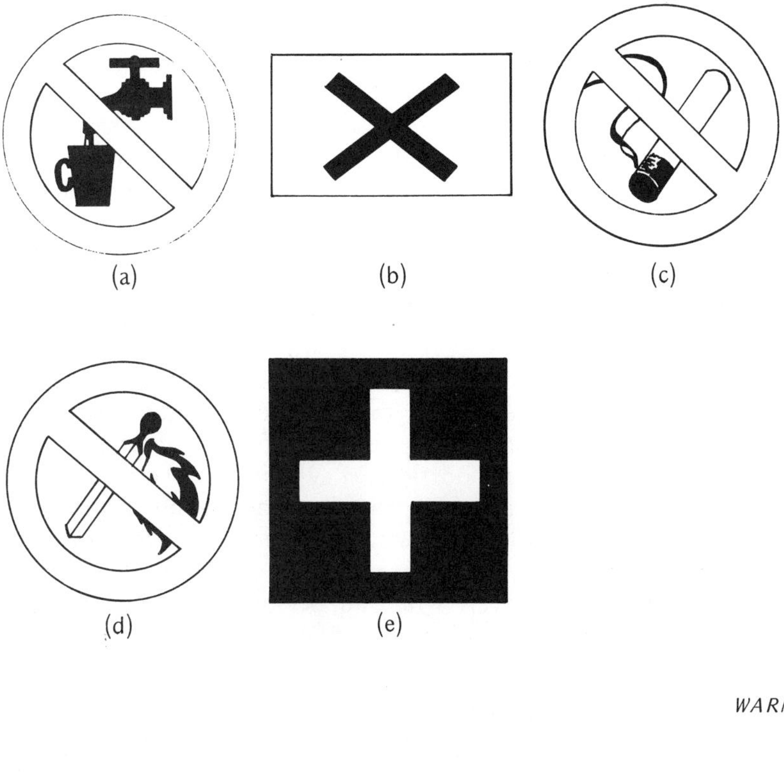

WARNING SIGNS

Figure 3-11:
(a) "Water not for drinking";
(b) "dangerous to health";
(c) "no smoking";
(d) "no open flame";
(e) "First Aid";
(Courtesy of Bel-Arts Products).

WARNING SIGNS 39 *

This sign (Figure 3-12) appearing on a door indicates that **radiotherapy** is being given in this area. Only specially trained personnel work in this area because they work with radioactive materials.

Radioactive materials give off invisible but penetrating rays capable of destroying body tissues. Unhealthy tissues are more easily destroyed by the rays than healthy tissues, of course, but healthy tissues can be damaged if care is not exercised. Obviously these materials are always handled carefully. Patients receive therapy which exposes them to just enough radiation to destroy unhealthy cells.

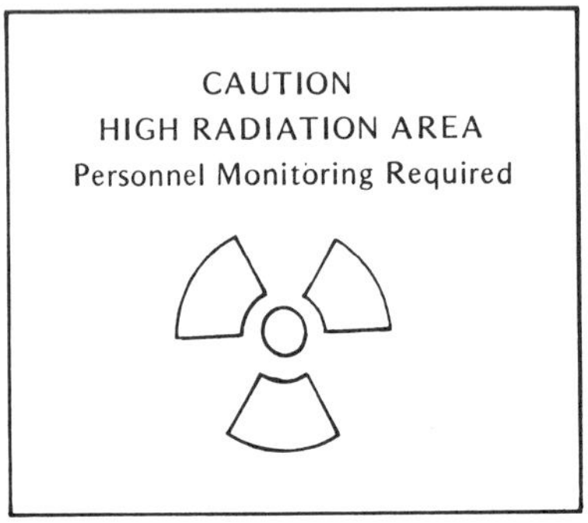

Figure 3-12: Radiation warning sign *(Courtesy of Picker Corporation).*

CAUTION
HIGH RADIATION AREA
Personnel Monitoring Required

This highly specialized branch of medicine is called "nuclear medicine." Very strict rules have been established by the government to protect both the staff and the patients being treated. Employees working in the treatment area wear specialized radiation sensitive indicators which change color according to degree of radiation exposure. Only workers using specified techniques and wearing a badge similar to the one pictured in Figure 3-13 can even enter this area. The symbol, then, acts as a clear warning to unauthorized persons to stay away. Persons who see it understand its meaning; it signals a definite message of "danger."

Figure 3-13: Film badge.

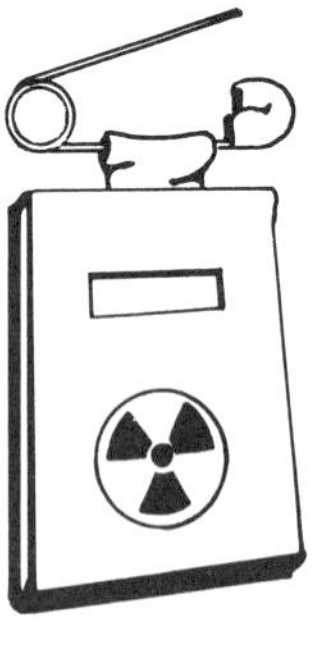

Another symbol that calls attention to "danger" is the one in Figure 3-14. Wherever it appears the skull and crossbones indicate that a substance is poisonous if taken internally. This symbol on a medicine bottle is a warning to everyone that it contains a drug that must be properly handled and controlled.

There are many dangers inherent in the operation of the highly technical services that a hospital provides. The hazards are minimized, however, when all personnel are aware of possible dangers and are prudent about avoiding them.

For example, pure oxygen is widely used in hospitals. It is also a gas which readily supports combustion. The chances of fire are always high when it is in use. It is very important, therefore, not to smoke or carry on any activity with flames or sparks which might cause a fire when oxygen is in use. Usually a "No Smoking" sign is present as a reminder. But the green triangle symbol for oxygen strongly reminds everyone of its nature and of the precautions that must be followed. Other signs with words add messages such as "Authorized Personnel Only," "Do Not Enter," and "Oxygen in Use." Now you know some symbols that are used that say the same thing as the words.

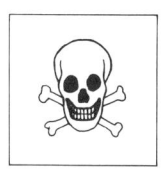

Figure 3-14: "Poison"

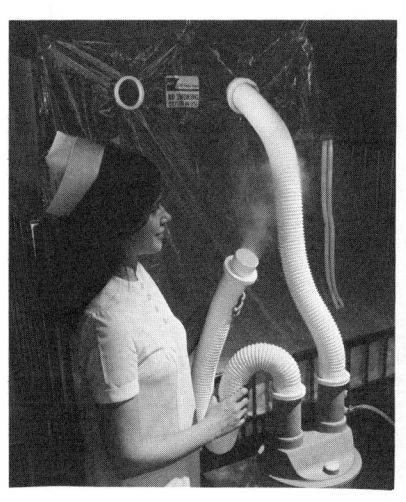

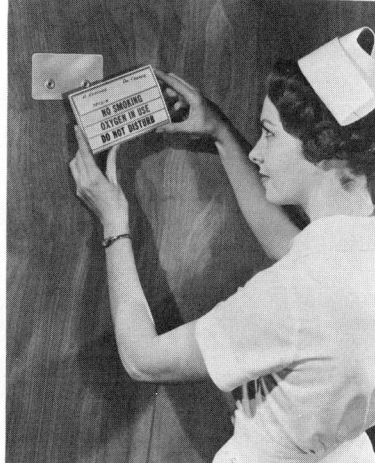

Figure 3-15: (left) Note the warning sign attached to the oxygen tent *(courtesy of Ohio Medical Products, Division of Airco, Inc.).*

Figure 3-16: (right) Signs are silent reminders of important messages *(courtesy of American Hospital Supply Corporation).*

Hospital Staff Identification

People who work on hospital staffs frequently wear name tags which give their name and title, but if you observe very carefully you may see other signs which also give you information. The type of uniform worn by certain health workers identifies their duties in a hospital.

Candy stripers were originally so named as such because of their red and white striped uniforms. Nurses usually dress in white and students from a particular nursing school usually all dress alike. There are no hard and fast rules today about uniforms, but very often within a given hospital the various types of health workers wear distinctive clothing. In many hospitals, nurses still wear caps as symbols of their status. A black banded cap may indicate a registered nurse and a blue "V" is representative in some hospitals of a licensed vocational nurse or licensed practical nurse.

Figure 3-17: The black band is frequently worn on the cap of a Registered Nurse

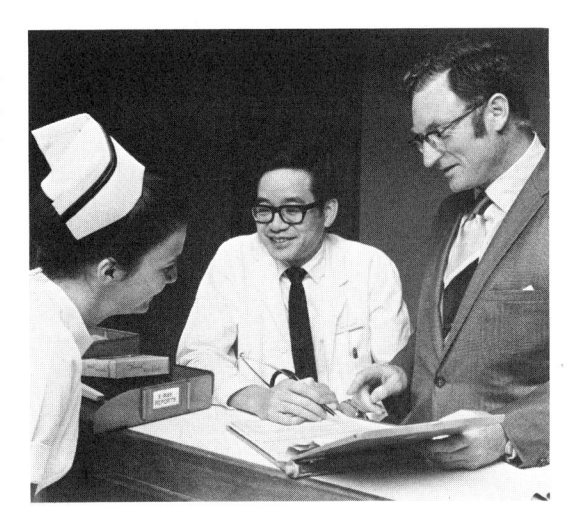

Look carefully at people's uniforms and you will see that many health workers wear a pin, a token of their particular profession and the school in which they received their education. Many of the pins will have a caduceus, a symbol of medicine, or a lamp, a symbol of nursing.

Figure 3-18: (a) Lamp; (b) Caduceus.

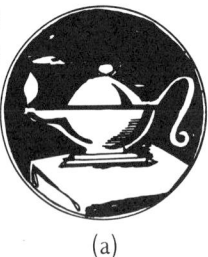

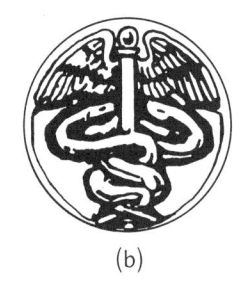

(a) (b)

An Important Symbol

Sterile (free from all living organisms) bandages must be instantly recognized because a person who has had surgery must be protected until healing is complete. The area of the **incision** (cut) is covered with a gauze called a **dressing** (bandage). It protects the incisional area from infection. Such dressings must always be free of germs and ready for use. But since germs are too small to be seen, it is impossible to see whether clean dressings are sterile or unsterile. To make sure, all dressings are packaged and marked with a special symbol. This is done by sealing packages of gauze with a sensitized tape that changes color when it is sterilized. Temperatures high enough to kill all germs also affect the tape. A single glance at the tape color lets you know whether the materials inside the package are safe to

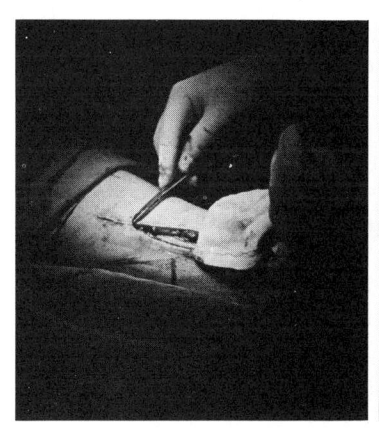

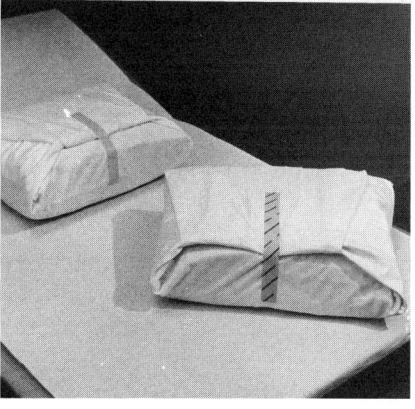

Figure 3-19: (left) A surgical incision being closed. It must be protected until healed

Figure 3-20: (right) Note the change in tape after sterilization *(courtesy of 3 M Company).*

use. The correctly colored tape is a silent sign of sterility. Figure 3-20 shows the tape before and after the sterilizing process.

Colors as Symbols

Colors are widely used in hospitals in a variety of ways. In some hospitals a sign in the lobby has a small colored block beside the name of each department. Colored lines or arrows on the corridor floors that match the lobby sign help people to find the department listed. They simply follow the matching colored line to its destination.

Sometimes color is used to identify the records of a particular physician's patients or the particular service that is providing care. Colored strips are affixed to a patient's record or to his bed. These call attention to a particular need such as a red strip indicating "reorder drugs." Tanks of medical gases are color coded for immediate identification; green for oxygen, blue for nitrous oxide, and orange for cyclopropane. Linen is also color coded for special departmental use; green for operating room, blue for obstetrics, white for use in the general care units.

In some hospitals, different colored inks are used to record the patient care given at certain times of the day or in certain situations. For example, information during the day hours of 7:00 a.m. to 7:00 p.m. may be recorded in blue, while information about the patient recorded from 7:00 p.m. to 7:00 a.m. is recorded in red. Information from the operating room is written in green and from the emergency room in brown. There are no absolute rules about the use of color, but once you become familiar with the color codes used in your facility a single glance at the symbolic color will give you immediate information.

Message Systems

Often it is necessary to locate a doctor, a special medical team, or a worker in a hurry. Each hospital has a rapid contact system known by all its staff. Some doctors carry a "bleeper"

WARNING SIGNS 43 *

call system as well. Similar to a radio receiver it transmits particular sounds when they are needed. That bleeper sound means very clearly "go to the nearest telephone, there is a message waiting for you."

Many hospitals install a paging system which is installed on each of the hospital units. A call board is strategically placed on the wall and a system of flashing lights appears. Each person who may be needed in a hurry is assigned a number. Then, when it lights up on the page system that person knows he is needed. The number is a symbol for the person's name.

An oral call system is also used in many hospitals. The name of the needed person is broadcast over the "page." The called person goes to the nearest telephone to obtain his message on hearing his name. This system is also sometimes used to alert whole groups of persons to an emergency situation. "Code Blue" or "Code 99" or "Code 66" are signals that some hospitals use to alert key personnel that a patient's heart has stopped (**cardiac arrest**). The emergency team rushes to the patient's room or emergency area ready to administer the needed assistance. It is very important that all personnel know and recognize these special signals, respond immediately if it is their responsibility, and stay out of the way if it is not. "Code Red" or "Doctor Red" are the signals that there is a fire and that fire control practices must be immediately put into effect. "Code Grey" or "Father O'Malley" are signals that a security officer is needed immediately.

It is obvious that code words do not mean the same to all persons hearing them. "Doctor Red" sounds like the name of a physician to any patient or visitor but for the hospital personnel it has a far different meaning.

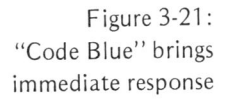

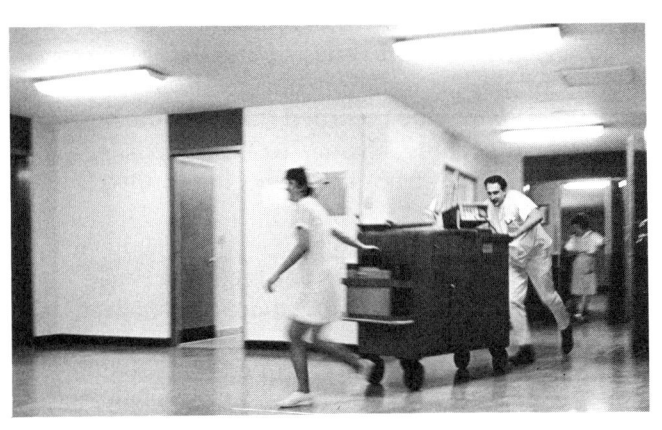

Figure 3-21: "Code Blue" brings immediate response

*44 NON-ORAL AND SYMBOLIC COMMUNICATIONS

Ringing bells, buzzers, and flashing lights are symbols of patient need. A patient sounds a buzzer to alert hospital personnel when he or she needs assistance. The buzzer sound usually is accompanied by a white light that flashes over the patient's bed, outside the room door, and at the nursing station. A red flashing light indicates the need for either emergency or immediate attention. Buzzer switches are located at the patient's bedside, bathroom, and treatment rooms.

Although patients are assigned to a specific bed for their hospital stay, they often leave that assigned area for treatments in other departments, surgery, or various tests. It is important that all personnel know at all times exactly where each patient is so that his care can be coordinated continuously. Each patient is listed on the board at the nursing station and tokens representing various departments are affixed in turn to the board to indicate the presence of the patient in a particular department.

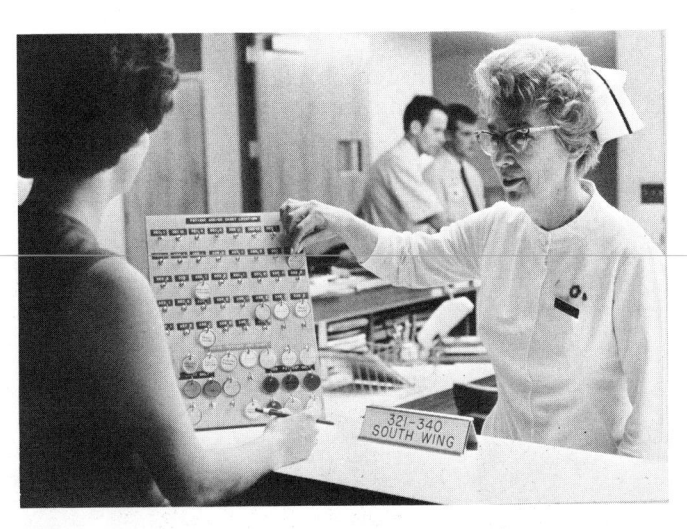

Figure 3-22: Patient location board

Symbolic Body Language

Body language is the way in which we express feelings and attitudes without saying a single word. Sometimes it is the expression on a person's face that sends a message. Sometimes it is the way a person uses his body, but generally it is a combination of both of these expressions that portrays a person's real feelings.

Examine Figure 3-23a to see how the person is expressing her feelings. The position of the arms and legs of the person in Figure 3-23a leaves little doubt that this person is happy. The

WARNING SIGNS 45 *

Figure 3-23:

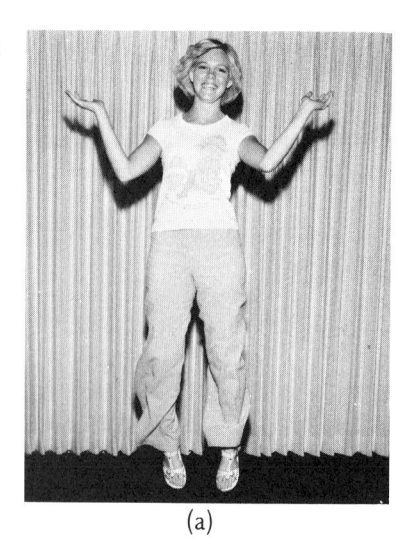

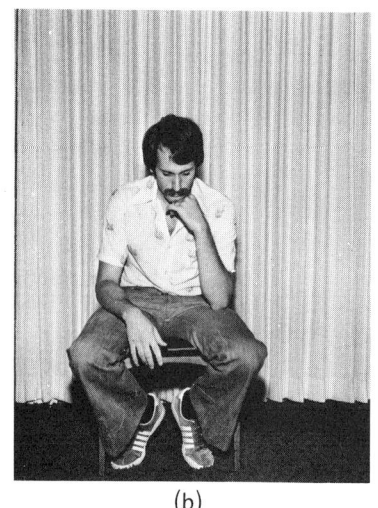

(a)   (b)

face reveals excitement and happiness. There is no doubt that facial expression and body stance reveal how people feel. Contrast the person in Figure 3-24a and Figure 3-24b. Are the feelings being expressed the same?

Figure 3-24:
(a) Happy or angry?
(b) worried or carefree?
(courtesy of Ayerst Laboratories).

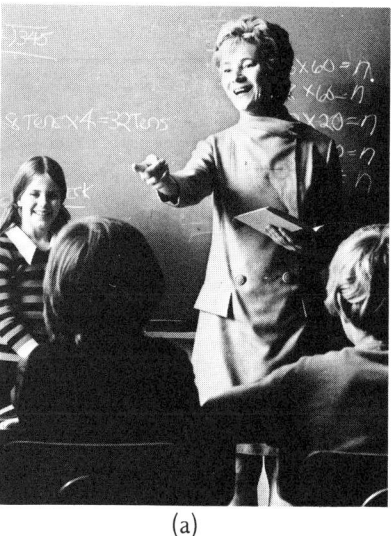

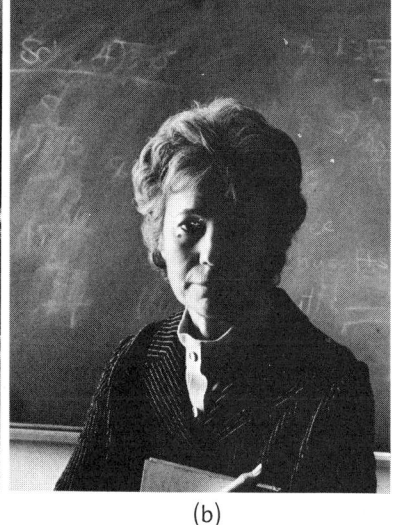

(a)   (b)

Patients offer clues of their inner feelings more subtly to the health worker. Look at the following pictures and try to label the attitude or feeling depicted.

* 46 *NON-ORAL AND SYMBOLIC COMMUNICATIONS*

Figure 3-25:

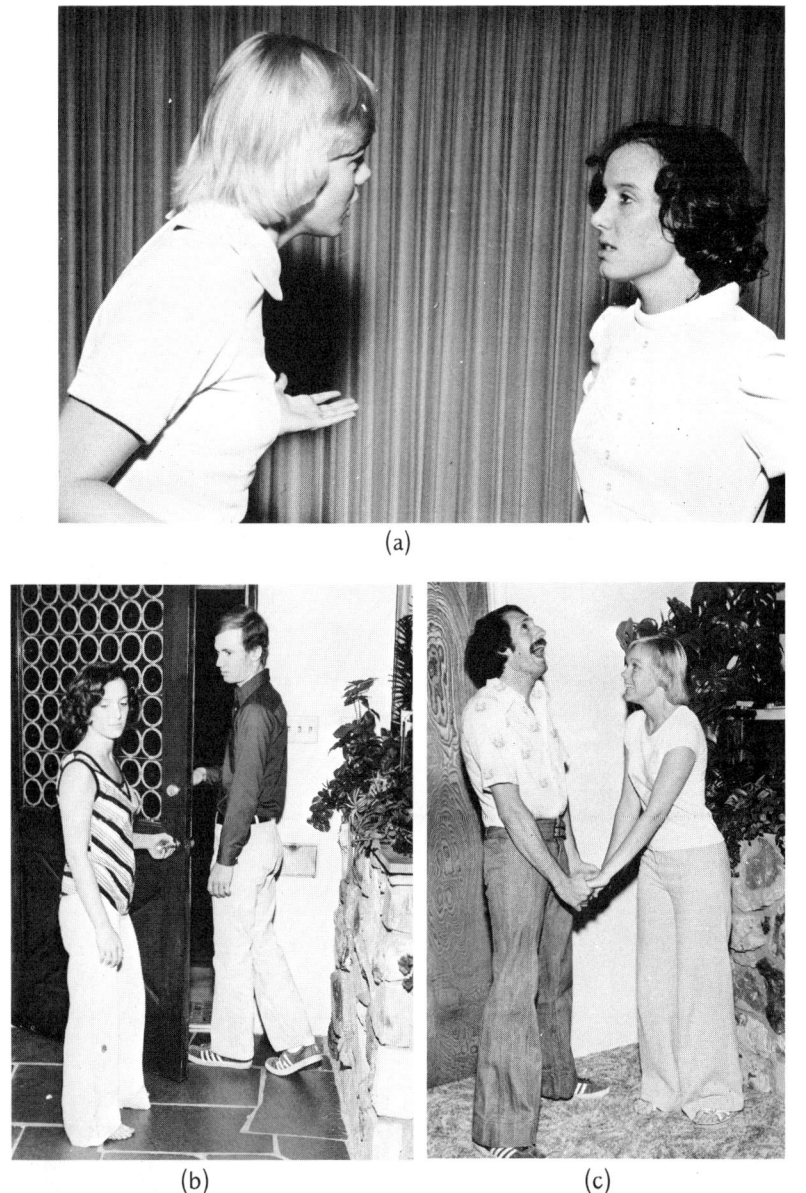

(a)

(b)   (c)

SUMMARY

Symbols are tokens, representations, signs, or objects which stand for something else. Symbols in the form of pictures, words, colors, and numbers play an important role in conveying important information to all health workers.

WARNING SIGNS 47 *

PRACTICE & REVIEW

A. Identify the professional logo by writing the name of the organization or profession it represents in the space provided.

1. _____

2. _____

3. _____

4. _____

5. _____

6. _____

7. _____

48 NON-ORAL AND SYMBOLIC COMMUNICATIONS

8. _____

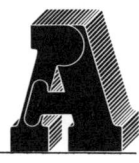

9. _____

B. Match the symbols reproduced here with the message in the column at the right.

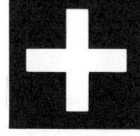

___ 1.   a. Dangerous to Health

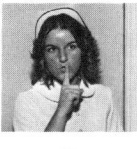

___ 2.   b. No Open Flame

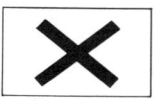

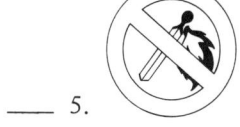

___ 3.   c. Quiet Please

___ 4.   d. First Aid

___ 5.   e. No Smoking

 f. This Area Accessible

WARNING SIGNS 49 *

C. What do these three signs mean?

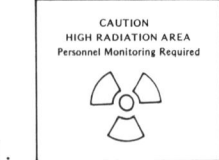

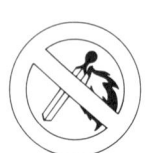

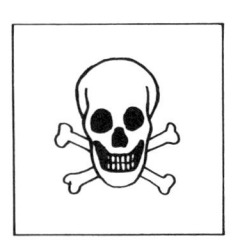

1. _____

2. _____

3. _____

* 50 NON-ORAL AND SYMBOLIC COMMUNICATIONS

After studying Chapter 4
Combining Word Forms
You should be able to:

* *Pronounce and define each of its new medical words and phrases and use the new technical jargon.*

* *Identify and define a prefix and a suffix.*

* *Combine prefixes and suffixes with basic words to form medical terms.*

PRONOUNCE THESE TEN COMBINING FORMS WITH YOUR TEACHER:

PREFIXES & SUFFIXES

cele (sēl)
cephal (sef'ah-l)
opthalm (of-thal'm)
paresis (pah-re'sis)
phleb (fleb')
phobia (fo'be-ah)
pneum (nu'm)
pseudo (su'do)
psycho (si'ko)
rrhea (re'ah)

Many medical words are formed by combining a basic term with prefixes (special beginnings) and with suffixes (special endings). Thus by altering combinations, specialized new words can be easily understood, recognized and learned. In this lesson there are approximately one hundred combining forms that can be used in literally thousands of different word combinations. They are used in medicine to communicate important details and subtle differences. For example, **cyte**, meaning cell, can be combined with numerous prefixes or suffixes to describe and identify the billions of cells in the body according to their differing functions: leukocyte, histiocyte, cytoblast, thrombocyte, fibrocyte, cytopenia, astrocyte, etc. As you can see the list has almost infinite possibilities.

A combining form is not always a suffix or a prefix but can also be a basic term to which either or both are attached. For example, the combining form "path" (pathy) may be used either as a prefix in the word pathology or as a suffix in the word adenopathy. The suffixes, prefixes, and combining terms

Figure 4-1: Blood cells formed in bone marrow.

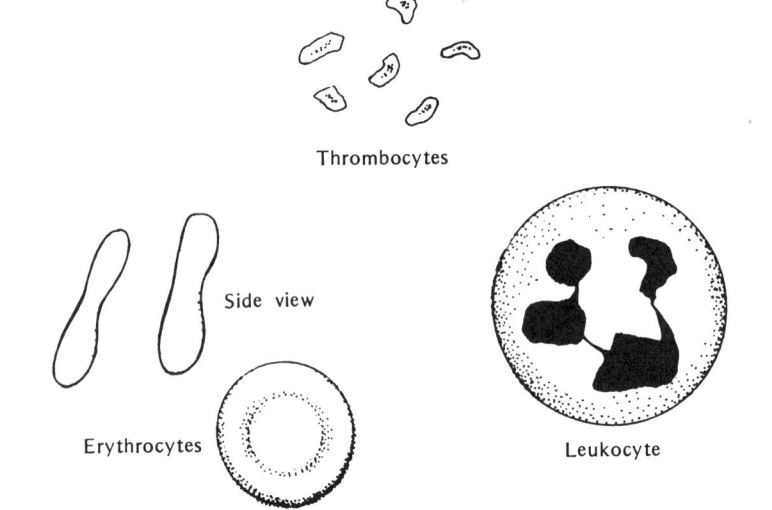

Thrombocytes

Side view

Erythrocytes

Leukocyte

in this lesson will help you make immediate use of your new knowledge.

List 1

Prefixes & Combining Forms	Pronunciation	Meaning
chondr-	kon'dr	cartilage
costa-	kos'ta	rib
epi-	ep'ĭ	above, upon
erythro-	e-rith'ro	red
hemo-	he'mo	blood
intra-	in'trah	within
leuko-, leuk-	lu'k	white
oss-, osteo-	ŏs, ŏs'te-o	bone
peri-	pĕr'e	around
thrombo-	throm'bo	clot

Suffixes & Combining Forms	Pronunciation	Meaning
-cyte	sit	cell
-blast	blast	bud, sprout

In a textbook you might read the following explanation:

Long bones of the body continue to grow in length and circumference until maturity. The **epi**physeal (**above** growing bone end) of the long bone is separated by cartilage from the long bone. It is responsible for the growth in length of the **oss**eous (bony) tissue. It is in this area that **chondro**cytes (cartilage cells) maintain a thin area of cartilage which is gradually replaced by **osteo**cytes as **oss**ification (converting to bone) takes place.

Bones grow in circumference because special **osteoblasts** (young bone-forming cells) found in the **periosteum** (outside covering of bone) continually lay down osseous (bone) tissue. In addition to providing strength and protection, osseous tissue has a **hemopoietic** (blood forming) function. Some of the **leuko**cytes (white blood cells) as well as **thrombo**cytes (blood clotting cells) and **erythro**cytes (red blood cells) have **intra**osseous (within bone) origin. The hemopoietic cells are found in the ends of long bones and in flat bones such as the sternum and ribs. These two bones are attached by way of **costa**l (rib) cartilage.

Figure 4-2: Long bone structure

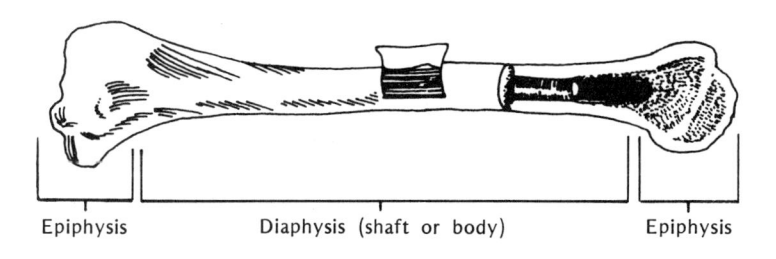

Epiphysis Diaphysis (shaft or body) Epiphysis

List 2

Prefixes & Combining Forms	Pronunciation	Meaning
ad-	ăd	to, toward, increase
aden-	ăd-en	gland
ante-	ăn'te	before, forward
bi-, bin-	bi, bin	two
dys-	dĭs	painful
hyster-	his-ter	uterus
metra-, metro-	mĕ'trah, mĕ'tro	uterus
neo-	ne'o	new
para-	păr'ah	around, near
pre-	pre	before

List 2 continued	Suffixes & Combining Forms	Pronunciation	Meaning
	-cele	sel	hernia or protrusion
	-oma	o'mah	tumor
	-pathy	păth'e	abnormality or disease
	-plasm	plăzm	stuff, substance
	-rrhea	re'ah	flow, discharge

Figure 4-3: (a) Normal position of uterus; (b) anteflexed position of uterus.

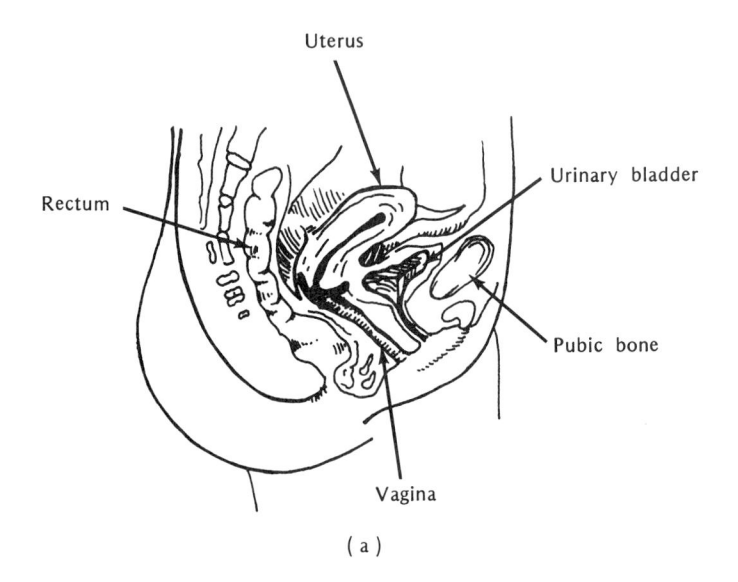

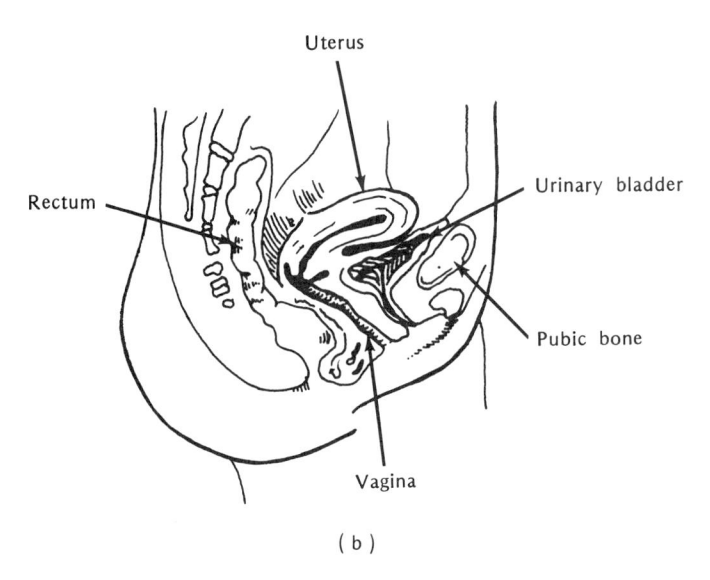

(a)

(b)

*54 COMBINING WORD FORMS

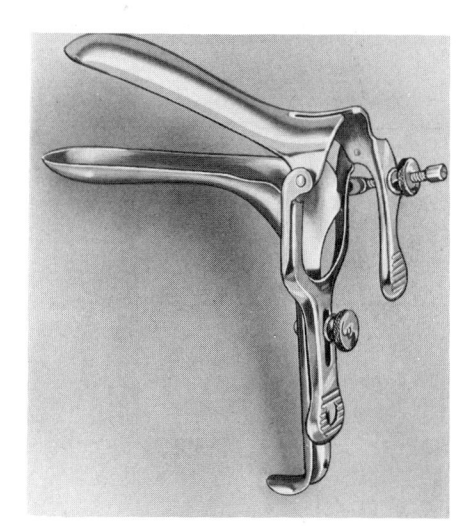

Figure 4-4: Bivalve vaginal speculum *(courtesy of Sherwood Medical Industries).*

These notes were made regarding Mrs. Jones following a pelvic examination by her physician:

Mrs. Jones is in for a **pre**-operative (before surgery) pelvic examination. Vaginal examination: digitally (with fingers) and using **bi**valve (two-valve) vaginal speculum reveals marked cysto**cele** (bladder protrusion or herniation, swelling) and recto**cele** (rectal protrusion). Condition accompanied by complaint of **dys**parunia (painful intercourse), dysmeno**rrhea** (painful menstrual flow) and metro**rrhea** (abnormal uterine discharge). Evidence of metro**pathy** (uterine abnormality). Uterus is severely **ante**flexed (bent forward or before). Large **neo**plasm (new growth or substance) felt in wall of uterus. Possible **ade**noma (glandular tumor). **Para**metric examination negative (near or around uterus). The adnexa (tubes and ovaries near or toward uterus) appear normal.

Impression:
Uterine neoplasm
Anteflexed uterus

Possible recommendation:
Pelvic exploration
Hysterectomy (removal of uterus)

List 3

Prefixes & Combining Forms	Pronunciation	Meaning
chole-	ko′le	bile; gall
cyst-	sĭst	bladder
denti-, dent-	děn-tĭ	tooth
derma-	der′mah	skin
laparo-, lapar-	lăp′ah-ro	loin; flank

COMBINING WORD FORMS 55

List 3
continued

Suffixes & Combining Forms	Pronunciation	Meaning
-asis	ah-sĭs	state; condition
-ectomy	ek′to-me	excision; removal
-itis	i′tĭs	inflammation
-lith	lĭth	stone
-otomy	ot′o-me	cutting into

Figure 4-5: Note the location of the organs described in diagnosis.

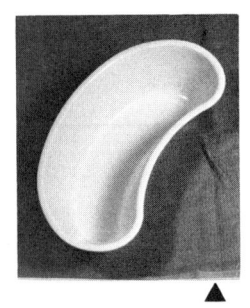

Figure 4-6: Emesis basin.

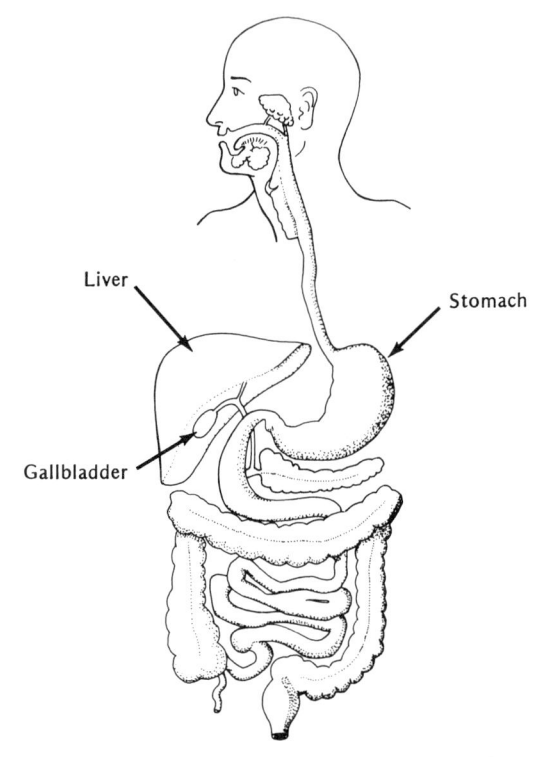

The following is a sample hospital nursing assignment:

Nurse: P. Monroe, L.V.N.
Patient: Mrs. Janice Price   **Room:** 472B
Diagnosis:
Cholecys**titis** (gallbladder inflammation)
Cholelith**asis** (gall stone condition)
Nursing Care:
    1. Surgical **derma**tological (skin) preparation for **lapar**otomy (surgery which cuts into the loin) and possible cholecys**tec-tomy** (removal of) and **lysis** (breaking up) of adhesions.

*56 *COMBINING WORD FORMS*

2. Vomiting. Record all **emesis** (vomiting).
3. Has false teeth. Be sure to provide **denture** (tooth) cup.

List 4

Prefixes & Combining Forms	Pronunciation	Meaning
ano-	an-o	bowel
arth-	ar'th	joint
bio-	bi'o	life
entero-	en'ter-o	intestine
gastr-, gastro-	gas'tr	stomach
gero-	jer'o	aged
gloss-	glos'	tongue
im-, in-	im, in	into; in, not
mast-	măst	breast
pan-	păn	all
phleb-	fleb'	vein
procto-	prok'to	rectum

Suffixes & Combining Forms	Pronunciation	Meaning
-phobia	fo'be-ah	fear
-somni	som'nĭ	sleep

This is a nursing summary prepared by a student as the basis for a discussion of pertinent nursing care:

Patient: Mrs. E. N. Dettone, 75 year-old female
Admitted: June 16
Admission Diagnosis:
1. **Gastroenter**itis (stomach and intestine inflammation).
2. **Anal** (opening to lower bowel) mass (growth).

On initial encounter this alert, cooperative **geriatric** (aged) lady appeared even older than her recorded age. Her hair was totally white and her face was drawn and fatigued. She stated she had been sick to her stomach and had had frequent "bloody" stools and some pain for the past four days. Her tongue was reddened and sore, giving evidence of a **gloss**itis (tongue inflammation) due to inadequate food and fluid intake. Diagnostic tests were carried out which included:
1. Gastric analysis.
2. **Procto**scopy (examination of rectum) and sigmoidoscopy (examination of the sigmoid colon).
3. Anal **bio**psy (taking some living tissue from the opening into the bowel).

COMBINING WORD FORMS 57 *

Figure 4-7: Note the body organs that are mentioned in the nursing summary.

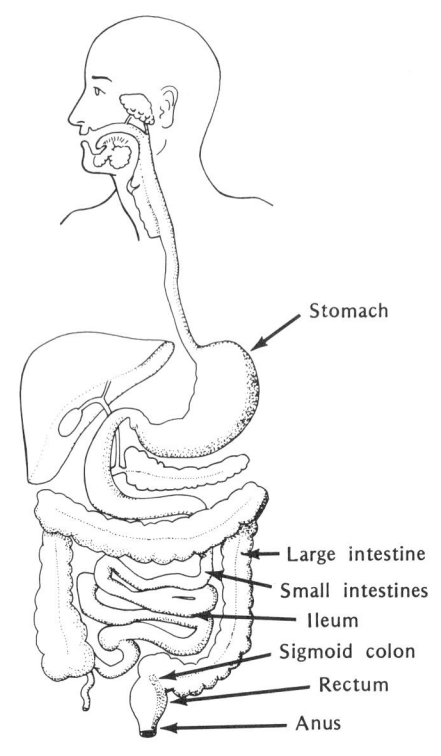

4. **Gastro**intestinal series (X-ray studies of stomach and intestines).
5. Stool culture.

One evening during her hospitalization Mrs. Dettone suffered an attack of anthro**phobia** (marked fear of flowers). When an arrangement was delivered to her roommate she became so disturbed and anxious that she experienced in**somnia** (not able to sleep) until the flowers were completely removed from the room. She revealed a past history of three pregnancies, followed each time by a **mast**itis (breast inflammation) so she was disappointedly unable to nurse any of her children. She had a **pan**hysterectomy (excision of the whole uterus) shortly after the birth of her third child some 33 years ago. At that time she had a **phleb**itis (vein inflammation) and was confined to bed for a week. Other than some **arth**ritis (joint inflammation) in her knee that "flares up" occasionally she has been remarkably well until her present problem.

Figure 4-8: Proctoscope (an instrument used to view the lower bowel).

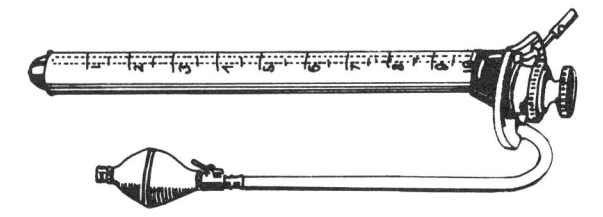

List 5

Prefixes & Combining Forms	Pronunciation	Meaning
a-, an-	a, ăn	without; not; deficient
ab-	ăb	away from
arterio-	ar-te′re-o	relating to a blood vessel
cardi-	kar′de	heart
endo-	en′do	within
hyper-	hi′per	above; excess of
hypo-	hi′po	under; deficiency of
my-	mi	muscle
poly-	pol′e	many
scler-	skle′r	hard
tachy-	tăk′e	fast
vas-	vas	vessel

Suffixes & Combining Forms	Pronunciation	Meaning
-oxia	ok′se-ah	pertaining to oxygen
-osis	o′sĭs	process; condition

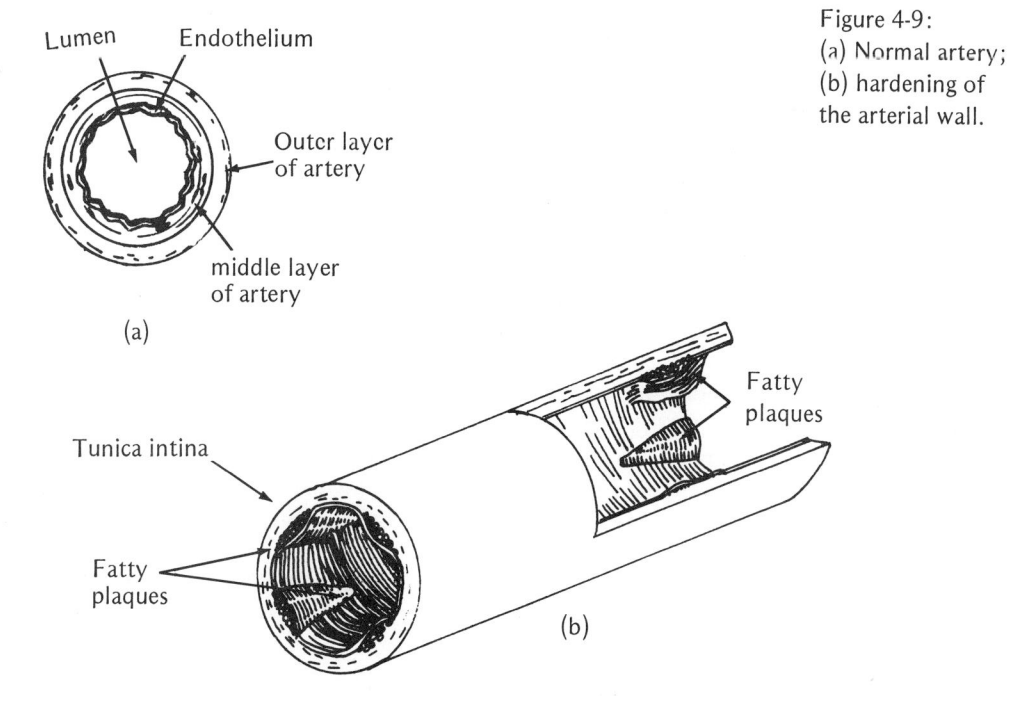

Figure 4-9:
(a) Normal artery;
(b) hardening of the arterial wall.

COMBINING WORD FORMS 59

Figure 4-10: Three layers make up the heart wall.

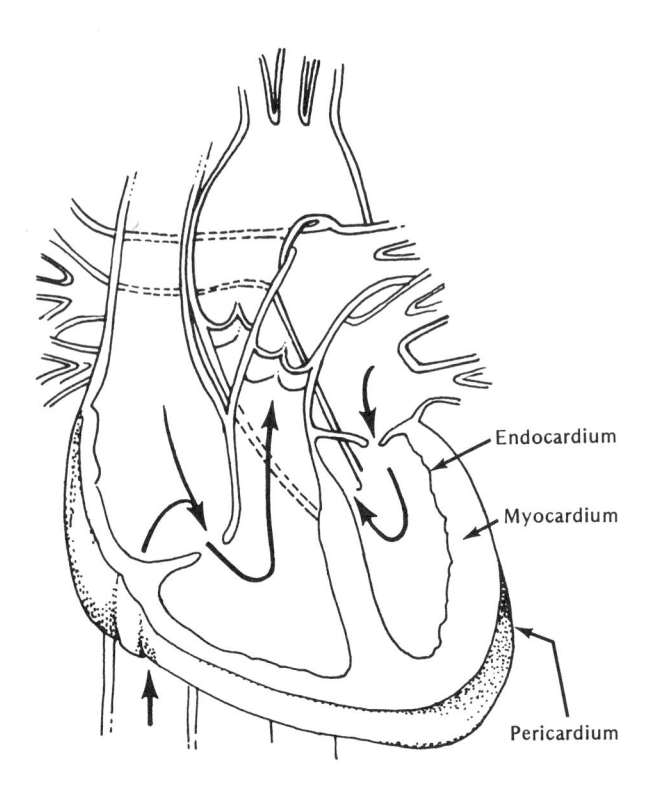

Endocardium
Myocardium
Pericardium

This is an example of an article which might appear in a family health magazine:

Arteriosclerosis (blood vessel hardening process) is a common health problem faced by much of the American populace today. Essentially, this condition affects the **endo**thelium (lining within) of the **vas**cular (blood vessel) system of the body. Arteriosclerosis is a **poly**vascular (many vessel) disease which narrows the arteries obstructing the flow of blood. **Cardi**ac (heart) attacks and **hyper**tension (high blood pressure) are frequently due to just such narrowing. **Tachy**cardia (fast heart) accompanies these conditions as the **myo**cardium (heart muscle) strives to deliver blood through the **ab**normally (away from normal) narrowed passageways. The **an**omaly (not normal) in blood flow results in insufficient oxygen reaching the tissues. This condition is called **hypo**xia (under supply of oxygen).

* 60 *COMBINING WORD FORMS*

List 6

Prefixes & Combining Forms	Pronunciation	Meaning
cephal—	sef'ah-l	head
crani-	kra'ne	skull
encephal-	en-sef'ah-l	brain
hemi-	hem'i	half
infra-	in'frah	below
neuro-	nu'ro	nerve
opthalm-	of-thal'm	eye
oto-	o'to	ear
pseudo-	su'do	false
psycho-	si'ko	soul; mind
sub-	sub	under

Suffixes & Combining Forms	Pronunciation	Meaning
-algia	al'je-ah	pain
-paresis	pah-re'sis	paralysis

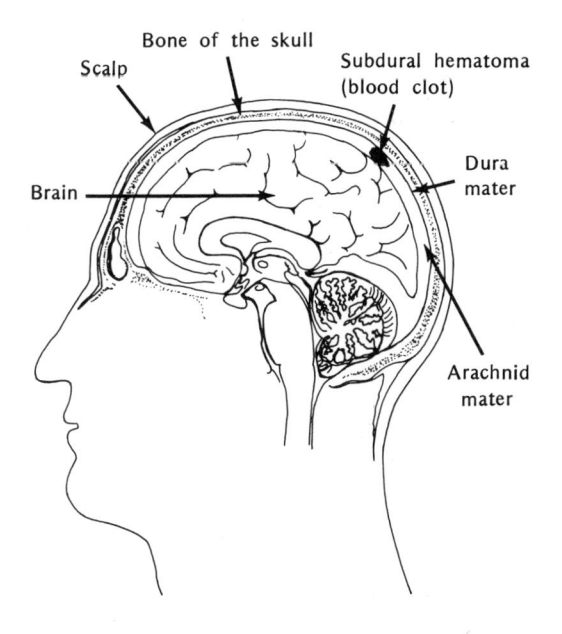

Figure 4-11: A subdural hematoma occurs when blood accumulates between two layers of the brain coverings.

COMBINING WORD FORMS 61 *

Angela Delang, R.N., on duty in a **neuro**surgical (nerve) unit found these diagnoses among her assigned patients:

Patient	Diagnosis
R. Dentom, rm. 702a	**Sub**dural hematoma (blood clot below the covering of the brain)
P. Henen, rm. 702b	**Infra**neision rt. eye (downward, below deviation of eye)
J. Davis, rm. 702c	**Cephal**algia/undetermined etiology (head pain, unknown cause)
R. Petofsky, rm. 703	Viral **encephal**itis (brain inflammation)
L. Crammer, rm. 704a	**Pseudohemi**paresis (false half-paralysis)
D. Murray, rm. 704b	Migraine headache of **psycho**somatic origin (caused by emotional or mind reactions)
B. Schmidt, rm. 704c	**Opthalm**odynia (nerve pain of the eye)
C. Connelly, rm. 704d	**Crani**otomy (skull which had undergone surgical cutting)
E. Perez, rm. 705	Left **oto**cleisis (closing of ear passage)

List 7

Prefixes & Combining Forms	Pronunciation	Meaning
ex-	eks	out
hydro-	hi-dro′	water
neph-	něf	kidney
py-, pyo-	pi, pio	pus
ren-	ren	kidney
retro-	ret′ro	backward
supra-	soo′prah	above
tox-	tŏks	poison
uro-, uria-	u′ro	urine

Suffixes & Combining Forms	Pronunciation	Meaning
-stomy	s'to-me	to create an opening
-plasty	plas'te	surgical correction

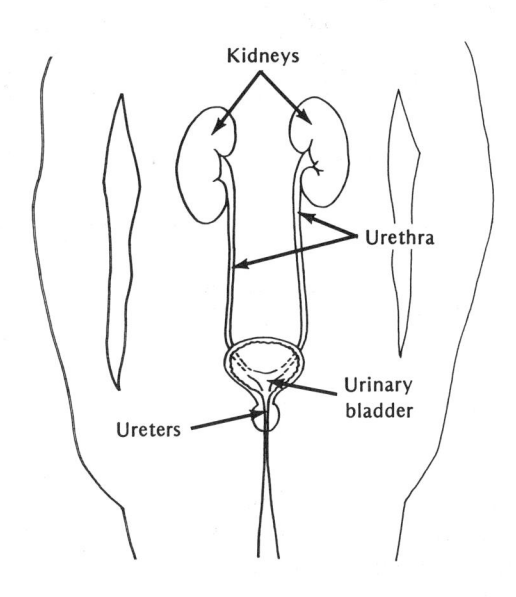

Figure 4-12: Organs of the urinary system.

This brief description will increase your understanding of urinary disease.

The urinary system is composed of two kidneys and two tube-like ureters found in the **retro**peritoneal (backward or behind the peritoneum) space, a urinary bladder in the pelvic cavity and a small tube, the urethra, which drains outside the body. The **suprare**nal (above the kidney) space is occupied by the adrenal (to or toward or near the kidney) glands.

Hydronephrosis (condition of water in the kidney) is one form of renal pathology in which the nephron (functioning kidney unit) is eventually destroyed by pressure as urinary stasis or stoppage develops. Hydronephrosis can develop when **ren**al calculi (kidney stones) block the ureter. If urine is not **ex**creted (put out) from the body properly, **tox**ic (poisonous) substances accumulate in the kidneys resulting in **neph**ritis (kidney inflammation). **Py**uria (pus in the urine) is one of the signs of nephritis. Surgical correction of this situation through nephro**stomy** (surgical drainage of kidney) may be necessary to reestablish adequate drainage from this organ.

Figure 4-13: (left) Internal normal kidney. Urine produced in the cortex is drained through the medulla into the pelvis and then into the ureter.

Figure 4-14: (right) Hydronephrosis.

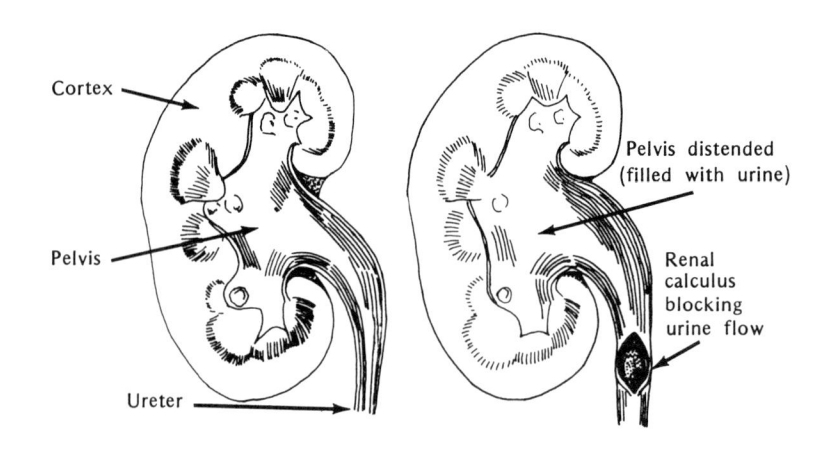

List 8

Prefixes & Combining Forms	Pronunciation	Meaning
anti-, ant-	an′tĭ	against
audio-	aw′de	hearing
centesis	sen-te′sĭs	puncture; perforate
inter-	in′ter	between
micro-	mi′kro	small
myc-, myco-	mi-k, mi-ko	fungus
pneum-, pneumo-	nu′m, nu′mo	air; lung
pyr-, pyro-	pi-re	fever
radio-	ra′deo	ray
thoraco-, thorac-	tho′rah-ko, tho′rahk	relating to chest or thorax

Suffixes & Combining Forms	Pronunciation	Meaning
-gram	gram	record
-logy	ŏl′o-je	study of
-scope	skop	examine

A ward clerk transferring orders for a particular patient to a cardex learns a great deal about that patient. For instance, she finds that the doctor suspects a **pneumo**nia (lung condition) caused either by a bacterial germ (pneumococcus) or by a fungus (**myco**tic). She realizes that the orders mean that she has to make arrangements with the **radiology** department (X-ray study) to take front or anterior (A), back or posterior (P) and

* 64 COMBINING WORD FORMS

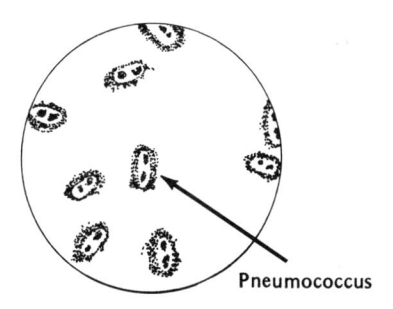

Figure 4-15: Pneumococci as seen under the microscope.

side or lateral X-rays of the patient's chest. She also knows that a sputum specimen has to be collected and examined under a **microscope** (an instrument to examine things too small to be seen by the naked eye). Again, copying orders into the record she notes that the patient is to be given aspirin for fever (**pyrexia**) and analgesics to relieve the chest pain he is experiencing between his ribs (**intercostal**) and that the **antibiotics** (against living organisms) are to be discontinued and probably changed. The ward clerk reads on: if fluid continues to be present in the chest the doctor will consider **centesis** (a procedure to puncture and drain) of the **thorax** (chest). She promptly makes arrangements for Mr. Robinson to have his ears tested in accord with the order for an **audiogram** (a hearing test of which a graphic record will be made).

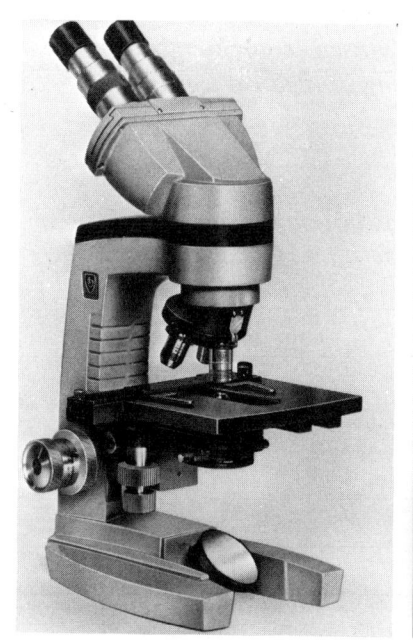

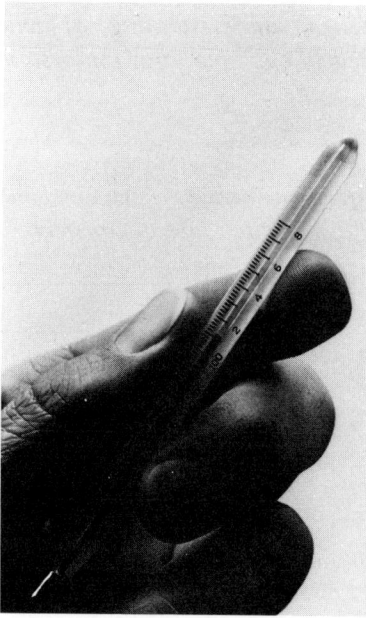

Figure 4-16: (left) Microscope *(courtesy of American Optical Corporation).*

Figure 4-17: (right) The temperature show illustrates pyrexea.

COMBINING WORD FORMS 65 *

Here are the orders as she actually received and transferred them:

October 17

1. Rule out pneumococcal pneumonia/mycotic pneumonia.
2. Schedule with radiology department for A/P and lateral thorax.
3. Aspirin, grs. x q 3° for pyrexia.
4. Continue analgesic for intercostal pain.
5. Discontinue present antibiotic drugs.
6. Sputum specimen to laboratory for microscopic examination.
7. Schedule for audiogram 10/19.
8. If chest fluid not decreased by a.m. would like to consult on thoracentesis.

SUMMARY   *Combining forms are very useful in medical communication. Prefixes and suffixes can be used together and with basic terms in many ways to form countless new words. A fundamental understanding of widely-used combining forms will greatly enhance your understanding of medical words.*

PRACTICE & REVIEW   *Explain and define the new combining terms you have been using. Remember, you learned how to pronounce them at the beginning of this chapter.*

1. cele _____
2. cephal _____
3. opthalm _____
4. paresis _____
5. phleb _____
6. phobia _____
7. pneum _____

8. pseudo _____

9. psycho _____

10. rrhea _____

Now, double-check the meaning of the terms above by studying the brief definitions given in the Glossary-Index at the back of this text.

Test yourself quickly before going on to learn other medical and professional terms. Use these short review exercises to practice for your new work in health services. Your teacher will also help by recommending various other Study Activities.

A. Match the prefixes at the left with the proper definition in the right-hand column:

  ____ 1. osteo-   a. intestine
  ____ 2. neo-   b. below
  ____ 3. chole-   c. new
  ____ 4. entero-   d. above
  ____ 5. cardi-   e. against
  ____ 6. hyper-   f. bone
  ____ 7. anti-   g. before
  ____ 8. ot-   h. ear
  ____ 9. infra-   i. gall bladder
  ____ 10. ante-   j. heart

B. Match the suffixes on the left with their definition in the right-hand column:

  ____ 1. -ology   a. abnormality
  ____ 2. -algia   b. process, condition
  ____ 3. -oxia   c. study of
  ____ 4. -scope   d. cell
  ____ 5. -osis   e. stone
  ____ 6. -oma   f. cutting into
  ____ 7. -otomy   g. pertaining to oxygen
  ____ 8. -cyte   h. pain
  ____ 9. -pathy   i. tumor
  ____ 10. -lith   j. examine

C. Carefully study the terms below. Then draw a single line under the prefixes and a double line under the suffixes:

1. toxic
2. gastric
3. proctoscopy
4. fibrocyte
5. epiphyseal
6. ossification
7. costal
8. bivalve
9. nephritis
10. parametric
11. craniotomy
12. pneumonia
13. osteocyte
14. hematosis
15. hypertension
16. myocardium
17. vascular
18. endothelium
19. anthrophobia
20. hydronephrosis

After studying Chapter 5
Common Medical Abbreviations
You should be able to:

* Pronounce and define each of its new medical words and phrases and use the new technical jargon.

* Name and give an example of the three systems of measurement.

* List the initials of eight health workers.

* List ten abbreviations used in a hospital.

* Name five common health problems and their abbreviations.

PRONOUNCE THESE TEN NEW WORDS WITH YOUR TEACHER: MEDICAL WORDS

anorexia (an″o-rek′se-ah)
auscultate (aw′skul-tat)
sphygmomanometer (sfig′mo-mah-nom′e-ter)
umbilicus (um-bĭl′ē-kus)
speculum (spek′u-lum)

liter (lēt-er)
deci- (des′ĭ)
centi- (sen′tĭ)
milli- (mil′e)
kilo- (kil′o)

Abbreviations are shortened forms of words. They are used by the very busy people in the health field to communicate accurately and to save time as they exchange ideas and orders with one another. Sometimes the abbreviation is part of the word such as O.B. (obstetrics) which is pronounced as two separate letters or Peds, a shortened form of pediatrics. The abbreviation **Peds** is pronounced as a single syllable. See Figure 5-1.

Sometimes, though, abbreviations are in the form of a series of letters. Most such abbreviations are standard, such as EEG, the electroencephalogram. Here the letters are the initials of combining terms: E for electric, E for encephalo (brain), and G for gram (recording). Hence, EEG is a recording of the electrical patterns of the brain. Another, ECG, stands for an electrocardiogram, a heart function test.

Figure 5-1:
The pediatrician examines the baby in the 'peds' department.

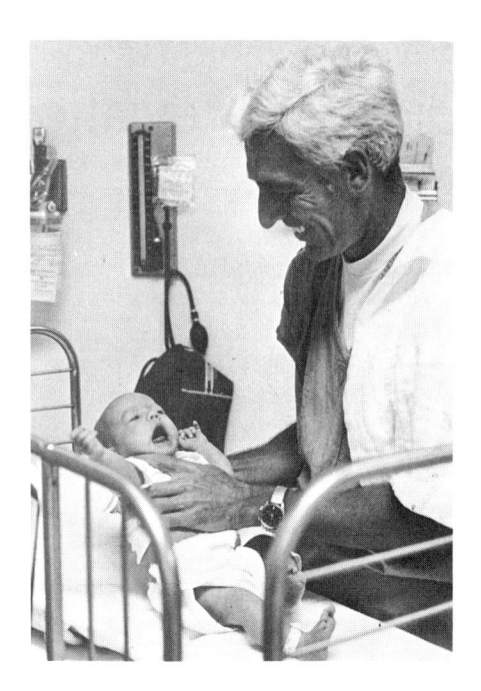

Figure 5-2:
This is an ECG strip. What test has been recorded?

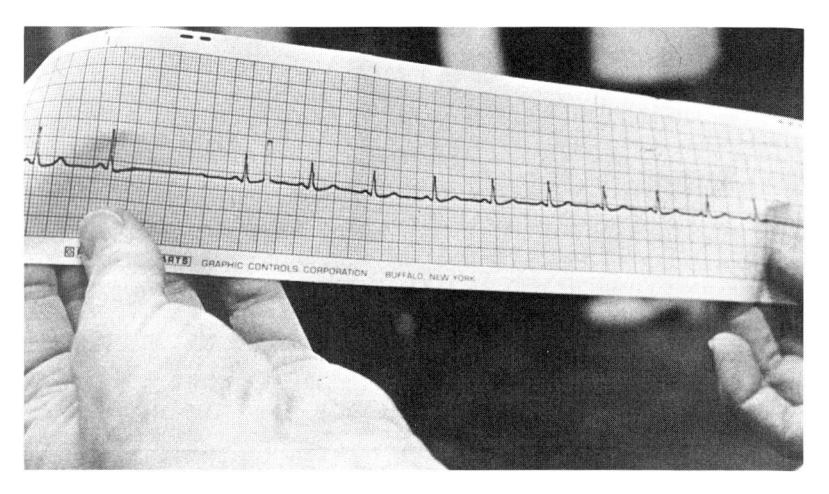

Other shortened words which are common have come into being primarily through usage. These are considered medical **jargon** (specialized vocabulary). For example, all hospital personnel recognize that a patient being readied for surgery will have an order to prepare or "prep" the skin before the surgery is performed. **Prepping** the skin usually includes removing all body hair with a razor and cleaning the skin with a special soap to cut down on the possibility of infection.

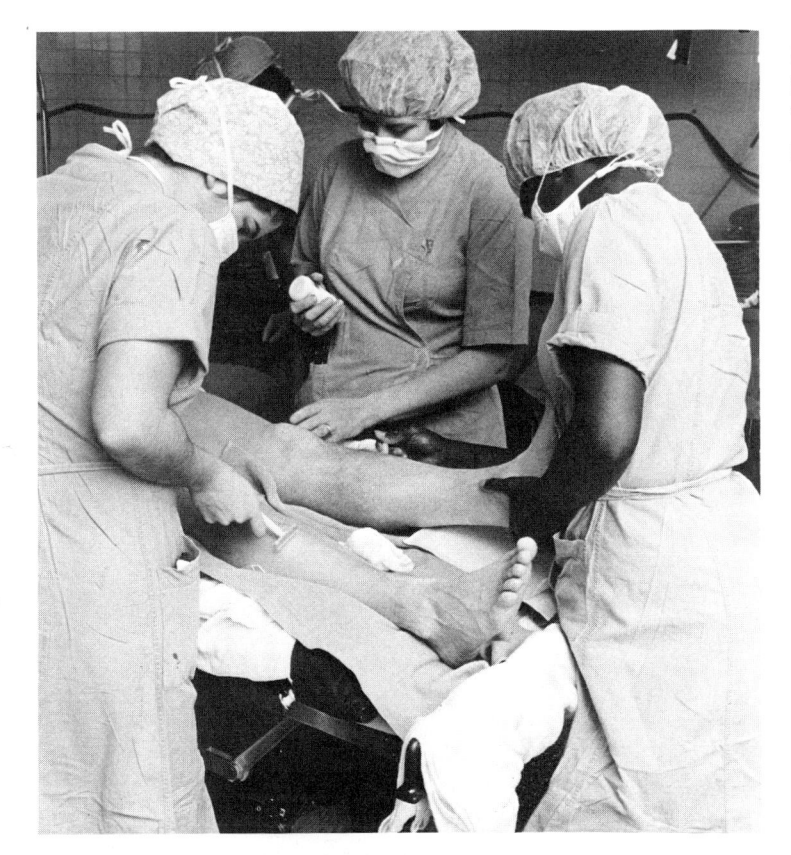

Figure 5-3: Surgical skin 'prep' prior to surgery.

Though frequently used, abbreviations are only safe and only of value if they are correctly understood. You can imagine the problem if a physician orders an EEG and the laboratory personnel perform an ECG, recording the electrical activity of the heart rather than of the brain. In fact, EKG is used by some medical staff to order an electrocardiogram simply because the sounds of "ee" and "see" in E*E*G and E*C*G can be confused easily. So, never be embarrassed to admit you do not recognize an abbreviation or do not understand the medical jargon. Be prompt in seeking clarification at *all* times since some abbreviations are non-standard and may vary from hospital to hospital and from one part of the country to another.

Abbreviations are used by every member of the health team when communicating with one another. But you must be careful when talking with patients. Although health workers are very comfortable using abbreviations, patients may become confused and unduly anxious when shortened forms are used in their presence.

HEALTH WORKER ABBREVIATIONS Health workers are often designated by both official and non-official initials such as those listed below:

R.N.	Registered Nurse
L.V.N.	Licensed Vocational Nurse
L.P.N.	Licensed Practical Nurse
N.A.	Nursing Assistant
H.A.	Health Assistant
M.D.	Doctor of Medicine
R.C.T.	Respiratory Care Therapist
R.T.	Radiologic Technologist
E.M.T.	Emergency Medical Technician
M.A.	Medical Assistant

Do you remember how each health worker functions on the health team?

Figure 5-4: (left) The R.N. is checking the report with the L.V.N.

Figure 5-5: (right) The R.C.T. helps the patient breath more easily with an I.P.P.B. machine (Intermittent Positive Breathing) *(courtesy of Puritan-Bennett Corporation).*

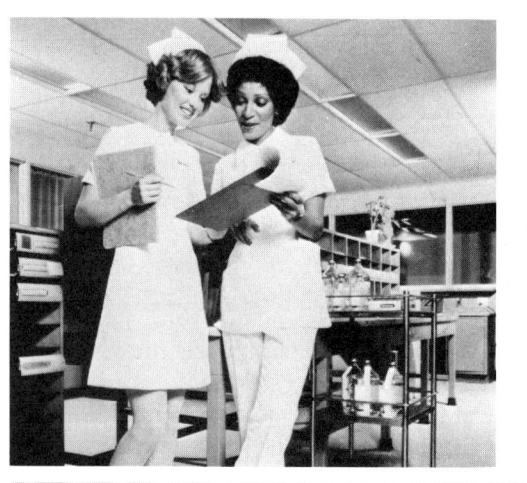

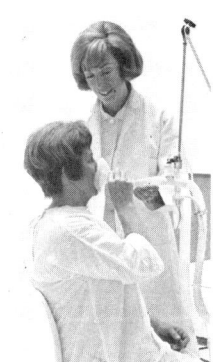

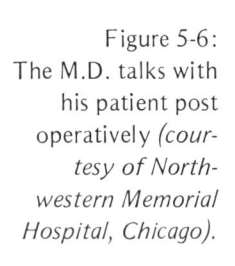

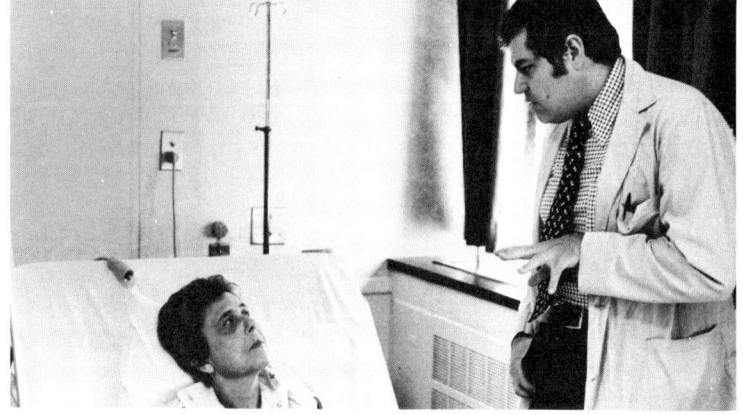

Figure 5-6: The M.D. talks with his patient post operatively *(courtesy of Northwestern Memorial Hospital, Chicago).*

*72 COMMON MEDICAL ABBREVIATIONS

HOSPITAL DEPARTMENT ABBREVIATIONS

Departments in the hospital are frequently designated by abbreviations or initials. Many you will recognize from previous lessons.

C.S.	Central Service (or Supply); area where supplies are prepared
E.R.	Emergency Room; area where emergency cases are treated
O.R.	Operating Room; area where surgery is performed
I.C.C.	Intensive Coronary (or Cardiac) Care for heart attack victims
Med/Surg	Medical and Surgical Service; care for patients with medical and surgical conditions
O.B.	Obstetrics; care for maternity patients
Peds	Pediatrics; care for sick children
Neuro	Neurology; care for patients with nervous system ailments
D.C.U.	Definitive Care Unit; an intermediate care unit between intensive care and general care
Psych	Psychiatry; care for those with emotional illness
Gyne	Gynecology; care for female reproductive problems
Rehab	Rehabilitation; area where restorative therapy is provided

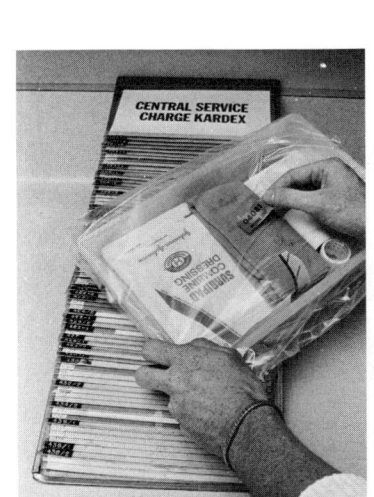

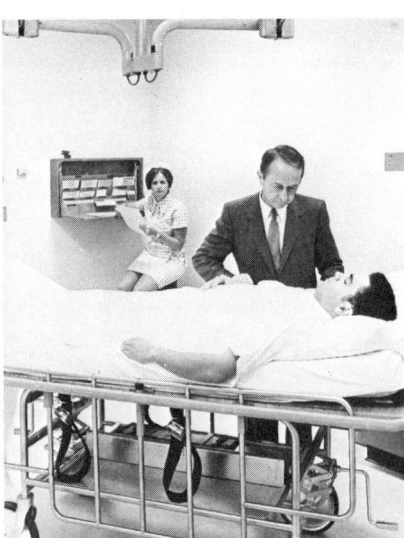

Figure 5-7: (left) The C.S. department packages, trays of supplies for the surg-unit.

Figure 5-8: (right) The LPN is ready to note the findings of the M.D. as he examines the patient in the E.R.

Figure 5-9: The Surgical Team performs surgery in the O.R.

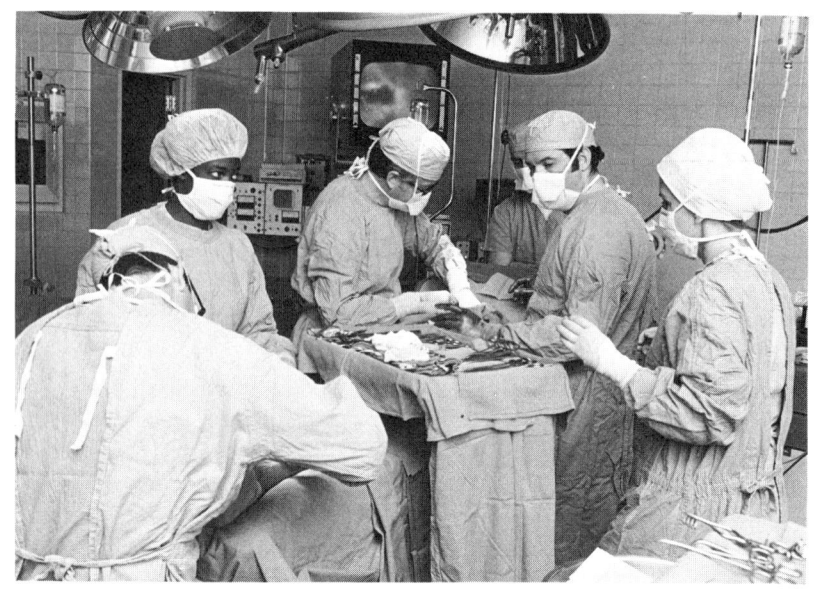

Figure 5-10: This young person is receiving rehab instruction to help him overcome the handicap of a developmental abnormality *(courtesy of The National Foundation March of Dimes)*.

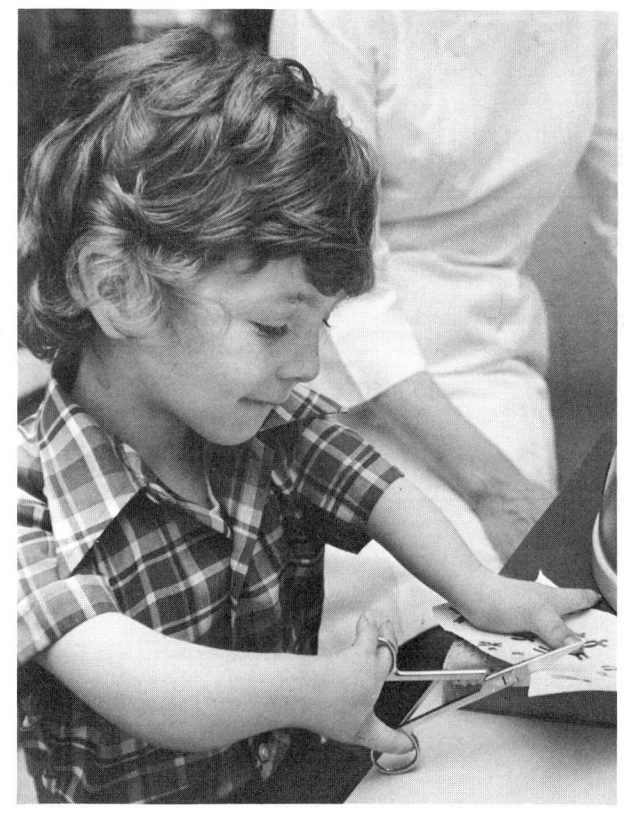

ABBREVIATIONS FOR TESTS

We have already seen that EEG and ECG are used in place of the long words electroencephalogram and electrocardiogram. Here are some other tests that are usually expressed in a similar way.

EMG	Electromyogram; a muscle function test
v.s.	Vital signs which include temperature, pulse rate, respiratory rate and blood pressure
T.	Temperature
P.	Pulse
R.	Respiration
BP or B/P	Blood pressure
V.D.R.L.	Venereal Disease Research Laboratory; test for syphilis
CBC	Complete blood count in which the different types of blood cells are checked
Hb	Hemoglobin; test to determine quantity of red matter in the erythrocytes
RBC	Red blood cell count
WBC	White blood cell count

As you work in the hospital environment with other health workers you will add many more abbreviations to your working vocabulary.

ABBREVIATIONS FOR COMMON HEALTH PROBLEMS

Some of the more common health problems are also designated with initials which are easily understood. Look at the following list and see if you can tell why the letters are used.

C.H.F.	Congestive Heart Failure; condition in which pumping action of the heart is ineffective
R.H.D.	Rheumatic Heart Disease; disease of the heart following rheumatic fever
A.S.H.D.	Arteriosclerotic Heart Disease; disease of the heart associated with changes in the arterial blood vessels
C.O.	Coronary Occlusion; disease of the blood vessels (*coronary*) which carry nourishment to the heart
C.V.A.	Cerebrovascular Accident; interruption of the flow of blood to the brain
H.V.D.	Hypertensive Vascular Disease; disease of the blood vessels associated with an elevated blood pressure

U.R.I.	Upper Respiratory Infection; infection involving the nose, throat, and windpipe which form the upper part of the respiratory system
P.I.D.	Pelvic Inflammatory Disease; inflammatory process involving the reproductive organs found in the lower part of the body
M.S.	Multiple Sclerosis; disease of young adults in which hardened areas form in the brain and spinal cord interfering with normal function
V.D.	Venereal Disease; any one of a number of diseases that are passed from person to person through direct sexual contact

THE PHYSICAL EXAMINATION

In each of the preceding examples the first letter of each word is used in the shortened form.

When a patient visits a physician's office, the patient's current complaint (**C.C.**), also referred to as present problem, is considered in relation to the **findings** (observations) made during the routine physical **exam** (examination). The physical examination is conducted by the physician in a back office with the assistance of the office nurse or medical assistant. Physicians offices usually have two areas; a **front office** or business office, and a **back office** where the actual care is given.

Figure 5-11: (left) The M.A. records the patient's weight in pounds as part of the physical exam in the M.D.'s office *(courtesy of American Association of Medical Assistants, Inc.).*

Figure 5-12: (right) The M.A. also records the B.P. as part of the V.S. before the patient sees the physician *(courtesy of American Association of Medical Assistants, Inc.).*

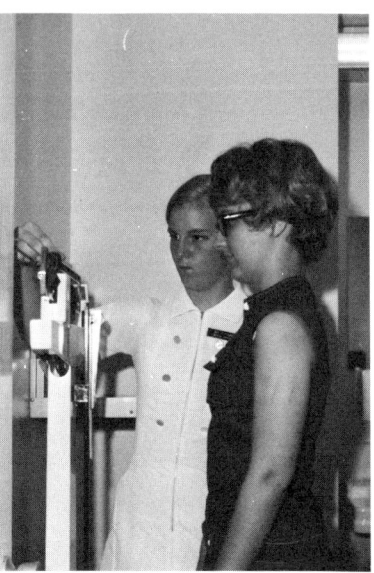

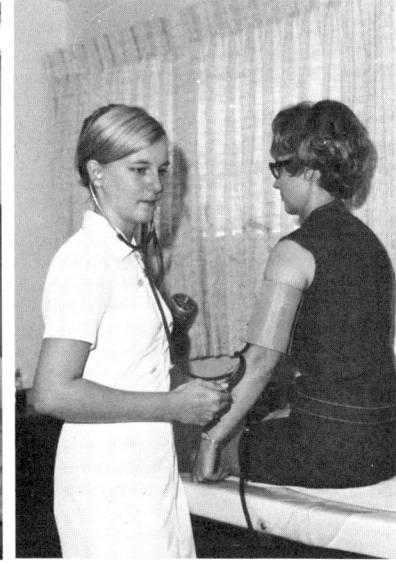

* 76 *MEDICAL WORDS*

BRONSON MEDICAL ASSOCIATES

Physical and History

Name: Anders, Johanna   Date: 6/8/XX
Age: 46   Ht. 67"   Wt. 132 lbs.
V.S.   T. 99.2   P. 82   R. 22   B/P 158/110
C.C. S.O.B. on exertion - insomnia 4 wks. duration
     c/o Tension
     Anorexia

M.H. Gravida VI   Para IV
(M) S D W   17 yrs.
F.H. States father died of "Old Age" Mother still living
     DX as diabetic, 3 brothers L & W

Present Findings:

Figure 5-13: The Physical and History form is started by the Assistant.

The medical assistant uses a variety of shortened forms as she assists in the examination of the patient and records both her observations and physician's findings. Before the physician sees the patient, the M.A., L.V.N., or R.N. who is assisting the physician with the back office work, determines the patient's height (**ht.**), weight (**wt.**), age, and vital signs (**v.s.**) which include T., P., R., and B/P. She may also elicit information about the C.C. or present illness (**P.I.**) and the patient's past history (**P.H.**). She may ask questions about the family history (**F.H.**) such as the health status of the parents and the number of brothers and sisters (**siblings**) and the state of their health. Depending on the nature of the current complaint, she may seek information about the patient's marital history (**M.H.**). The form the assistant hands to the doctor, to which he will add the findings of the physical examination, may look like Figure 5-13.

For your easier review and learning the abbreviations used by the medical assistant are summarized in the list in the margin.

Dx
diagnosis

C.C.
current complaint

S.O.B.
shortness of breath

C/O
complains of

F.H.
family history

M.H.
marital history

M. S. D. W.
married, single, divorced, widowed

L & W
living & well

ht.	**"**	**v.s.**	**P.**	**wks.**
height	inches	vital signs	pulse	weeks
wt.	**lbs.**	**T.**	**R.**	**P.I.**
weight	pounds	temperature	respiration	present illness

THE PHYSICAL EXAMINATION

Other terms the assistant might use would include **insomnia**, sleeplessness; **anorexia**, loss of appetite; **gravida**, number of pregnancies; **para**, number of pregnancies carried to delivery.

Using his hands to feel (**palpate**), his eyes to see (**inspect**), and his ears to hear (**auscultate**), the physician examines the patient to determine the presence of any abnormalities and to establish a diagnosis for the present **complaint** (problem or illness). The medical assistant helps with this exam and makes notations about the physician's findings.

The patient may need to assume different positions during the examination, depending upon the area of the body being assessed. The most common positions included in a general **physical** (the word exam is often deleted) include: the semi-sitting position (**Fowler's**); the **horizontal recumbent** or **supine position**, with the patient lying on her back; the **lithotomy position**, usually used for pelvic examinations; the **proctologic position**, for rectal examinations; **Trendelenburg's position** with the patient's head lower than her body; **prone position**, places the patient face down on her abdomen. Figures 5-14a,b,c,d,e illustrate some of the positions assumed by the patient during the physical examination.

Figure 5-14:
(a) The semi-sitting or Fowler's position;
(b) recombent or supine position;
(c) lithotomy position;
(d) proctologic;
(e) trendelenberg
(courtesy of American Hospital Supply Corporation).

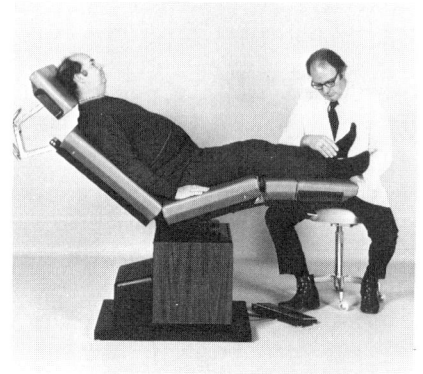

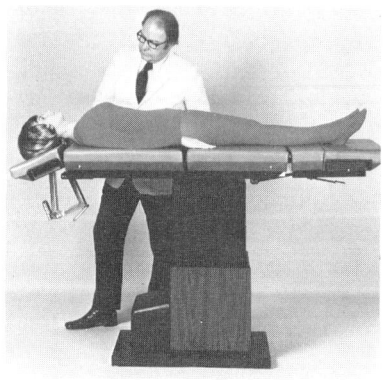

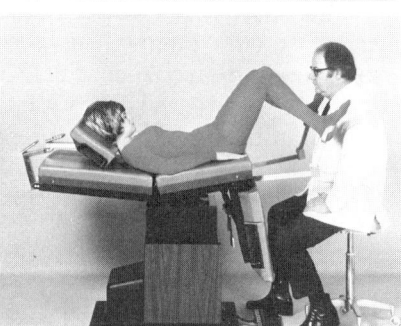

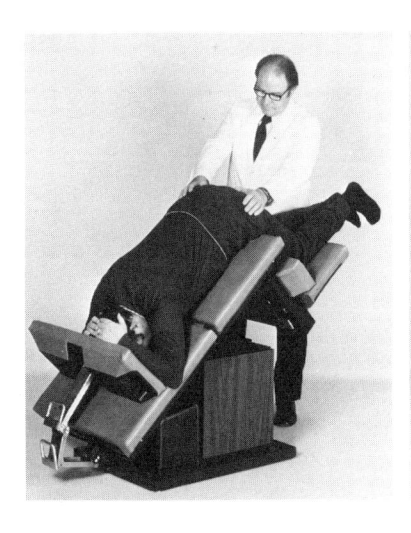

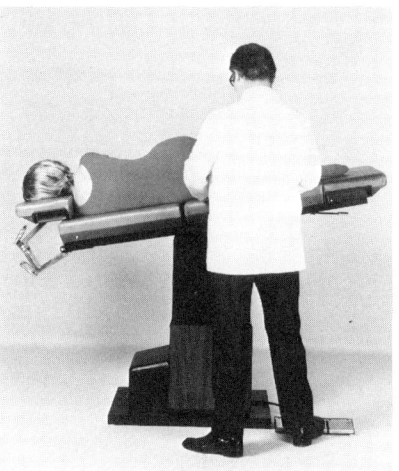

Several **instruments** (medical tools) used in examining patients include: a **sphygmomanometer** (instrument to measure blood pressure), a **thermometer** (to measure the temperature), an **otoscope** (ear viewer), an **opthalmoscope**, (interior eye viewer), a **percussion hammer** (for tapping), a **stethoscope** (to listen with), various **speculums** (instruments for enlarging a body opening), a tongue depressor, and a small flashlight.

The medical assistant observes and assists as the doctor examines the patient in a systematic manner. To correctly note the findings, the medical assistant must be familiar with the body landmarks the doctor uses as he/she proceeds. After the physical examination the M.A. transfers the notations of the findings to the physical and history form.

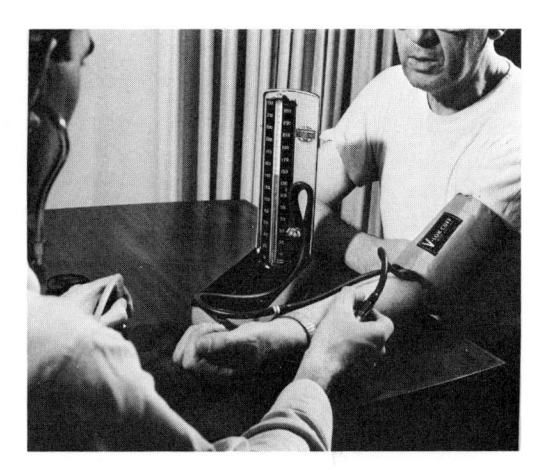

Figure 5-15: Sphygmomanometer *(courtesy of W.A. Baun Co., Inc.)*.

THE PHYSICAL EXAMINATION 79 *

Figure 5-16: (left) Percussion hammer *(courtesy of Ameri-Hospital Supply Corporation).*

Figure 5-17: (right) Stethoscope *(courtesy of Curtin Matheson Scientific, Inc.).*

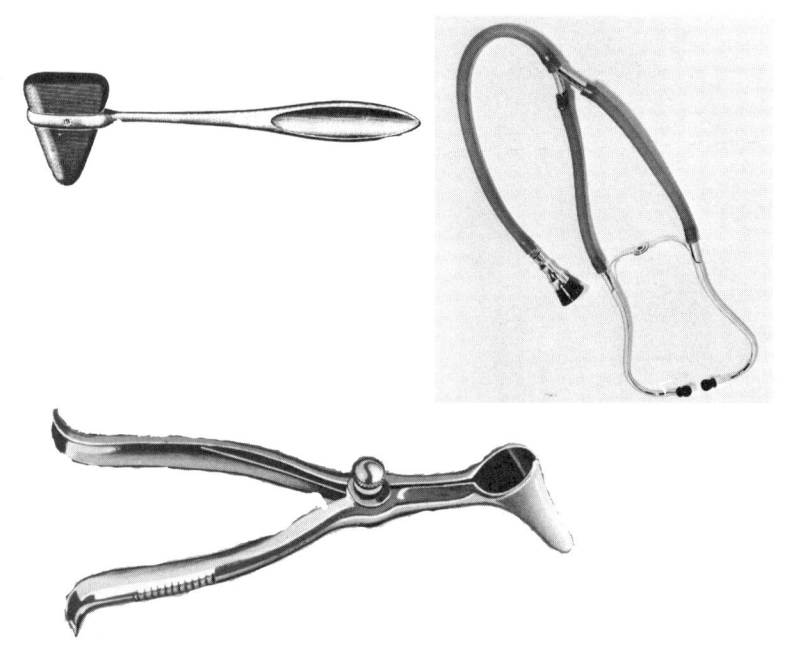

Figure 5-19: (a) Anal speculum *(courtesy of Sherwood Medical Industries).* (b) some instruments used in the physical exam.

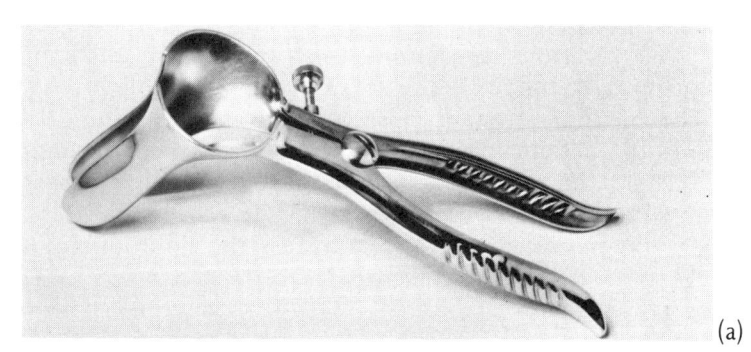

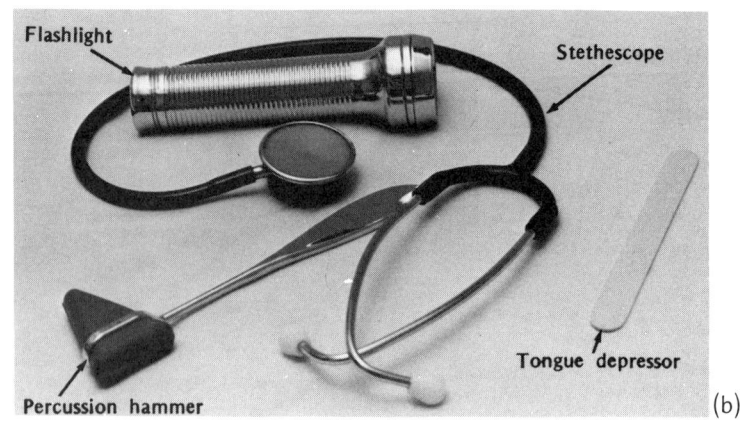

(a)

Flashlight Stethescope Tongue depressor Percussion hammer

(b)

* 80 MEDICAL WORDS

A knowledge of body planes and anatomical parts enables all health personnel to use specific terms and abbreviations in common. Regardless of the position assumed by a patient, the health worker describing a body part does so by first making a mental "translation" to its anatomic position.

BODY PLANES AND LANDMARKS

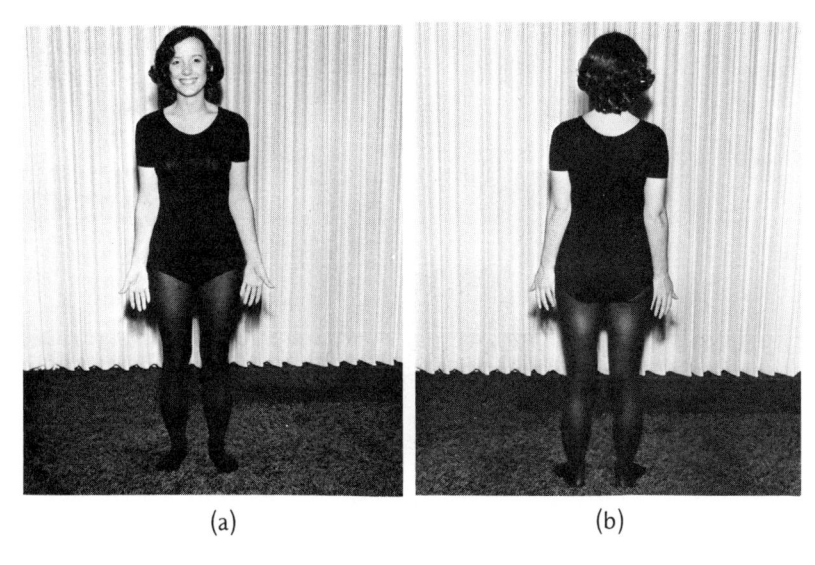

Figure 5-20:
(a) anatomical position: body erect, feet flat, palms forward. Anterior view;
(b) anatomical position. Posterior view.

(a)   (b)

In medicine planes are formed by imaginary lines which divide the body. The **midsagittal** (midline) plane divides the body into right (**R**) and left (**L**) halves. The **transverse** plane divides the body into upper (**superior** or **cranial**) and lower (**inferior**) sections, and the **coronal** plane divides the body into back (**posterior** or **dorsal**) and front (**anterior** or **ventral**). The term **medial** locates structures nearer the midline and **lateral** those away from the midline.

The arms and legs (**appendages**) are connected at the shoulders and hips to the body (**trunk**). The part of the appendages closest to the point of attachment are described as **proximal**. Those farthest away are **distal**. The axial trunk is divided into a **thorax** (chest) and an **abdomen** (between the thorax and pelvis). The surface of the abdomen is further divided into four sections (**quadrants**). The section over the naval (**umbilicus**) is called the umbilical area. Other areas are the right upper quadrant (**RUQ**), left upper quadrant (**LUQ**), and the right lower quadrant (**RLQ**) and left lower quadrant (**LLQ**).

Several other terms help us identify, locate and name body areas and parts. They are identified on the diagrams in Figures 5-24, 5-25, and 5-26.

Figure 5-21:
(a) Imaginary planes divide the body;
(b) imaginary planes divide the body. Note the terminology.

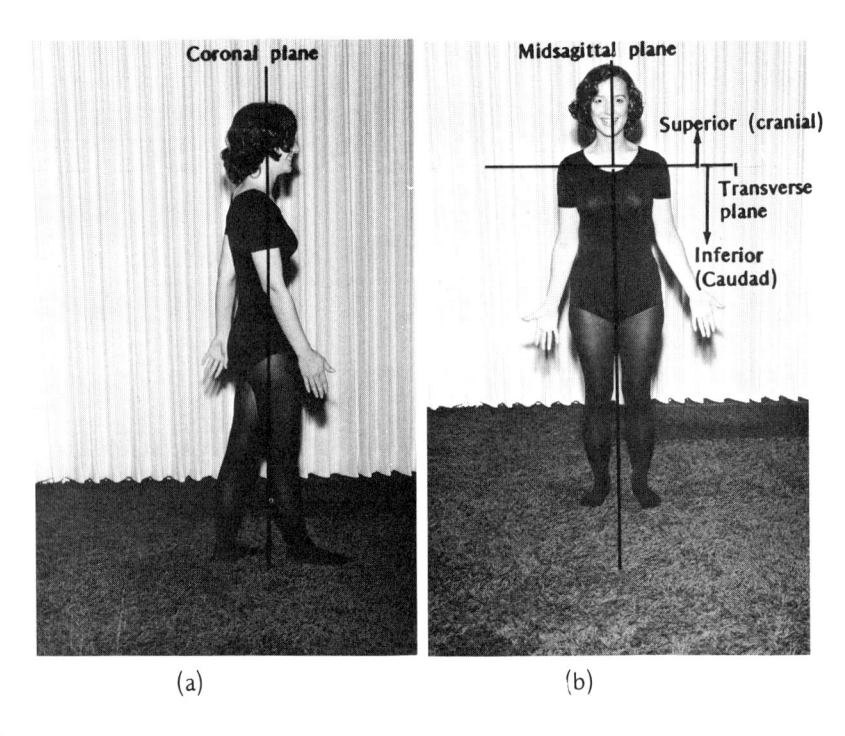

Figure 5-22: Descriptive terms for body parts

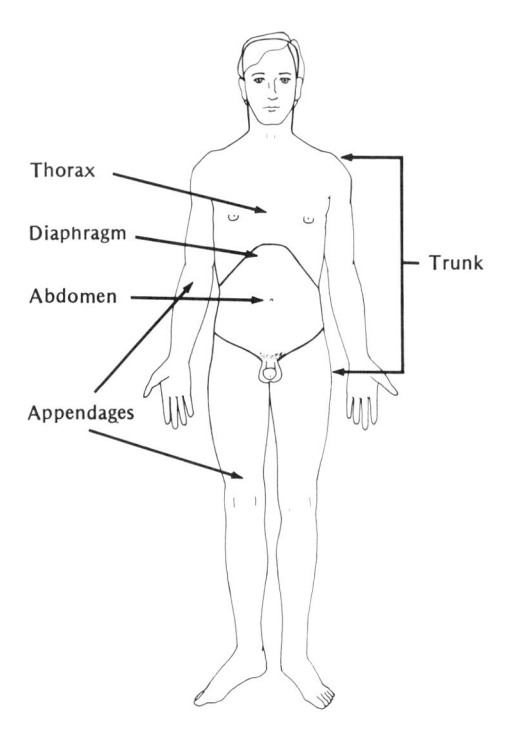

*82 MEDICAL WORDS

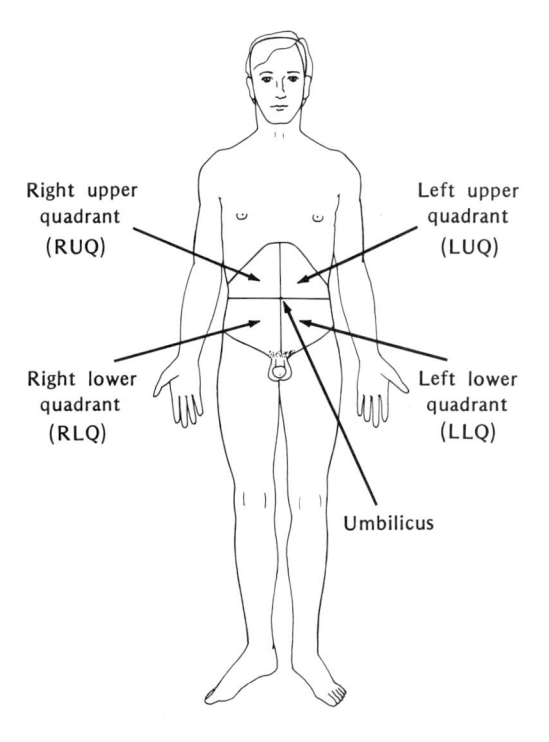

Figure 5-23: Abdominal quadrants.

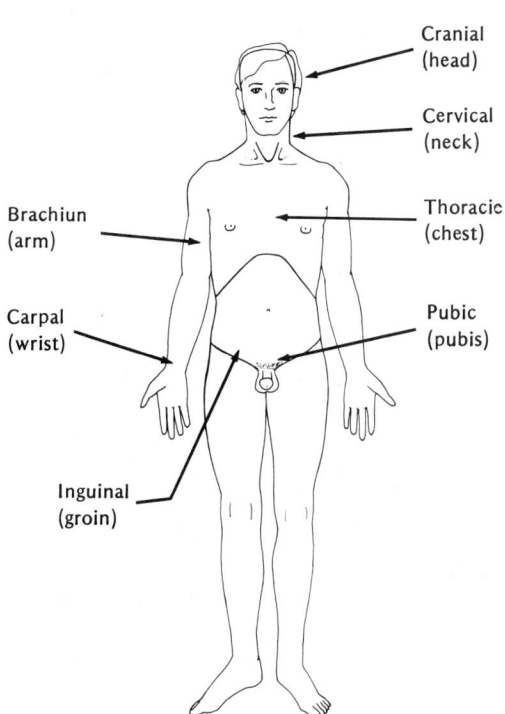

Figure 5-24: Terms pertaining to body parts or areas: Anterior view.

BODY PLANES AND LANDMARKS 83 *

Figure 5-25: (left) Arms have been abducted to expose Axilla.

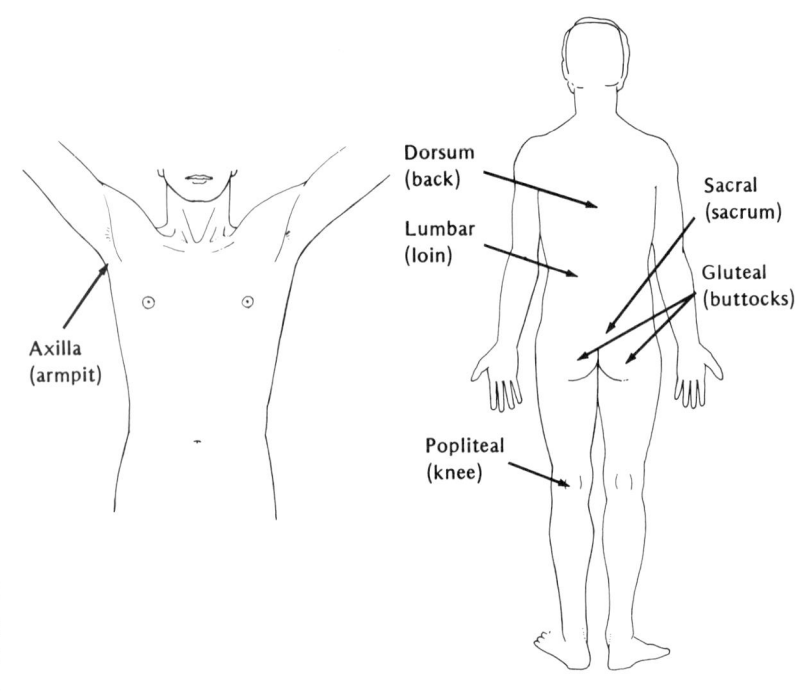

Axilla (armpit)

Dorsum (back)
Lumbar (loin)
Sacral (sacrum)
Gluteal (buttocks)
Popliteal (knee)

Figure 5-26: (right) Terms pertaining to body areas: Posterior view.

Look at the diagram to learn the location of each area.

After the physical examination is completed, the physical and history sheet might look like Figure 5-27a.

As you can tell from the information (**data**) on the physical and history form, the patient is to be admitted to the hospital for surgery. The medical assistant may make the formal arrangements with the hospital admissions office.

Learning of the expected admission, the hospital **floor nurse** (staff member) contacted the doctor for orders. The following orders were given for Mrs. Anders to the floor nurse over the phone.

* * *

Orders Telephoned by Physician to the Floor Nurse

My patient, Mrs. Johanna Anders, who is 46, is to be admitted to the East seventh floor for surgery day after tomorrow for abdominal **laporotomy** (exploratory operation) and **biopsy** (tissue sample). She has a mass in her right lower quadrant which I think is probably a neoplasm. I want to rule out the possibility of a malignancy. I want an intravenous infusion started right away of five percent dextrose and water, one thousand milliliters. Let it run at forty drops per minute. Put her on a low sodium diet and force fluids. I want an intake and output record kept. Take her vital signs twice a day and this afternoon she can be out of bed as she wishes. I have **booked** (reserved)

* 84 MEDICAL WORDS

Present Findings: Figure 5-27 (a).

Physical Exam

General	Well nourished, somewhat dehydrated 42 yr. old ♀
Skin	Dry, pale.
HEENT	Neg., no masses.
Neck	Neg.
Chest	Neg.
Lungs	Neg.
Heart	Neg.
Abdomen	Firm moveable, palpable mass app 10 cm in diameter in RLQ.
Genitalia	
Lymphatics	
Blood Vessels	
Locomotor	
Extremities	
Neuro	
Rectal	
Vaginal	Palpable mass in RLQ.
Diagnosis	Mass RLQ, mod hypertension, anxiety syndrome. Admit to hospital for biopsy. Provisional Dx: Neoplasia RLQ R/O malignancy.

Anders, Johanna
721 E. Second St.
Alhambra, PA
J. Bronson, M.D.

BODY PLANES AND LANDMARKS 85 *

Figure 5-27 (b).

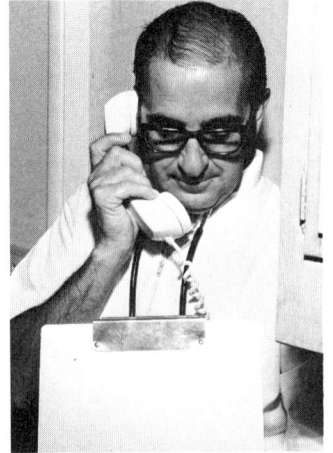

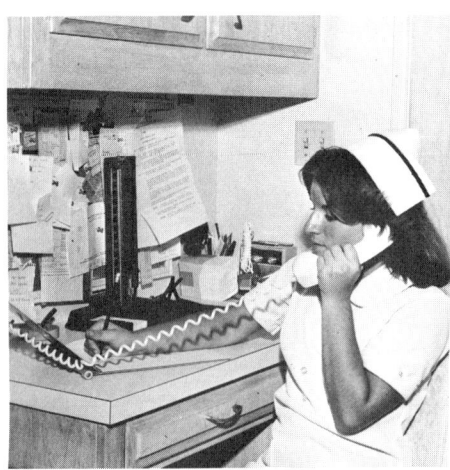

Figure 5-28: The floor nurse takes the orders from the physician.

the operating room, too, for day after tomorrow at eight o'clock in the morning. Prepare the abdominal skin tomorrow night and give her a soap suds enema before she goes to sleep tomorrow night. She can have five grains of aspirin every four hours for headache as she needs it. Give her valium, two milligrams, three times a day by mouth. Let her have a 100 milligram capsule of nembutal for sleep tonight. Oh, yes, do the routine urinalysis and complete blood count, and I have scheduled her for an electrocardiogram tomorrow.

* * *

These are the orders as written by the floor nurse.

Name *Anders, J.*	Age *46*	Date *6/18/00*
Dx *Mass RLQ*	*R/O Neoplasia*	*Abd. Lap. and Biopsy*
Orders		
1. Admit to E-7		
2. I.V. 1000 ml 5% D/W 40 gtts/min. stat		
3. LoNa diet		
4. F.F. I & O		
5. v.s. B.I.D.		
6. O.O.B. ad lib this /P		
7. O.R. II @ 8/A 6/20		
8. Abd. prep + S.S.E. @ H.S. 6/19		

* 86 *MEDICAL WORDS*

Orders
9. ASA, grs. V p.m. Headache q4° prn
10. Valium 2 mg tabs T.I.D. p.o.
11. Nembutal Cap $\bar{\imath}$ 100 mg @ H.S.
12. U.A. & C.B.C.
13. E.C.G. 6/19

V.O. Dr. J. Bronson B.H.

These orders will be transferred to several other forms serving to communicate the doctors orders to the entire staff. Make a careful comparison of the two forms of medical communication.

In order to correctly carry out these orders, the staff must understand the abbreviations and shortened forms used by the nurse. In addition they must correctly identify measurements for the medications to be given.

All the staff members must be familiar with Roman numerals, abbreviations, shortened forms and time frame indicators to understand the orders. The shortened forms and initials to be understood are:

I.V.	intravenous; given directly into a vein
D/W	dextrose and water; a solution of sugar water
LoNa	a diet with low salt content
F.F.	force fluids; encourage the patient to drink
I & O	intake & output; measure all fluid the patient takes and eliminates
abd.	abdominal *lap*; laporotomy (exploratory operation)
O.O.B.	out of bed (the patient may get up)
ad lib	as desired; as often as patient wishes
S.S.E.	soap suds enema (a procedure to clear the lower bowel)
UA	urinalysis; examination of a urine *spec.* (specimen)
/min	per minute
p.r.n.	whenever necessary
V.O.	verbal orders

CBC, ECG, O.R. and v.s. are initials you should recognize. Do you?

TIME AND MEASUREMENTS Numbers, letters and symbols are used to express time and measurements. Look at the lists in the margin.

TIME REFERENCE

Hd or **Hor. decub.**
at bedtime

Bid
twice a day

H.s.
hour of sleep (bedtime)

p̄
P.M. (after noon)

ā
A.M. (morning)

q
4° every 4 hours

q.o.d.
every other day

t.i.d.
three times a day

q.i.d.
four times a day

hr. or **h.**
hour

stat
at once

a.c.
before meals

p.c.
after meals

q.d.
every day, daily

noct
in the night

q.n.
every night

MEASUREMENTS

ml (milliliter)
a measure of liquid

mg (milligram)
a measure of dry weight

grs (grains)
a measure of dry weight

cap (capsule)
dose-sized container for medicine

QUANTITIES

q.s.
as much as required

aa̤
equal part of each

s̤s
one half

tab
tablet

amt
amount

oz.
ounce

qt.
quart

pt.
pint

tsp.
teaspoon

Tbsp. or **T.**
tablespoon

DIRECTIONS

s.o.s.
if necessary

d.c.
discontinue

per
through

M
mix

NPO
nothing by mouth

non rep
do not repeat

Sig or **S**
label

℞
take

c̄
with

s̄
without

The most common Roman numerals used in medicine are one through ten. Check those listed here to be sure you are familiar with them:

ROMAN NUMERALS

1	I	6	VI
2	II	7	VII
3	III	8	VIII
4	IV	9	IX
5	V	10	X

Now reread the orders as the nurse wrote them and see if they make more sense.

The measurements probably are the most difficult to understand. In medicine, three different systems of measurement are used. They are the household, apothecary, and metric systems. As a health worker you will learn to convert from one system to the other. But remember the conversions are into approximate measurements. You will become very proficient in the conversions because you will encounter these systems of measurement every day in your work. For now, simply try to learn a few basic relationships since symbols and abbreviations are often used to express measurements in medicine. You may already be familiar with some of the common household measurements and their abbreviations that are listed below.

Measurement Systems Used in Medicine

HOUSEHOLD MEASURES

WEIGHTS (dry)

oz
ounces

lbs
pounds

VOLUMES (liquid)

gtts
drops

oz
ounces

pt.
pint

qt.
quart

LENGTHS

in. or "
inches

APOTHECARY MEASURES

WEIGHTS (dry)

gr
grain

scruple

ounce

lb.
pound

VOLUME (liquid)

m
minim

f
fluidram

f
fluidounce

pt.
pint

qt.
quart

ROMAN NUMERALS 89 *

	Comparative Values (approximate)	
HOUSEHOLD		APOTHECARY
drop	=	minim
60 drops (1 tsp.)	=	1 fluidram
32 fluid ounces	=	1 quart

Metric System

The metric system is the most important since it is used almost universally in all scientific work, including the medical field. It deals in length, area, capacity, volume, and weight measurements. Metric measurement units are based on the decimal system and are expressed in multiples and fractions of 10. The basic unit for length is the **meter (m)**, for dry weight the **gram (gm)**, and for liquid volume the **liter (litre or l)**.

Numerical prefixes are applied to each basic unit as follows.

Prefix	Equivalent
deci- = (d)	0.1 or 1/10 of the unit
centi- = (c)	0.01 or 1/100 of the unit
milli- = (m)	0.001 or 1/1000 of the unit
kilo- = (k)	1000 x the unit

For example: 1/10 of a meter = 1 decimeter (**dm.**)
1/10 of a gram = 1 decigram (**dc.**)
1/10 of a liter = 1 deciliter (**dl.**)

Prefix	Meter	Gram	Liter
deci-	decimeter (dc)	decigram (dg)	deciliter (dl) 1/10
centi-	centimeter (cc)	centigram (cg)	centiliter (cl) 1/100
milli-	millimeter (mm)	milligram (mg)	milliliter (ml) 1/1000
kilo-	kilometer (km)	kilogram (kg)	kilometer (kl) 1000 x

In actual usage 1 **c.c.** (cubic centimeter) is used interchangeably with 1 milliliter (ml). Most often **linear** (length) measurements utilize centimeters, dry weights customarily use milligrams and kilograms, liquid volumes generally utilize milliliters and liters.

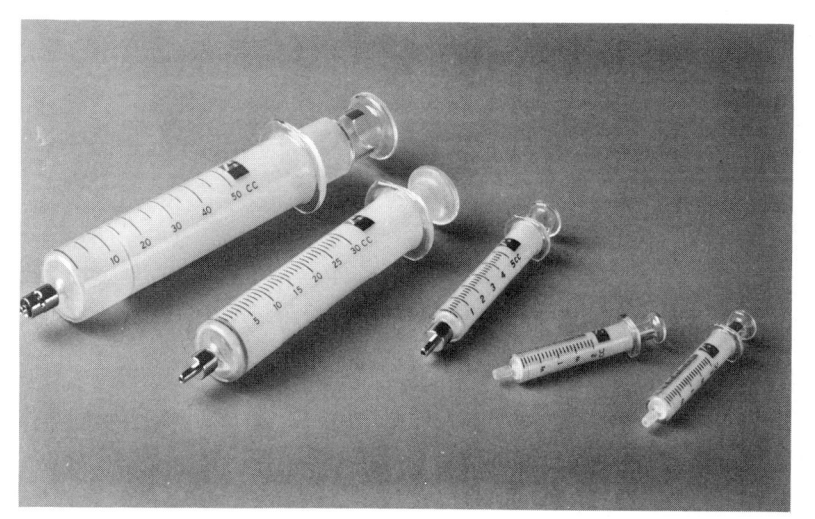

Figure 5-29: Syringe with c.c. calibrations: c.c. or ml is a metric measurement *(courtesy of Scientific Products, Div. of American Hospital Supply Corporation).*

Let us take these most common measurements and relate them to the other systems that are also in use. Remember that in the metric system the measurements are multiples or fractions of three basic units; the liter for liquid volume, the gram for dry weight, and the meter for length.

TABLE OF COMPARATIVE VALUES (approximated)

METRIC	HOUSEHOLD	APOTHECARY
Liquid Volume		
1.060 ml (milliliter)	1 gtt.	1 m
1 ml, cc (cubic centimeter)	**15 gtts.**	15 m
4.5 ml (milliliter)	**1 tsp.**	1 f
1000 ml (milliliter)	32 f	1 qt.
Dry Weight		
1 kg (kilogram)	2.2 lbs.	
Lengths		
2.54 cm (centimeters)	**1 inch**	
25.4 mm (millimeters)	1 inch	

The **underscored terms** in the table of comparative values indicate the most commonly applied measurements.

Look at each of the following figures. They are containers which you will see in the hospital. Notice that the calibrations are in the metric system.

Figure 5-30: Which two sytems of measurement are shown on this ruler?

ROMAN NUMERALS 91 *

Figure 5-31: (left) This medicine cup has measurements for ounces and centimeters *(courtesy of Bel-Arts Products).*

Figure 5-32: (right) A medicine glass; what measurement might be used in place of ml? *(courtesy of Curtin Matheson Scientific, Inc.).*

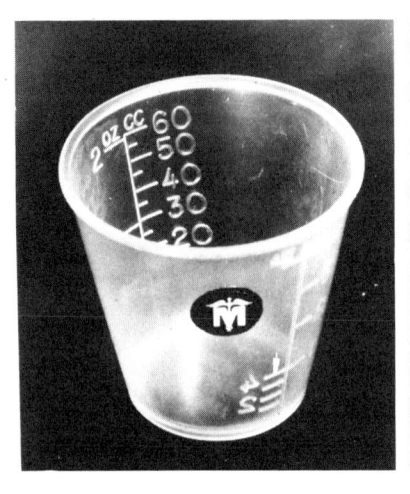

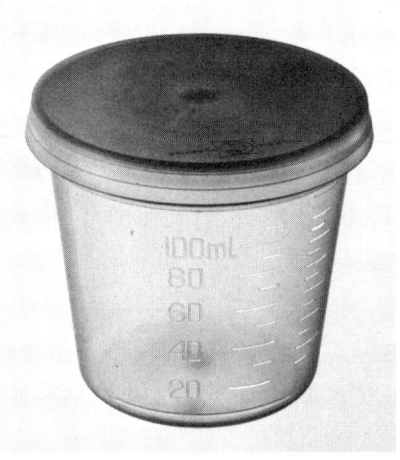

Figure 5-33: (left) How much fluid can be measured in this graduate cylinder? *(courtesy of Bel-Arts Products).*

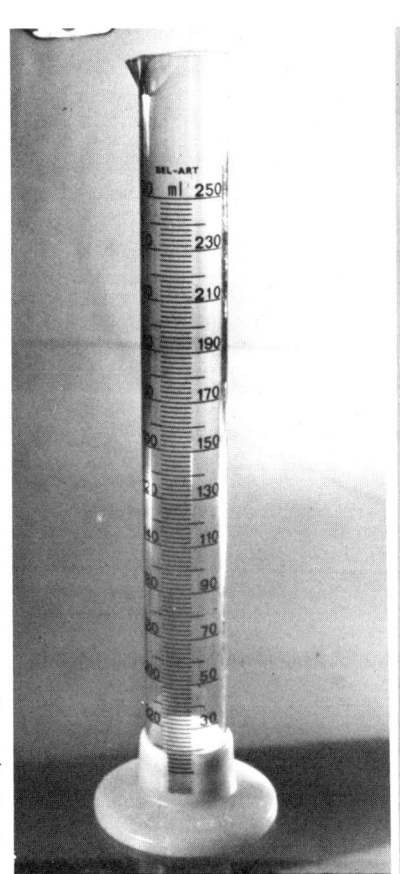

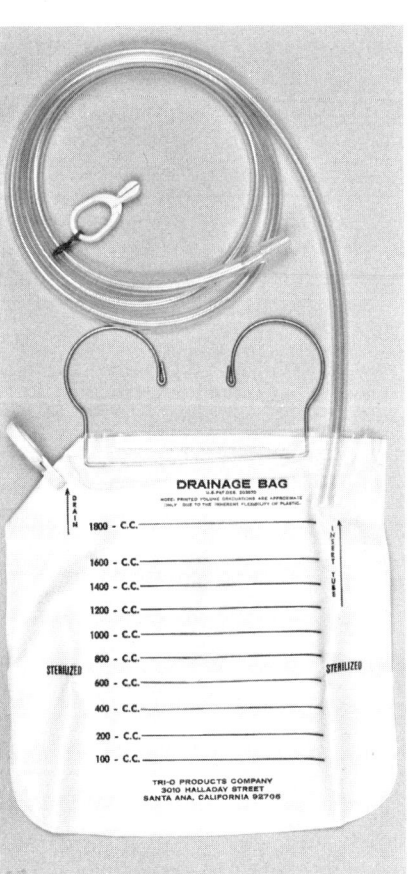

Figure 5-34: (right) Urinary drainage bag. What system of measurement is used? *(courtesy of American Hospital Supply Corporation).*

*92 MEDICAL WORDS

SUMMARY

Medical abbreviations are a commonly used communication too. They may be initials or shortened forms of the words. Not all abbreviated forms are standard. It is therefore mandatory that each person be <u>absolutely sure</u> of the correct meaning of each shortened form being used.

PRACTICE & REVIEW

Explain and define the new special terms you have been using. Remember, you learned how to pronounce them at the beginning of this chapter.

1. anorexia _____
2. auscultate _____
3. sphygmomanometer _____
4. umbilicus _____
5. speculum _____
6. liter _____
7. deci- _____
8. centi- _____
9. milli- _____
10. kilo- _____

Now, double-check the meaning of the terms above by studying the brief definitions given in the Glossary-Index at the back of this text.

Test yourself quickly before going on to learn other medical and professional terms. Use these short review exercises to practice for your new work in health services. Your teacher will also help by recommending various other Study Activities.

A. Write the abbreviation for each of the following places or procedures:

1. Central Service _____
2. Emergency Room _____
3. Operating Room _____
4. Intensive Coronary Care _____
5. Temperature _____
6. Complete Blood Count _____
7. Electromyogram _____

ROMAN NUMERALS 93 *

8. Hemoglobin _____

9. Blood pressure _____

10. White blood cell count _____

B. Write the name of the health problem expressed by each set of letters below:

1. C.H.F. _____
2. P.I.D. _____
3. C.O. _____
4. M.S. _____
5. V.D. _____

C. On the Physical and History Sheet, a number of abbreviations are used. Give their meanings.

1. M.H. _____
2. c/o _____
3. lbs. _____
4. Dx. _____
5. S.O.B. _____
6. C.C. _____
7. P.I. _____
8. P. _____
9. " _____
10. V.S. _____

D. Interpret the following orders in the spaces provided below:

Order: *Medication to be taken*

1. Ac _____
2. T.I.D. _____
3. prn _____
4. Q.O.D. _____
5. H.S. _____

*94 *MEDICAL WORDS*

Order: *The amount of medication to be taken is*

6. tab II _____

7. Tab s̄s̄ _____

8. Cap I _____

9. _____

10. ā ā _____

Order: *Take as directed*

11. d.c. Tomorrow _____

12. Non rep _____

13. c̄ water _____

14. s̄ alcohol_____

15. s.o.s. _____

Order: *The measured amount to be taken is*

16. 5 mg _____

17. 2 grs _____

18. _____

19. 4 ml _____

20. 2 m _____

After studying Chapter 6

Basic Medical Asepsis

You should be able to:

* *Pronounce and define each of its new medical words and phrases and use the new technical jargon.*

* *Name five microorganisms.*

* *List five common communicable diseases.*

MEDICAL WORDS

PRONOUNCE THESE TEN NEW WORDS WITH YOUR TEACHER:

pseudopodia (su″do-po′de-ah)
antigen (an′ti-jen)
commensalism (ko-men′sal-izm)
Escherichia coli (esh″e-rik′e-ah) (ko″li)
fomites (fo′mi-tezs)

immunity (i-mu-ni-te)
morbidity (mor′bid′i-te)
saprophytes (sap′ro-fits)
enterotropic (en″ter-otrop′ik)
bacteriostatic (bak-te″re-o-stat′ik)

One of the very first **techniques** (methods of procedure) that all health personnel must learn is that of handwashing. They must learn this because hands not properly cleansed can easily transfer unclean material from either the nurse to the patient or from the patient to the nurse herself or else serve to transfer unclean material from patient to patient through the nurse.

Sepsis means infection and **asepsis** means without infection. Correct handwashing is the foundation of the aseptic technique designed to prevent infection and its transfer. **Contamination** (soiling by contact) occurs when microorganisms are transferred from one source to another. It can easily occur if a person is unfamiliar with the concepts of **microbiology** (the study of microorganisms).

MICROORGANISMS

Microorganisms or **microbes** are forms so small that they are seen only with a microscope. They are more simple forms of life than man, but they do have definite form and structure. Most microbes belong to the plant or animal kingdoms but some are classified in a separate kingdom called Protista.

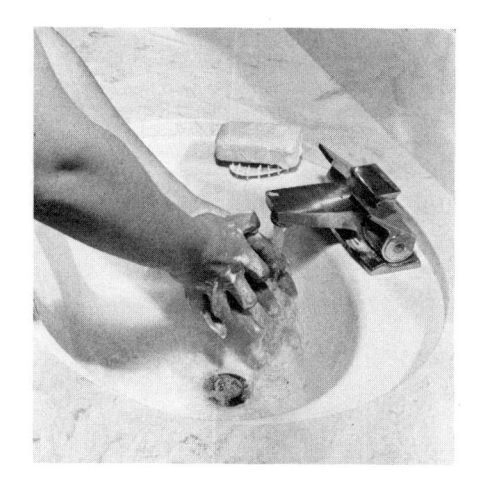

Figure 6-1: Proper hand washing is fundamental to medical asepsis.

The six basic classifications are:

    yeasts   bacteria   viruses
    molds   rickettsiae protozoa

Yeasts and molds are in the plant kingdom and are studied in the special branch of microbiology called **mycology**. The bacteria, rickettsiae and protozoa are classified as protista. Most microbes are helpful to the ecology and are **non-parthogenic** (non-disease producing). Some, however, are **pathogenic** (disease producing) for man; they are sometimes called germs. The non-pathogens far outnumber the pathogens. The primary concern in medicine are the pathogens and their affect on the human body.

Many special terms are used in describing the different microbes and their pathologic effect. Since so many **infections** (invasion of the body by pathogens) are caused by bacteria and viruses, and since so many of the same terms and expressions are used in relation to all the microbes, our attention will be focused on these two groups.

Viruses

Viruses are ultramicroscopic (too small to be seen with the ordinary microscope) forms that can invade any part of the body. Because of their extremely small size, they are difficult to study. They also have special growth requirements which make it very difficult to maintain them in the laboratory. They cannot remain outside a living cell and survive. They are therefore known as **obligate intracellular parasites** which means they must live within a living cell. Diagnosis of viral diseases is usually made on the basis of the patient's signs and symptoms rather than on specific laboratory techniques.

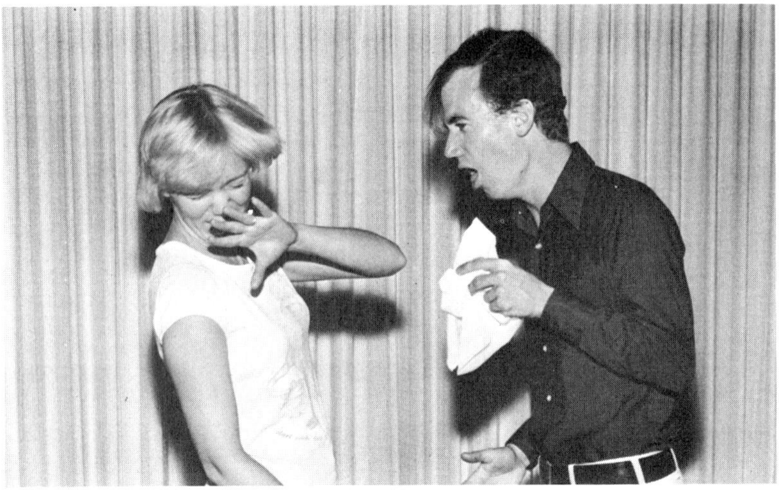

Figure 6-2: The microorganisms pass from the portal of exit of one person to the portal of entry of another.

Most pathogens—viruses and others—have specific ways in which they enter the body to cause disease. These special ways of entering are called the **portals of entry** and the special ways of leaving are called the portals of exit. For example, **pneumotropic** (turning toward, affinity for) viruses affect the lungs. They enter the body by way of the upper respiratory tract and leave the body through the same route. The portals of entry and exit for the pneumotropic viruses are the **secretions** (the products of glandular activity) and **excretions** (waste materials) of the respiratory **tract** (passageway) that leads to and from the lungs.

One way to classify viruses, then, is according to the part of the body infected or to their portal of entry or exit.

Table 6-1

Type of Virus	Bodily Part Affected	Example of Disease
Viscerotropic	Internal organ like the liver	Hepatitis (inflammation of the liver)
Enterotropic	Intestinal tract & later the nervous system	Poliomyelitis (Infantile Paralysis)
Dermotropic	Skin	Measles, a childhood disease
Neurotropic	Nervous system	Hydrophobia (Rabies)

Viruses cause many of the highly **communicable** (easily passed from person to person) diseases of childhood. Each year we see many such cases of measles, chicken pox, and mumps.

* 98 *BASIC MEDICAL ASEPSIS*

The **morbidity** (number of cases) rate for these diseases is relatively high in childhood but the **mortality** (death) rates are relatively low. These communicable diseases have both a common name and a medical name. All are caused by viruses. Look at the chart which follows to learn the common and proper name for some of the childhood infectious diseases which are communicable.

Table 6-2

Common Name	Medical Name	Type of Virus
Measles (7 day or regular)	Rubeola	Dermotropic
German measles (3 day)	Rubella	Dermotropic
Chicken pox	Varicella	Dermotropic
Small pox	Variola	Dermotropic
Mumps	Parotitis	Viscerotropic
Infantile Paralysis	Poliomyelitis	Enterotropic

Communicable diseases may remain present in a particular community with a few cases occurring all the time. The condition is then called **endemic**. Measles is an endemic disease. When such an infectious disease spreads rapidly among large numbers of people it is called an **epidemic**. Every few years we see epidemics of measles striking large numbers of children. When a communicable disease spreads widely it becomes **pandemic**. Flu, a pneumotropic viral disease, is frequently pandemic during the fall, winter, and spring months. **Antibiotic** (life destroying or growth suppressing) drugs are effective for controlling many infectious diseases. However, antibiotics are generally ineffective against the viral diseases. Treatment of persons with viral infections is supportive and utilizes the patient's own inner body defenses to effect recovery.

The Bacteria

At one time bacteria were considered to be the simplest form of plant life. Today, however, they are believed to be among the primitive one-celled forms that do not fit readily into either plant or animal life. They are called **protista** (simplest organisms).

Bacteria have rigid walls which give the various kinds a characteristic shape. Those bacteria that are rod shaped are called **bacilli** (bacillus is singular). Those that are round are called **cocci** (coccus is singular), and those that are shaped like

Figure 6-3: Bacterial shapes.

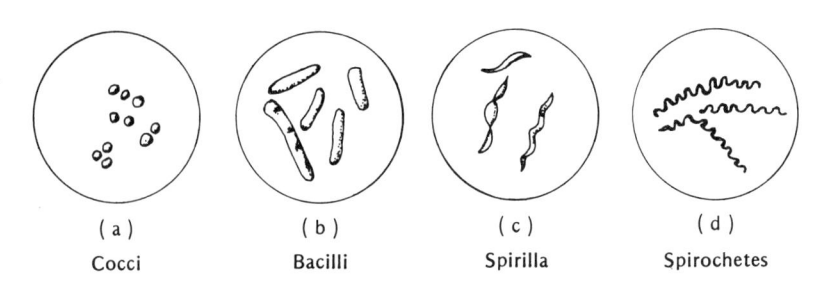

(a) Cocci (b) Bacilli (c) Spirilla (d) Spirochetes

flexible spirals are known as **spirilla** (spirillum), while those that resemble a corkscrew and are tightly coiled are known as **spirochetes** (spirochete).

Pathogenic forms occur in each shape of bacteria. They invade the body and cause infectious diseases. Most have a specific portal of entry and exit. Bacteria are larger than viruses. They are measured in **microns**. Its symbol from Greek is μ (pronounced mu). A micron is equal to .001 mm, so you can only imagine how very small they really are. The head of a pin is equal to 1 mm and we are dealing with forms that have a diameter of 1/1000 of mm or less. Imagine one thousand of these organisms stretched across the head of a pin. But they can be seen with the compound microscope, can be kept alive in the laboratory, and can be more easily studied than viruses because they can be **stained** (colored).

Many kinds of bacteria and other organisms live together in the environment; in water, soil and food. Some live on **organic** matter (matter which has had life or is living) and are called **heterotrophs**. Heterotrophic organisms that live on dead organic matter are called **saprophytes**. Heterotropic organisms that require living matter for their nourishment are called **parasites**. A few saprophytes such as the bacteria which cause **tetanus** (lockjaw) and **botulism** (a serious form of food poisoning) are pathogenic for man. Some organisms live on **inorganic** matter (matter which never had life) and are called **autotrophs**. They are non-pathogens. Both types of organisms make an important contribution to the ecological systems of the world.

The term used to explain the relationships which exist between organisms in the ecological system is **symbiosis**. The organisms in the environment live in a symbiotic relationship with each other. Symbiotic relationships are not always the same. Terms used to express the type of symbiosis which exists include **commensalism** (one organism derives benefit from the other but does no harm), **mutualism** (each derives benefit), and **parasitism** (one derives benefit at the other's expense).

Normal Flora

Communities of organisms can be found living on and in the human body in symbiosis with each other and with the body which acts as host for these organisms. Different areas of the body have a normal variation in population and this is called the **normal flora**. Certain organisms which form part of the normal flora of the intestinal tract such as the bacterium, *Escherichia coli*, are commensals as long as they remain in the intestinal tract. When they find their way out of the tract and enter a break in the skin, they cause an infection. Organisms that behave in this way are not true pathogens. They are called **opportunists** since they cause disease only when a special opportunity occurs. Some organisms that are part of the normal intestinal flora derive benefit from the body but live in mutualism because they also help in the manufacture of vitamins which are important to the body's health.

Medicine is primarily concerned with the parasites which live at the expense of the body. True pathogens belong to this group and are responsible for most of the infectious diseases. The **gonococcus**, which causes the infectious, highly communicable disease of **gonorrhea**, is an example.

IDENTIFICATION OF BACTERIA

Many techniques are used to identify the specific bacterium that causes a particular infection. Sometimes more than one organism is involved (**mixed infection**) but usually one organism is responsible and it must be identified so that proper therapy can be instituted.

Morphology

As we learned, different bacteria have different shapes so the shape of the organisms is an important characteristic. The way in which the bacteria are arranged is also a clue.

Those using the prefix **diplo-** occur in pairs. The gonoccus is a diplococcus. Those clustered together are prefixed by **staphylo-** (cluster) such as the *Staphylococcus epidermidis*, an organism commonly found on the skin. Those growing in chains use the prefix **strepto-** such as the *Streptococcus hemolyticus*, a **virulent** (strongly pathogenic) organism which causes scarlet fever.

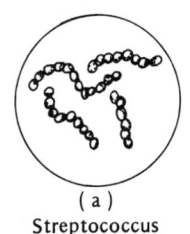

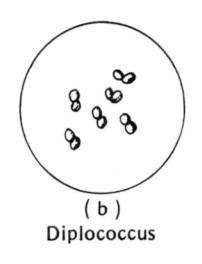

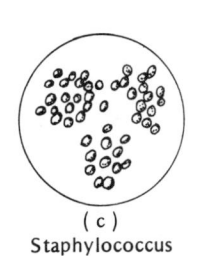

Figure 6-4: Bacterial morphology.

(a) Streptococcus   (b) Diplococcus   (c) Staphylococcus

Other special characteristics of an organism also help to identify the microbe. These include the presence of **capsules** (an extra covering) or its **mobility** (ability to move) or its ability to form **spores** (forms resistant to destruction). Capsules make it more difficult to destroy the organism either with drugs such as antibiotics, or **chemotherapeutics** (special chemical drugs).

Methods of mobility vary with the **species** (type of microbe). Some have long whip-like appendages called **flagella**, some have tiny moveable hairs called **cilia**, and some like the protozoa move by extending part of themselves forward and then allowing the remaining cell to flow into the projected part. This form of locomotion is known as **pseudopodia** or false feet.

Figure 6-5: Means of microbial mobility.

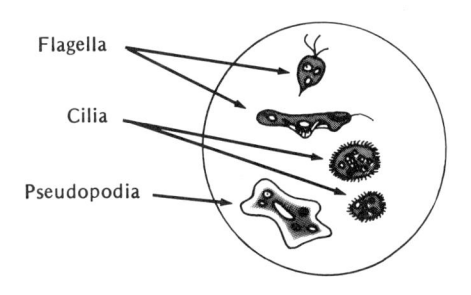

Laboratory Culture

When conditions are unfavorable, some bacteria such as the tetanus organism (*Clostridium tetani*), are able to consolidate their living material in such a way that they become highly resistant to destruction. They form spores. Such spores are **non-vegetative** (non-active or reproducing) but they can sustain the life of the organism until conditions become favorable.

In the laboratory bacteria are grown in special containers on a material known as **media**. The growth of the organism on the media is called a **culture**. Cultural characteristics which can be used to help identify the organism include the color and size of the colonies, the type of media required, and the presence of bacterial products produced.

There are many kinds of culture media; some are solid with a gelatin base, and others are liquid. The media is usually prepared in test tubes or poured into **petrie dishes** (a flat, covered dish).

Since microbes are so small, they need very little media on which to grow. Many different substances such as blood, protein, or sugar are added to the basic media to provide special nutrition for various microbes. Samples of infectious material (also called a culture) are taken from the patient and introduced into the culture media. At each spot where a single bacterial

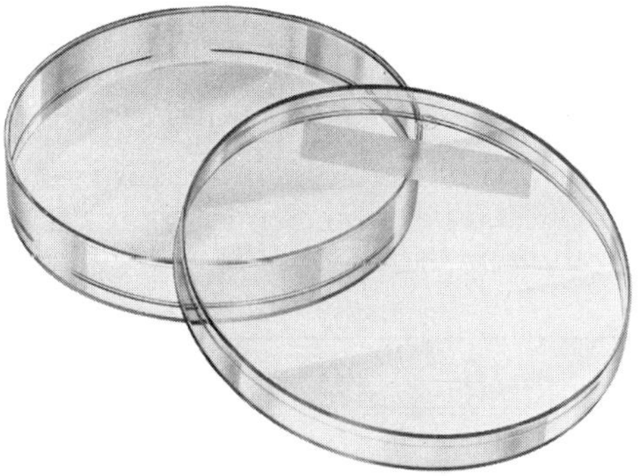

Figure 6-6: The petri dish is filled with media for the growth of microbes *(courtesy of Curtin Matheson Scientific, Inc.).*

microbe lands, a **colony** (a mass of organisms) big enough to be seen will develop as the organism reproduces itself by simply dividing in half (binary fission). In suitable media, binary fission can occur every 20 minutes so that the numbers produced in a 24-48 hour period can be phenomenal.

Different organisms produce differing colony characteristics, such as a color or shape which further aids in the identification. As the colony increases, products enter the media which can be identified. Some are **enzymes**, chemicals which influence chemical reactions and are necessary for microbial growth. Others are poisonous products such as **toxins**. Bacteria do not all produce the same enzymes or toxins and so the presence of a specific enzyme or toxin in the media may be used to identify the organism forming the colony.

Many bacteria have two names, one common and one proper. For example, the mycobacterium tuberculosis is also called the **tubercle bacillus** because a wall called a *tubercle* is formed around it when it enters the body. Look at the table to see some of the proper and common bacterial names.

Table 6-3

Proper Bacterial Name	*Common Bacterial Name*	*Disease*
Neisseria gonnorrhea	Gonoccus	Gonorrhea (clapps)
Diplococcus pneumoniae	Pneumococcus	Pneumonia & other infections
Mycobacterium tuberculosis	Tubercle Bacillus	Tuberculosis
Neisseria meningitidis	Meningococcus	Epidemic Meningitis
Treponema pallidum	Syphilis Organism	Syphilis

BODY DEFENSES

The constant presence of so many pathogens and opportunists in and on the body poses the constant threat of possible infection. But the healthy human body has a series of mechanisms which prevent infection from happening more often than it does. These mechanisms are known as the outer and inner body defenses.

Table 6-4

INFECTION-PREVENTION MECHANISMS

Outer Body Defenses	Inner Body Defenses
Intact skin	Inflammation (non-specific)
Enzymes	Phagocytosis (non-specific)
Mucous membrane	Fever & leukocytosis (non-specific)
Vibrissae	Antibody formation (specific)
Cilia	

The primary outer body defense is an intact skin. As long as there are no breaks in the skin, organisms find it difficult to penetrate and invade the underlying tissues. Skin secretions also contain a **bactericidal** (bacteria killing) enzyme called lysozyme which keeps bacterial counts low. The same secretion is found in tears, whose constant washing action helps protect the delicate tissue (**conjunctiva**) which covers the eyes and lines the eyelids.

Parts of the body which open to the outside are lined with a special tissue called mucous membrane. This moist tissue produces a sticky substance called **mucus** which traps microbes before they can get deeply into the body. This membrane also produces a mild acid and protects the mouth and anus, the beginning and end of the gastrointestinal tract, the uretheral **orifice** (opening) into the urinary tract, the vaginal orifice to the vagina leading into the female reproductive tract, and the nasal orifice into the respiratory tract. Tiny hair-like processes, **cilia**, constantly beat the mucus-trapped particles toward the exterior to be expelled.

Short, coarse hairs, **vibrissae**, guard the nasal orifice to screen foreign particles. Microbes are very sensitive to extremes in acidity and alkalinity. The presence of acid may be either **bacteriostatic** (inhibit bacterial growth) or bactericidal. Cells in the stomach produce hydrochloric acid (HCL) which is bactericidal. Sneezing and coughing actively propel materials out of the respiratory tract.

Inflammation

When something foreign to the body, an irritant, enters the

tissue, the body protects itself in non-specific ways through the inflammatory response. The purpose of this series of non-specific events is to restrain the irritant, remove it if possible, and to repair any damage that has been done by the irritant. The presence of an inflammation is indicated by certain signs and symptoms. The body area is red, hot, swollen, painful, and function is lost. We speak of that part as inflamed and used the suffix, -itis, with the name of the part. For example, an inflamed skin would be a **dermatitis**, an inflamed appendix is an **appendicitis**.

Microbes are frequently the irritant causing the inflammation. Certain microbes attract large numbers of white blood cells to the area. These are **pyogenic** or pus producing organisms. When pyogenic organisms are active the resulting **pus** (WBC, organisms, and tissue debris) forms an **exudate** (accumulation of fluid). This comes about because white blood cells rush to the area since they are able to surround an irritant, pulling it through their cell walls, and then destroying it. This special ability to consume foreign particles is called **phagocytosis**.

Inflammations due to pyogenic organisms and exhibiting the characteristic signs and symptoms are considered **acute** (sudden and severe). Sometimes, however, an irritant stimulates a lower grade response that continues over a longer period of time. It is then called **chronic** (long and continued). For example, the gonococcus stimulates an acute response but the tubercle bacillus engenders a chronic process. Sometimes the invading organism is so virulent that the body is overwhelmed. Then the inflammatory response can neither stop the multiplication of the microbes nor prevent their destruction and spread. The body then responds with a secondary defense which includes elevation of temperature (**pyrexia**) and an increase in the numbers of circulating white blood cells (**leukocytosis**). If these measures fail, the microbes may enter the blood stream and be carried to other parts of the body (**bacteremia**) or they may enter the blood stream and begin to reproduce (**septicemia**) which is a very serious condition.

Antibodies

The body has another protective mechanism that gradually develops in the presence of certain foreign irritants (**antigens**). This internal defense mechanism is known as antibody formation. **Antibodies** are protective substances which are developed in the body in response to the presence of an antigen. Different types of antibodies are produced in response to specific antigens. They neutralize the antigens or make them more susceptible to the action of **phagocytes** (cells capable of **phagocytosis**).

Antibodies are named according to their manner of inactivating antigens. See Table 6-5.

Table 6-5

Antibody	Action on Antigen
Agglutinins	cause antigens to clump together
Opsonins	make antigens sticky
Cytolysins	dissolve antigenic cells
Antitoxins	neutralize antigenic toxins
Viral neutralizing	make viruses inactive

Immunity

The formation of antibodies make a person **immune** (resistant) to further invasion by specific antigens. **Immunity** is the resistance possessed by a person to damage by antigens. First contact with an antigen makes an individual either less susceptible or more resistant (immune) to infection in subsequent contacts. This type of immunity is known as **naturally** (without artificial means) **acquired** (developed) **active** (self-produced) **immunity** (resistance).

Naturally acquired active immunity is only one type of immunity that can be developed. Other types of immunity include: naturally acquired passive immunity, artificially acquired passive immunity, and artificially acquired active immunity.

Notice in each of these types of immunity certain words are repeated. "Naturally" and "artificially" refer to the way the antigen is contacted. "Active" and "passive" refer to the source of the immunity.

Naturally means that the antigen is contacted by association with a person who has an **active** (current) case of a disease. Or it can mean that antibodies are transferred from a mother to her unborn child.

Artificially means coming in contact with either an antigen or an antibody through artificial means, such as an injection with a needle under the skin.

Active means that a given person develops his/her own antibodies in response to specific antigens.

Passive means that necessary antibodies are developed outside a given person's body and are then introduced into the body in some way.

Table 6-6

Type of Immunity	Agent	Method
Naturally Acquired Active Immunity	antigens	comes in contact with an active case, builds up own antibodies
Naturally Acquired Passive Immunity	antibodies	passes from mother to child before birth
Artificially Acquired Active Immunity	antigens	are injected or swallowed, builds own antibodies
Artificially Acquired Passive Immunity	antibodies	antibodies injected (sick person temporarily uses someone else's antibodies)

Vaccines (weakened antigens), **toxoids** (weakened toxins), and **antitoxins** (those derived from animals), and **gamma globulin** (blood protein containing antibodies) are all administered by health personnel to help patients develop immunity. Vaccines and toxoids (acting as antigens) promote active immunity. Antitoxins and gamma globulin (as antibodies) provide passive immunity.

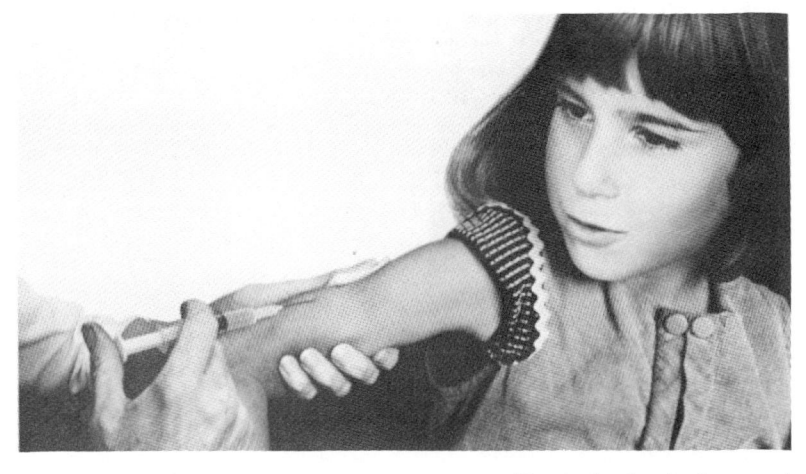

Figure 6-7: Vaccines are given to promote artificially acquired active immunity *(courtesy of Allied Chemical Corporation)*.

EXTERNAL CONTROL OF MICROBES

Vaccines and gamma globulin may afford the body internal protection but are of no value in controlling the spread of microbes outside the body. The methods employed for this control center around either the destruction or inhibition of the pathogens and the prevention of their distribution.

Heat and chemicals are the primary ways in which microbes are inhibited or destroyed. Most pathogens are **mesophilic** (middle loving), growing best at body temperature or only slightly higher. Cold is bacteriostatic for them, inhibiting or retarding their growth but extreme heat is bactericidal, providing the temperature is high enough and is maintained for a sufficient period of time.

The **autoclave**, a machine which boils water and produces steam under pressure can be used to sterilize materials. If the temperature is kept sufficiently high for a certain length of time, the articles will be **sterilized** (be made sterile). A **sterile** article is one that has no living organisms at all. An article is either sterile or not sterile; there is no in-between status.

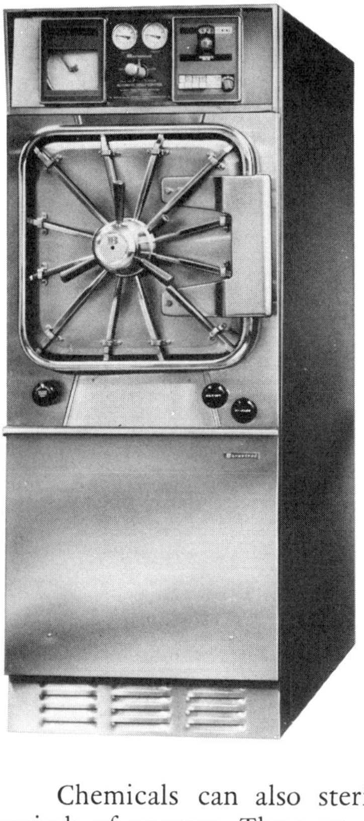

Figure 6-8: An autoclave *(courtesy of Curtin Matheson, Inc.)*.

Chemicals can also sterilize but they require very long periods of contact. They are more commonly used to **disinfect** (destroy pathogens) articles. A disinfected article has no pathogens, but non-pathogens may be present. **Disinfectants** (substances which disinfect) may be damaging to living tissues so disinfectants are used on **fomites** (inanimate objects on which

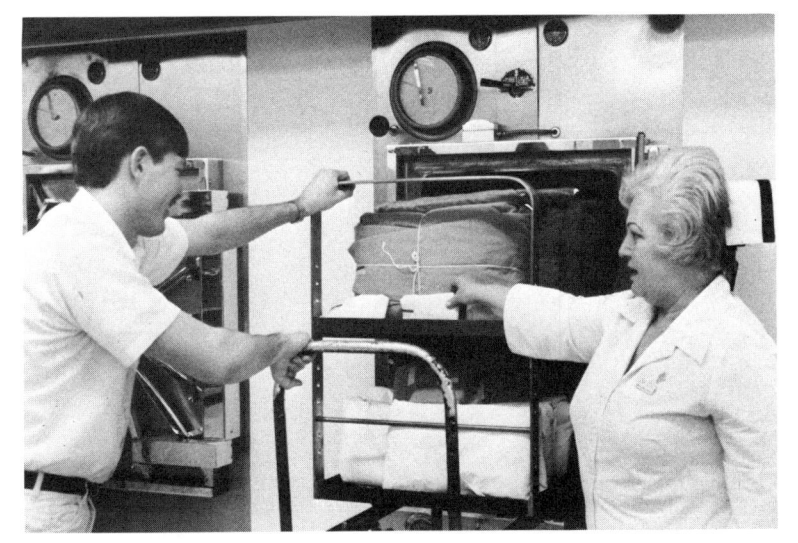

Figure 6-9: The staff of the Central Service preparing to sterilize linens for the Operating Room in the autoclave.

infectious materials may be found), such as bedpans, basins, and glassware. **Antiseptics** are anti-infection agents used in or on living tissues. This type of agent is used on breaks in the skin to prevent infection.

Pasteurization is a technique used for milk and beer and other food and drink. It preserves them and makes them safe to drink or eat. In this process, the temperature is raised high enough to destroy pathogens and cut down on non-pathogens. It does not produce a sterile product, but a safe one.

Control of microbes through control of transmission utilizes principles associated with portals of entrance and exit. Some organisms need a **vector** (an animal carrier) in their transmission, while others can be transferred through contaminated **fomites**. Fomites are non-harmful objects, such as clothing, that can harbor and transmit pathogens.

Knowledge of these facts is important. Applied to techniques for handling a specific microbe they can prevent the spread of that organism from an infected person to a susceptible host. For example, Staphylococcus epidermidis can cause a local infection such as an abscess. By covering the abscessed area with a bandage the doctor prevents the infectious disease from being spread to another individual by means of the exudate since the portal of exit through the skin is thus controlled. The nurse caring for this patient may, in her turn, have a small cut on her finger. By bandaging that finger she protects her portal of entry. Similarly, malaria, a protozoal disease caused by the *Plasmodium vivax*, is transferred from one person to

Figure 6-10: (left) Antiseptics are anti-infection agents used on living tissue.

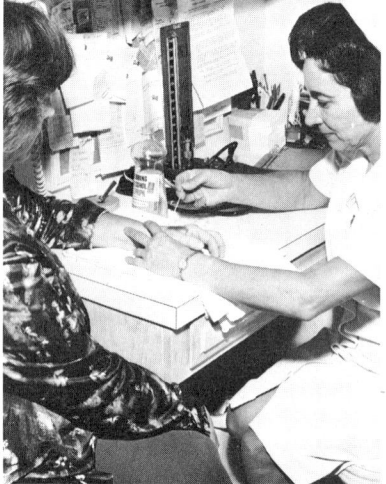

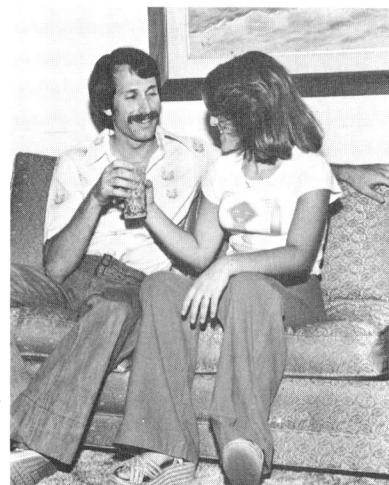

Figure 6-11: (right) A shared drinking glass can act as a fomes.

Figure 6-12: The bandage on the nurse's finger protects the portal of entry.

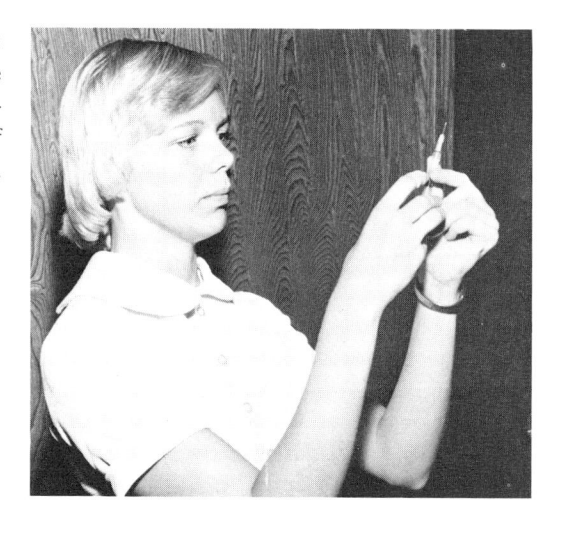

another by the anopheles mosquito, a vector. By destroying the breeding places of the mosquito and, therefore, the mosquitos, health workers control the spread of that disease.

Each time a health worker employs aseptic techniques such as washing his hands properly or using adequate time and temperature for sterilization, he is preventing infections and the spread of infectious microbes.

NOSOCOMIAL INFECTIONS

Infections acquired while in the hospital are called **nosocomial** infections. Unfortunately, some people do enter the hospital to be treated for one illness and become infected with

*110 *BASIC MEDICAL ASEPSIS*

another disease. To prevent this very undesirable event, elaborate precautions must be carried out by all staff. The precautions include proper housekeeping practices and careful aseptic techniques practiced by all personnel—beginning with hand washing—and carried out meticulously in the sensitive work areas such as obstetrics and surgery. For example, people entering and leaving the delivery suite and operating room even change their clothes.

SUMMARY

Infectious disease is a major health problem. In this chapter you have had an opportunity to familiarize yourself with terms associated with the basic concepts of microbiology and some common infectious and communicable diseases. Health workers play an enormously important role in the treatment and control of infectious disease through basic aseptic techniques.

PRACTICE & REVIEW

Explain and define the new special terms you have been using. Remember, you learned how to pronounce them at the beginning of this chapter.

1. pseudopodia _____
2. antigen _____
3. commensalism _____
_____
4. *Escherichia coli* _____
5. fomites _____
6. immunity _____
7. morbidity _____
8. saprophytes _____
9. enterotropic _____
10. bacteriostatic _____

Now, double-check the meaning of the terms above by studying the brief definitions given in the Glossary-Index at the back of this text.

Test yourself quickly before going on to learn other medical and professional terms. Use these short review exercises to practice for your new work in health services. Your teacher will also help by recommending various other Study Activities.

A. Complete the twelve statements below by writing in the correct word:

1. When many people, in a community, are infected with a communicable disease at one time, it is called an _____.
2. The _____ rate indicates the number of deaths due to a specific disease.
3. Viruses which affect the viscera are called _____.
4. Those chemical compounds whose name means "life destroying" and which are used to control certain microbes are called _____.
5. Microorganisms that can be colored are _____ for better microscopic viewing.
6. Soiling an object by transferring harmful organisms to it is known as _____.
7. Disease-producing organisms are called _____.
8. Heterotropic organisms that live on dead matter are called _____.
9. The normal microbial population found on the body is known as the normal _____.
10. When more than one organism is involved in an infection, it is called a _____ infection.
11. Resistant forms of some microbes are called _____.
12. Whip-like appendages which provide some organisms with mobility are called _____.

B. Briefly define the terms or prefixes below insofar as they describe something about the shape or growth patterns of microbes:

1. coccus _____
2. bacillus _____
3. spirillum _____
4. strepto- _____
5. staphylo- _____

C. Match the common name of the communicable disease at the left with its medical name in the right-hand column:

____ 1. seven day measles   a. variola
____ 2. German measles   b. Rubeola
____ 3. chicken pox   c. Rubella
____ 4. small pox   d. varicella
____ 5. Infantile paralysis   e. parotitis
                                     f. poliomyelitis

After studying Chapter 7
The Patient: Focus of Concern
You should be able to:

* *Pronounce and define each of its new medical words and phrases and use the new technical jargon.*

* *List five categories of disease.*

* *Name five acts that constitute a legal situation.*

PRONOUNCE THESE TEN NEW WORDS WITH YOUR TEACHER: MEDICAL WORDS

antipyretics (an″ti-pi-ret′ikz)
exacerbation (ĕg-zas″er-ba′shun)
ischemia (ĭs-ke′me-ah)
obstructed (ob-struk′ted)
atresia (ah-tre′ze-ah)
herniorrhaphy (her″ne-or′ah-fe)
cholecystectomy (ko″le-sĭs-tek′to-me)
expertise (ek-sper-tez)
dysarthrosis (dĭs″ar-thro′sĭs)
urinalysis (u′rĭ-nal′ĭ-sĭs)

The center of medical activity is neither the doctor, the nurse, nor the technician. Important as each of them are, it is the patient, the person being treated for disease, who is the focal point of professional health care.

The patient is a very special person. Like all workers in the medical field you will be taught to provide skilled care and support for him or her. Patients are individual persons and are unique in their responses to their current stress. It is very important that you as a health worker always keep the fact of a patient's individuality in mind. Whatever role you have in health work, you will have many opportunities for direct or indirect communications to or about each patient.

At one time the name "patient" was applied only to those already **overtly** (openly) sick with some disease and "in" a hospital for treatment. But today there is a definite trend toward **preventative health care** (keeping people well). This mode of health care attempts to keep people out of the patient category or at least keep them from becoming more seriously ill and only "out-patients."

Figure 7-1:
The patient; the focus of concern.

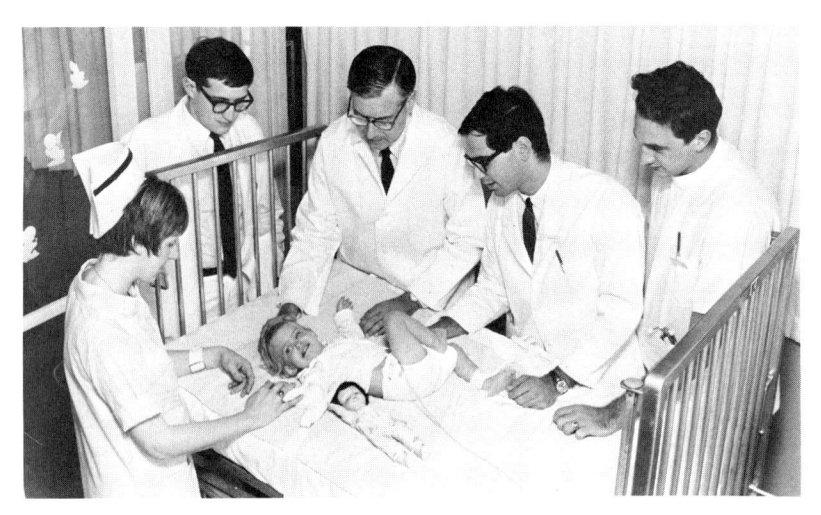

To achieve this goal, minor health problems are identified and treated before they can develop into major conditions requiring the more intensive care provided inside a hospital by a hospital staff. For example, contrast the case histories of R. Hansen and J. Sutton. Both of these people qualify for the title "patient" but they differ from one another in one important aspect—the stage when their condition was first recognized and diagnosed. Both men are in their mid-fifties, have high-pressure jobs, family responsibilities, and suffer from **hypertension** (high blood pressure).

Mr. Hansen, an executive in a book publishing firm, first became aware of his elevated blood pressure when he felt dizzy at work, momentarily losing consciousness. Later that day at the insistence of his wife, he visited his doctor and was found to have greatly elevated blood pressure. He was admitted to the hospital with a provisional diagnosis of "hypertension, possible stroke." Following two weeks of treatment which included bed rest, dietary management, and drug therapy, he was discharged with instructions for **follow-up** (continued) care.

Mr. Sutton, an assembly worker, felt well and had no history of major illness. The industrial nurse at his plant, in cooperation with the plant union, conducted a three-day blood pressure check and hypertension information program. Mr. Sutton's blood pressure was found to be elevated moderately and since he is a member of a **high risk** group (those persons with a greater likelihood of developing a specific condition), he received instructions on weight control and dietary management and was referred to a doctor for follow-up care.

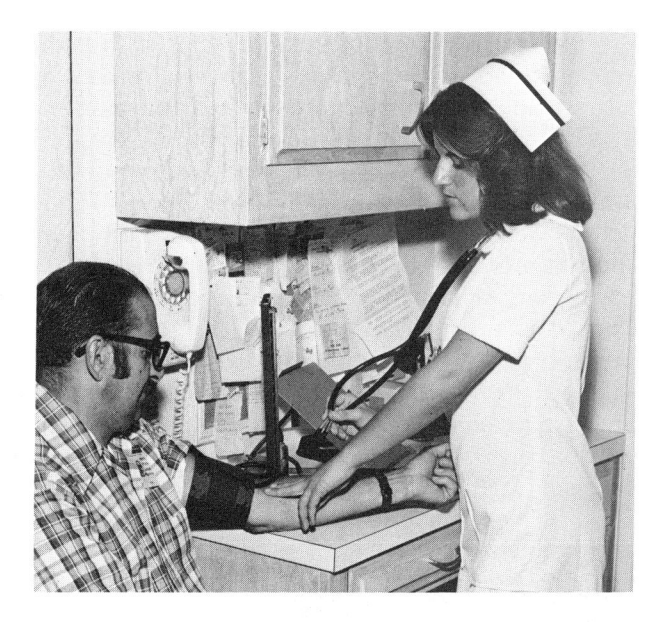

Figure 7-2: The industrial nurse practices preventative medicine by conducting a hypertension information program.

Mr. Hansen became an in-patient at the hospital but Mr. Sutton was able to remain out in the community carrying on his daily activities because of early diagnosis.

A patient then is not only a person confined to a hospital but is any person who can benefit from professional health **expertise** (expertness). You may also see from the case histories that the extent and duration of care required will also vary greatly.

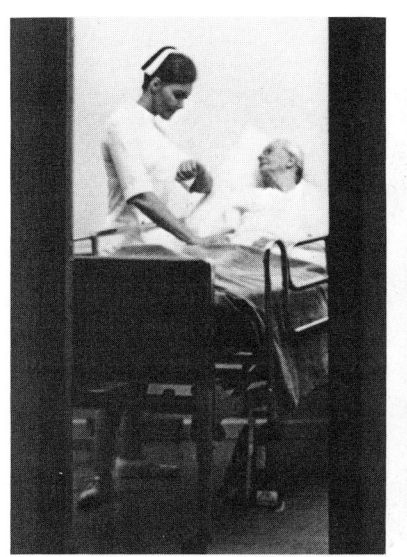

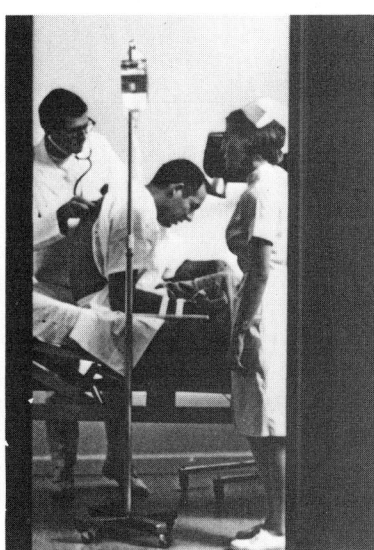

Figure 7-3: (left) This acutely ill patient is suffering from pneumonia *(courtesy of Eli Lily Company)*.

Figure 7-4: (right) Congestive heart failure is a chronic condition *(courtesy of Eli Lily Company)*.

MEDICAL WORDS 115 *

Patients may be acutely ill persons, such as those with heart attacks who must receive hospital care, or they may be chronically ill, such as those who have a chronic condition like arthritis, that may be treated at home or in the physician's office.

Some patients need physical care while others need emotional support and counseling. Some come for special therapy such as **dental** (tooth) care or rehabilitation from catastrophic illness, others for diagnostic tests such as blood counts. Some patients are confined to bed and require continuous care by a team of health workers in a health facility. Some patients are **ambulatory** (up walking) and living independent lives. They make appointments with professional health workers for help in some aspect of self care, such as planning a special diet. Remember that this latter type of patient is being called a **client** with increasing frequency.

Figure 7-5: Emotional support and counseling is part of medical care.

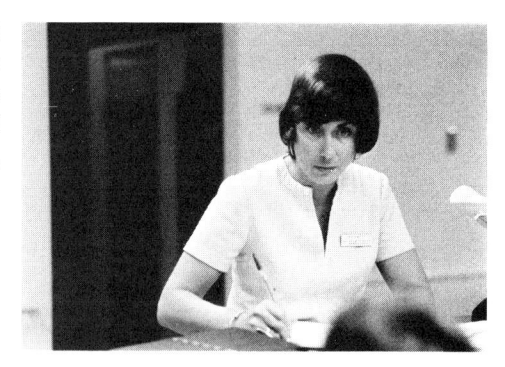

Figure 7-6: (left) This patient is ambulatory and visiting a clinic for special help he needs for a hearing defect *(courtesy of The National Foundation March of Dimes).*

Figure 7-7: (right) This patient is receiving help with diet planning *(courtesy of The National Foundation March of Dimes).*

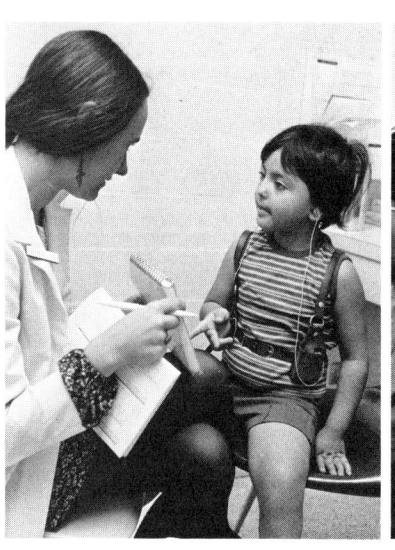

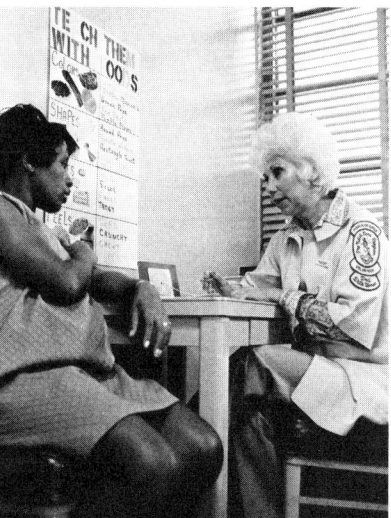

* 116 *THE PATIENT: FOCUS OF CONCERN*

Patients come in all ages, shapes, and sizes. Sometimes the words we use with "patient" give us a clue as to their identity. For example, look at the following list:

PERSONAL CHARACTERISTICS

Identifying Characteristics	Terms
Race	black/white/brown/yellow
Location in the community	in/out
Type of therapy	medical/surgical
Age	*geriatric* (aged)/pediatric
Weight	obese/malnourished
Part of body involved	gall bladder/stomach
Ability to verbalize	*aphrasic* (unable to speak)/vocal
Ability to understand	*aphasic* (unable to comprehend)/alert
Stage of illness	acute/chronic

Figure 7-8: (below) Mr. Clark, a patient with an infected gall bladder, in 208B *(courtesy of Eli Lilly Company).*

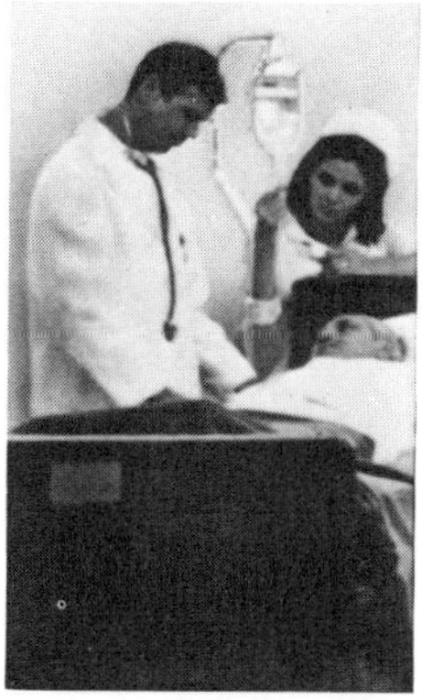

Helpful though they are, terms of characterization only give a fragmented view of the patient. Patients are complex wholes. A co-worker may refer to the patient as "the gall bladder in 208B" using hospital jargon, but this is improper and lacks dignity. Be careful that you do not fall into the same trap. To recognize the patient as "Mr. Clark, with the infected gall bladder, in 208B" takes a little longer to communicate but it is a worthwhile expenditure since it recognizes the patient as a person.

People under stress do not hear or see as well. Their attention is often poor, and they tend to forget what is said or misinterpret explanations. You will have to speak slowly and distinctly, avoiding jargon and shortened forms. Make explanations clear, choosing simple words. Repeat important parts and ask the patient for a return explanation. This gives you an opportunity to clarify any misunderstandings or problems. Remember, words do not always mean the same things to all people. An unhurried attitude will encourage the patient to actively participate. It gives both the patient and you the health worker an opportunity to clarify important points.

EXPLANATION TO PATIENT

PROFESSIONAL COMMUNICATIONS

Professional people have a variety of ways in which they communicate information about the patient and his care. Some communications are oral and some are written. Some are formal, some informal. All are important.

Oral Communications

Formal oral communications are spoken directly by one health worker to another. They concern the patient and his progress or care. A written notation is helpful if it is made during or shortly after the conversation, since it can serve as a reminder of salient points and can be used for continued reference.

Telephone Techniques

When answering the telephone always give your location, name and designation. For example, "Five South, Mrs. Franks, Ward Clerk speaking." This immediately identifies you to the caller as someone to whom information can be given, or it allows the caller to ask for someone else to assist him. If you are making the call, identify yourself as soon as the telephone is answered. Make sure that the party who answers is the proper person for the message. Then give the message, directions, or instructions in a brief, clear manner. Be courteous; it pays.

Telephones, in a health facility, as with any business, are for business purposes only and must never be used for personal communications.

Figure 7-9: (left) Oral communications are given directly from one medical assistant to another *(courtesy of American Association of Medical Assistants, Inc.)*.

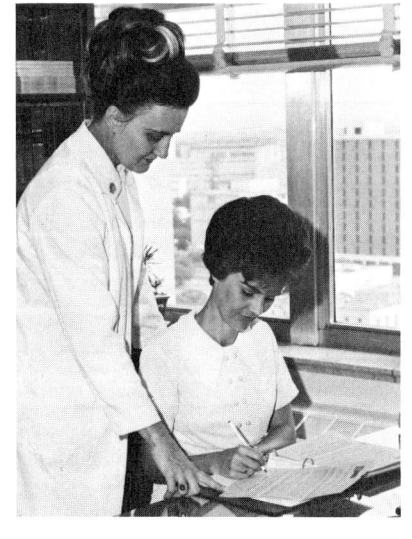

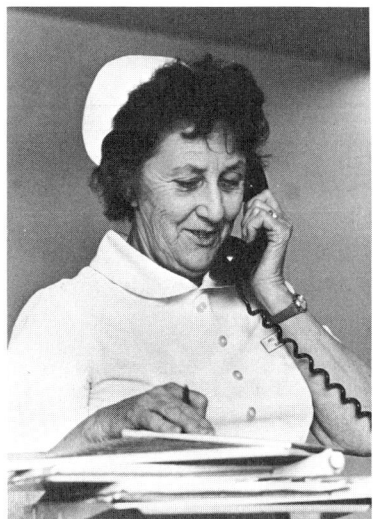

Figure 7-10: (right) Telephones in a health facility are for business only.

ORDERS FOR PATIENT CARE

Orders regarding patient therapy are formal, whether oral or written communications. They are frequently transmitted over the telephone. Two points must be remembered in this situation. First, be sure you have the authority to accept formal

*118 *THE PATIENT: FOCUS OF CONCERN*

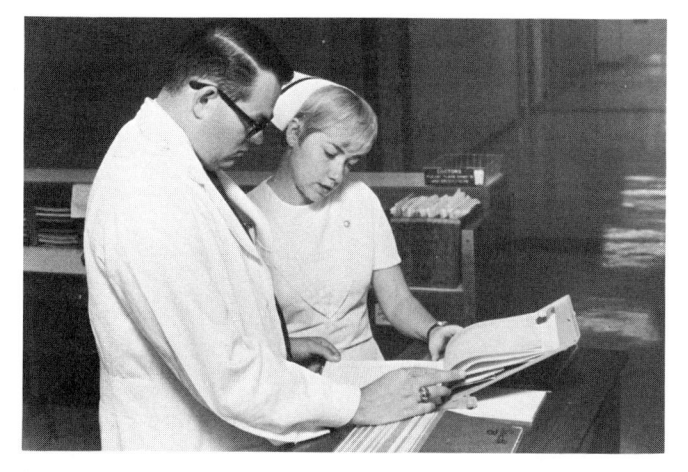

Figure 7-11: Orders for patient care are formal, oral and written communications

directions for patient care. Not all health workers have the **legal** (permitted by law) authority to accept such orders. Secondly, if you may legally take orders over the telephone, the orders must be accurately recorded, clarified, and signed as **T.O.** (telephone orders), and initialed by the receiver. For example, see the following:

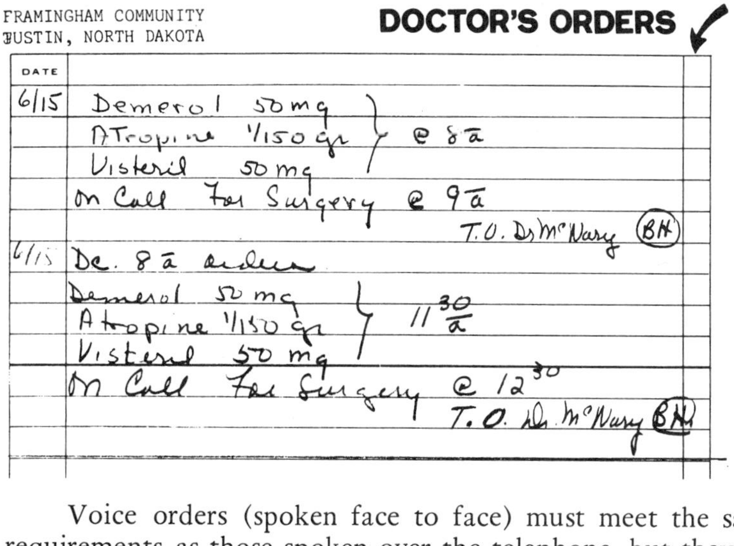
FRAMINGHAM COMMUNITY
JUSTIN, NORTH DAKOTA

DOCTOR'S ORDERS

DATE	
6/15	Demerol 50 mg }
	Atropine 1/150 gr } @ 8 ā
	Visteril 50 mg }
	On Call For Surgery @ 9 ā
	T.O. Dr McNary (BH)
6/15	Dc. 8 ā orders
	Demerol 50 mg }
	Atropine 1/150 gr } 11 30 ā
	Visteril 50 mg }
	On Call For Surgery @ 12 30
	T.O. Dr. McNary BH

Figure 7-12:

Voice orders (spoken face to face) must meet the same requirements as those spoken over the telephone, but they are signed **V.O.** (voice orders).

REPORTING ON PATIENT CARE

Patient care is given on a continuous basis. Hospital staffs usually work on a **shift** (a segment of working hours) basis: the **A.M. shift** (7:00a–3:30p), **P.M. shift** (3:00p–11:30p), and the

Figure 7-13: The report is an oral communication between staff members at change of shift

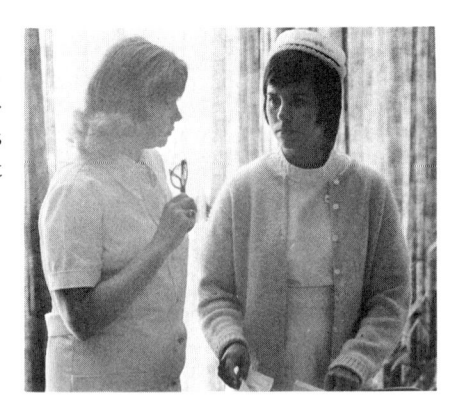

Night shift (11:00p-7:30a). Notice that the shifts overlap so that off-going staff members can have enough time to communicate information about the patients to the on-coming staff. This form of oral communication called **report**, includes information about each patient's progress and any unusual or **untoward** (unfavorable) events that have happened during the shift. The report is used to give directions for additional care to be given in the coming hours.

In this report, the name, location, and diagnosis of each patient should be presented; followed by a brief, but complete, summary of staff observations during the **tour of duty** (period of responsibility) just completed. A health worker is said to be "on duty" when he/she assumes responsibility for the patient. The information transmitted in the report in this way is usually noted on a pad or a report sheet for future reference by members of the on-coming shift.

HOSPITAL ASSIGNMENTS Each member of the team has specific responsibilities. An assignment sheet is usually posted somewhere in the unit giving these directions. The team member takes the assignment, reviews the patient needs, and develops a plan to carry out the indicated activities during the on-duty time.

Legal Responsibilities Hospital records are legal documents and their accuracy is a legal matter—as well as information. This subject is more thoroughly explained in Chapter 20.

Health Worker Responsibilities Taking care of a sick person is a tremendous responsibility and probably one of the most rewarding. For the protection of the patient, each person working with the patient must be competent, caring and responsible; *and* everything must be done in a legal way. The health worker is responsible for each of his own actions. Each health discipline has a framework of activities which are legally and professionally within the scope of normal

Figure 7-14:

ASSIGNMENTS   7:00 — 3:30   1 — NORTH

Team A	Team B
Team Leader G. Gregory R.N.	Team Leader P. Sennett R.N.
Rms. 7, 8a - K. Paul R.N. Meds	Rms. 18, 19 - R. Benson R.N. Meds
Rms. 2, 4, 5 - E. Hugo L.V.N.	Rms. 16, 17, 20 - S. Daye R.N.
Rms. 6, 9, 10, 11 - D. Sato L.V.N.	Rms. 21, 22, 23 - T. Kelly L.V.N.
Rms. 12, 14, 15 - O. Jones L.V.N.	Rms. 24, 25, 26, 27 - M. Wade L.V.N.
Nursing Assistants	**Nursing Assistants**
P. Smith assist Paul/Hugo	R. Rular assist Benson/Kaye
J. Dana assist Sato/Jones	L. Scotch assist Smith/Hogan

practice. A health worker who is aware of the normal **parameters** (boundaries) of his field and remains within them has no problem fulfilling his legal and professional responsibilities successfully.

LEGAL CONSIDERATIONS

A **crime** is a deliberate commission or omission of an act forbidden by law. Health workers must not commit crimes either deliberately or out of neglect. If a worker steals drugs for his own use or to sell, it is a deliberate illegal act or a crime of commission. If a worker sees someone else stealing and fails to report the action to his supervisor, he is guilty of **aiding and abetting** (assisting) a criminal. He is then guilty of a crime of omission as well.

Today we hear a great deal about malpractice. **Malpractice** means a neglect of professional duty or a failure of professional skill that results in injury, loss or damage. Starting an I.V. is considered to be within the scope of professional nursing practice. If a nursing assistant starts an I.V., using improper techniques, and the patient is injured, the nursing assistant is guilty of malpractice. Starting I.V.'s is not within the scope of a nursing assistant's regular responsibilities. Similarly, a physician is expected to recognize the signs of ordinary illness. If a patient with overt signs of coronary heart attack presents himself to an emergency room for care and is discharged by the physician in charge without adequate treatment, the physician is guilty of malpractice.

Negligence is neglect of duty by one who knows how or should know how to properly carry out his functions. Remember that each health discipline has boundaries and expectations for its members. Each worker is expected to be competent in certain skills, to recognize his/her limitations, and to exercise normal prudence in making judgments. For example, all nursing personnel know that side rails must be kept up on the beds of unconscious patients. If a nurse fails to carry out this procedure and the patient falls, the nurse is guilty of negligence.

If a health worker makes an untrue and damaging statement about a patient, that health worker is guilty of **slander**. If that same statement is put in writing, that worker is guilty of **libel**. We know, for instance, that patients suffering from diabetes mellitus sometimes act confused and **disoriented** (inability to recognize time, place or person) as the level of sugar in their blood rises. A case in point: an orderly observed a patient enter the hospital waiting room and was overheard commenting to a fellow worker that the person was "drunk." That was a clear case of slander. The man, a diabetic, was later admitted for care. If the orderly's observation and comment had become part of the hospital record, it would have been libel as well.

ETHICS

The code of medical ethics (right behavior toward the sick and all health workers) is a set of rules to which all health workers voluntarily ascribe. There is no legal binding force here. The authority is moral. As a health worker, this same code will guide you as you develop relationships with patients and co-workers.

Members of the health team are **privileged** people (given unusual opportunities). As privileged people, they have opportunities to learn much of a private nature about the patient and his illness. This is "privileged information" and must not be revealed to outsiders. It may be discussed with co-workers only in the context of the patient's care. Health workers do not indulge in **gossip** (idle talk) about the patient since that also violates the ethical code.

Private information gained as you carry out your duties

may never be used in any way for personal gain. For instance, if one of your patients is critically ill and you are privileged to be present as his will is being discussed or written, you are bound not to reveal this information to anyone. This holds true even if someone should attempt to entice you to divulge your knowledge.

Loyalty is also part of the ethical code in health care. Hospital problems, or problems which exist between co-workers are never shared with the patients or discussed in front of them. The role of the health worker is to support and protect the patient, helping the patient cope with his problems—not to involve the patient in any dilemmas faced by the health worker. The very foundation of the medical ethical code is the premise that human life is precious and that the preservation of life and promotion of health are the primary goals of all health workers. Moreover, there is in this premise the implied desire to help people to best live a quality life. Each act of the health worker must be directed toward these goals. Each worker is ethically bound never to participate in any activity that would be contrary in results.

Updating skills and keeping abreast of the ever-expanding knowledge base is a professional responsibility of all health workers. Each person must make sure that he is always competent to carry out his expected responsibilities. Participation in the medical profession means dedication to a continuing learning process.

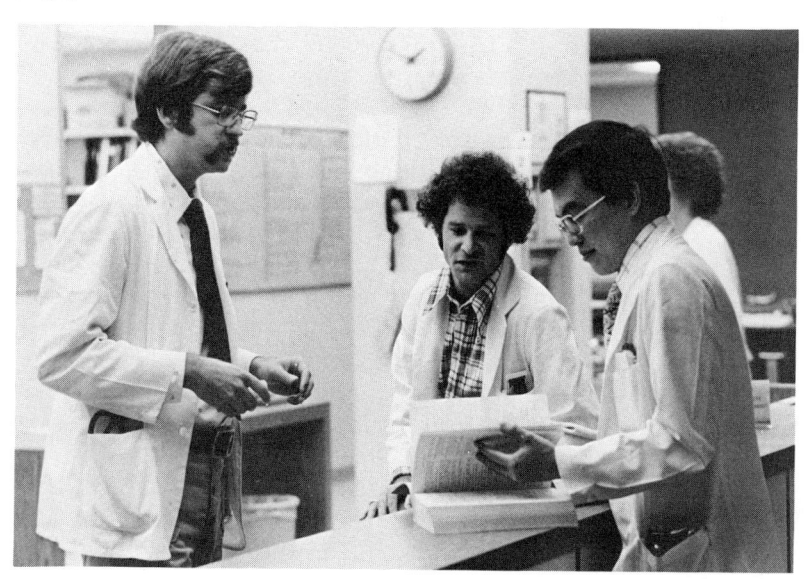

Figure 7-15: These interns are checking the latest publications in a continuous process to update their knowledge base.

Confidence in the value of any therapy is greatly influenced by the confidence the patient feels in the health worker. Not everyone can be successful in the health field. Success requires not only demonstrable skills but those perhaps less tangible, personal qualities which raise the patient's expectations by inspiring confidence. Good grooming, a friendly receptive approach, good manners, and tact are extremely important in generating a response of trust in the ability of the health worker to help the patient.

A health worker who is able to convey the impression that he is open, accepts the patient as a person first, and is not judgmental or critical, will more rapidly establish a working **rapport** (mutual understanding) than one who fails to communicate this impression.

DISEASE

At the beginning of this unit we identified the patient as a person with a disease or illness. At such times the person is under the stress of anxiety as well and requires special attention and help in establishing and maintaining successful relationships and interactions. That is what all the health team concentrates on. Remember, **disease** (departure from health) is a term which literally means "without ease." Broadly, disease implies that any normal functioning of the body has been disrupted. **Pathology** is the study of the disease process and the deviations from normal structure (**anatomy**) and function (**physiology**) which occur.

A disease may be evidenced in changes that can be seen in the tissues (**lesions**). If a lesion is present, the condition is classified as an **organic disease**. When no lesion is evident the disease is **functional**.

Tumors (neoplasms) are considered organic diseases even though the **primary** (original) lesion is microscopic. In certain types of **neoplasm** (new growth), secondary tumors develop in distant sites. This spread is known as **metastasis**. Metastatic lesions are characteristic of **malignant** (life threatening) neoplasms. Non-malignant neoplasms which do not metastasize are called **benign** (of mild type). The **etiology** (cause) of neoplasms is not fully understood. Some **dysmenorrhea** (painful menstruation) may be of organic origin, but frequently it is considered a functional disorder since no cause for the abnormality can usually be proven.

Many different categories of diseases are recognized. These include infections, traumas, neoplasms, nutritional diseases, ischemias, hypoxias, and birth defects. **Infectious diseases** are the result of the invasion by microorganisms. **Traumas** (injury) can result from hard blows, chemicals, radiation, and temperature extremes. **Fractures** (broken bones) and burns are in this category.

Nutritional diseases consist of those situations in which essential **nutrients** (foods) are either lacking, resulting in **malnutrition** (poor nutrition), or in those cases of faulty **metabolism** (the utilization of nutrients by the body), such as diabetes mellitus. In diabetes mellitus, the body is unable to metabolize or use **carbohydrates** (sugars) for energy in the normal way. In other cases, **ischemias** (diminished blood flow) and **hypoxias** (diminished levels of oxygen) are the etiology of another major pathology. Tissues deprived of these vital elements cannot function effectively. Such tissues **atrophy** (decrease in size and function) and eventually become **necrotic** (death of cells).

Children born with clubbed feet or internal problems such as bowel **atresia** (congenital absence of a body opening) are said to have **congenital** (present at birth) defects. When the congenital abnormality is the result of a **genetic defect** (one passed from parents to offspring), it is known as an **inherited** disease. Sickle cell anemia is such a condition.

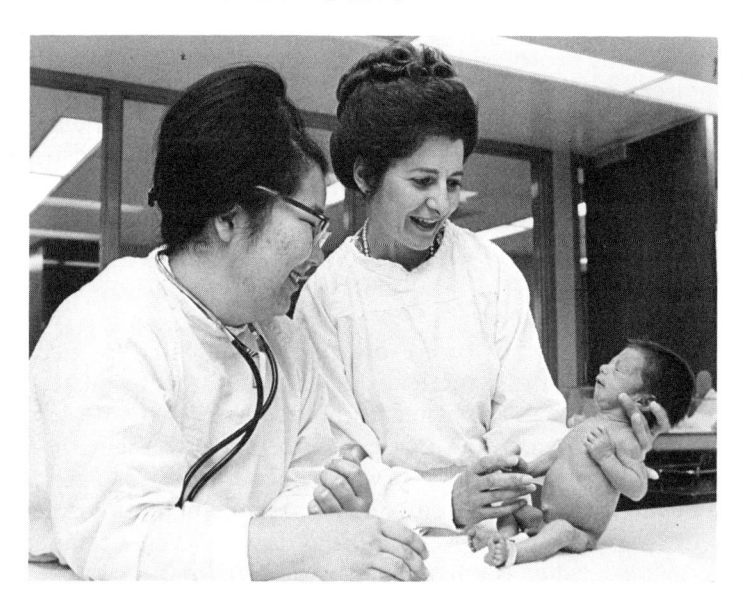

Figure 7-16: The neonatologist examines the newborn for congenital defects.

The presence of a pathologic condition is usually **manifested** (made known) in **signs** (seeable or observable characteristics) and symptoms. Signs are **overt** (open, not hidden). For instance, a **flushed** (reddened) face and rapid pulse are signs.

DISEASE 125

Symptoms are subjective; that is, they are felt by the patient but are not detectable to the observer. Being in pain, feeling hot or **nauseated** (sick to one's stomach) are all subjective phenomena experienced by the patient and are therefore symptoms. Actual vomiting (emesis) is a sign, however.

Disease patterns vary and the patient may suffer repeated **episodes** (incidents) of the same condition. They frequently experience periods of **exacerbation** (increased severity of symptoms) and **remission** (decreased severity of symptoms). Patients suffering from arthritis tend to experience periods of exacerbation when the joints become inflamed, painful and deformed (**dysarthrosis**). In between exacerbations, the patient's symptoms **abate** (diminish) and he is said to be in remission. It is necessary to know normal anatomy and physiology before the principles of pathology can be fully applied and understood. Later chapters in this book will provide a foundation for that understanding.

THE DIAGNOSIS

The physician makes a diagnosis by carefully compiling a history and examining the patient, and then correlating the symptomology and laboratory findings. To establish the **definitive** (final) diagnosis, the physician begins with the physical examination, using both direct visualization procedures, such as **cystoscopy** (procedure for looking into the bladder), and indirect procedures, such as the ECG. Next, laboratory methods are used to examine specimens taken from the patient, such as **urinalysis** (examination of urine) and blood chemistries. The physician then applies his expertise to the findings and establishes the diagnosis and prognosis. Then he plans the therapy. All this information must be summarized and communicated to the nursing staff so that orders can be properly followed.

THERAPEUTIC REGIMES

Treatment is based on four principal approaches: the symptomatic, drug, surgical, and radiation therapy. The symptomatic approach is designed to reduce the general discomfort of the symptoms of the disease and to promote the natural repair processes of the body. Rest is encouraged. **Analgesics** (pain relieving drugs) are given to control pain and **antipyretics** (fever reducing drugs) are given to bring down elevated temperatures. A balanced diet is encouraged with sufficient proteins to meet restorative needs.

Drug therapy includes the use of specific drugs as antibiotics and antivirals, and other chemicals that can control infections. It also includes the antitoxins that specifically neutralize the toxins produced by certain microbes. Drugs are also given to alter the specific physiology of the body. For example, some drugs are used to control neoplastic growth while others, like digitalis, are given to patients with **tachycardia** (abnormally fast rhythm) to slow the heart rate.

Surgery uses operative techniques to remove a diseased part. For example, when an **appendectomy** (removal of the appendix) or **cholecystectomy** (removal of the gall bladder) or **gastrectomy** (removal of the stomach) are performed, the diseased part is removed. Surgery is also employed to improve the function of an organ that is **obstructed** (blocked). For example, when the normal air passage is blocked from above, a **tracheotomy** (surgical opening into the trachea) is performed. **Gastrotomy** (surgical opening into stomach), **hysterotomy** (surgical opening into uterus), and laparotomy are all commonly performed surgeries.

A surgical repair of a body part is also of therapeutic value. Surgical repair procedures are named by combining the suffix **-orrhaphy** (repair of) with the name of the anatomical part. For example, a **herniorrhaphy** is performed to repair a **hernia** (protrusion of a part through an abnormal opening).

Replacement surgery exchanges donor tissue for diseased tissue, or replaces the diseased part with a **prosthesis** (artificial part).

Radiation therapy is most frequently employed in cases of neoplasia because cells that are abnormal and rapidly growing are more easily destroyed by radiant energy.

All medical therapy is designed to improve a specific health problem or to prevent further damage and to assist the patient in reaching optimum health and independence.

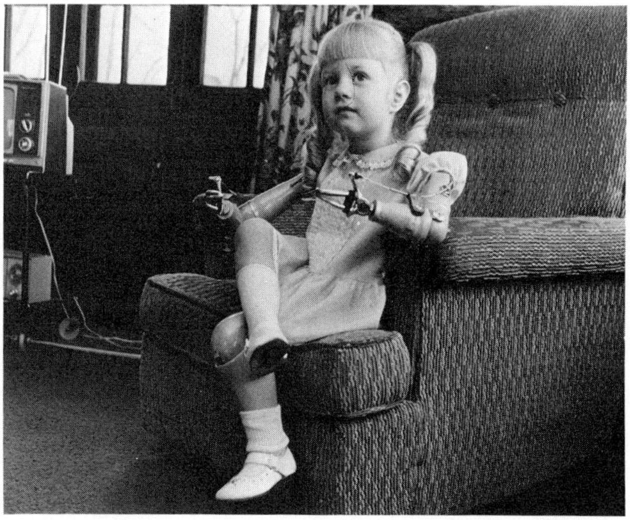

Figure 7-17: Phocomelia is a congenital abnormality requiring prostheses to replace the missing limbs *(courtesy of The National Foundation March of Dimes).*

SUMMARY   *Patients are people who are ill and must be given care. Hospitals provide that care on a 24-hour basis by having personnel work shifts of duty as they carry out accepted patient care procedures.*

The specific pathology experienced by the patient determines the therapeutic regime that will be instituted in his behalf.

PRACTICE & REVIEW   Explain and define the new special terms you have been using. Remember, you learned how to pronounce them at the beginning of this chapter.

1. antipyretics _____
2. exacerbation _____
3. ischemia _____
4. obstructed _____
5. atresia _____
6. herniorrhaphy _____
7. cholecystectomy _____
8. expertise _____
9. dysarthrosis _____
10. urinalysis _____

Now, double-check the meaning of the terms above by studying the brief definitions given in the Glossary-Index at the back of this text.

Test yourself quickly before going on to learn other medical and professional terms. Use these short review exercises to practice for your new work in health services. Your teacher will also help by recommending various other Study Activities.

A. Underline in each of the following sentences the word or words you learned in this chapter:

1. The patient was permitted to get out of bed and be ambulatory.
2. The urologist performed a cystoscopy in order to observe the bladder for lesions.
3. "What he said was untrue. That's libel!"
4. The hypertension clinic is a preventive health care facility.
5. Privileged information must be held in confidence.
6. After all the laboratory reports were in, the doctor made a definitive diagnosis.

7. Disease is often manifested in physical signs and symptoms such as a flushed face or emesis.
8. Malignant tumors are characterized by metastasis of tumor cells to other sites.
9. Because the trachea was obstructed, a tracheotomy was required.
10. After his release from the hospital, the patient was referred to the diabetic clinic for follow-up care.

B. Match the terms on the right with the correct statement on the left:

_____ 1. Refers to tooth   a. hypertension
_____ 2. Study of function   b. gossip
_____ 3. Pathological tissue changes   c. prosthesis
_____ 4. Elevated blood pressure   d. atrophy
_____ 5. Artificial part   e. lesion
_____ 6. Unfavorable   f. physiology
_____ 7. Decrease in size or function   g. anatomy
_____ 8. Insufficient oxygen   h. trauma
_____ 9. Idle talk   i. dental
_____ 10. Injury   j. asphasic
                                        k. untoward
                                        l. hypoxia

C. A word has been omitted from the five statements below. Select the words which best complete them from this list:

episode   necrotic   prosthesis
aphasic   geriatric   overtly
congenital   pediatric   malpractice

1. The ischemia was so severe that the tissues became _____ .
2. He reported only one _____ of nausea.
3. Because the patient was _____ she could not understand what was being said.
4. The _____ service gives care to the elderly.
5. The patient was crying out and _____ agitated.

After studying Chapter 8

Human Development

You should be able to:

* *Pronounce and define each of its new medical words and phrases and use the new technical jargon.*

* *Make a chart showing the organizational pattern of the human body.*

* *Identify ten body structures.*

MEDICAL WORDS
PRONOUNCE THESE TEN NEW WORDS WITH YOUR TEACHER:

alleles (ah-lel′s)
intercellular (in″ter-sel′u-lar)
diaphragm (di′ah-fram)
differentiate (dif″er-en″she a′t)
interstitial (in″ter-stich-al)
retroperitoneal (ret″ro-per″i-to-ne′al)
heterozygous (het″er-o-zi′gus)
meninges (mĕ-nin′jez)
cesarean section (sĕ-sa′re-an)
arachnoid mater (ah-rak′noid) (ma′ter)

Health workers take care of people—and people are very complex, highly structured organisms. The basic physical unit of human structure is the cell. Millions of these cells combine to constitute the body. These cells function both **independently** (alone) and **interdependently** (in concert with others) as tissues, organs and systems. The study of cells is called **cytology**.

CELLS–BASIC UNITS OF HUMAN STRUCTURE

Although there are many different kinds of cells in the body, they have certain characteristics in common. Each has a cell wall, cytoplasm, nucleus, and organelles. The cell wall (**cell membrane**) controls the movement of materials into and out of the cell. The **cytoplasm** composes the bulk of the cell material outside the nucleus. It is in the cytoplasm that the work of the cell is accomplished. If it is a mucous cell, it is here that mucus is produced. Various cell **organelles** (organ-like structures) are located in the cytoplasm and carry out cellular functions. For example, the **mitochondrion** (a cellular organelle) is composed of delicate membranes which produce energy for the cell. Other

Cells → Tissues → Organs → Systems → Man

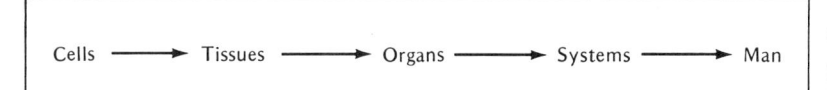

Figure 8-1: Organizational pattern of the human body.

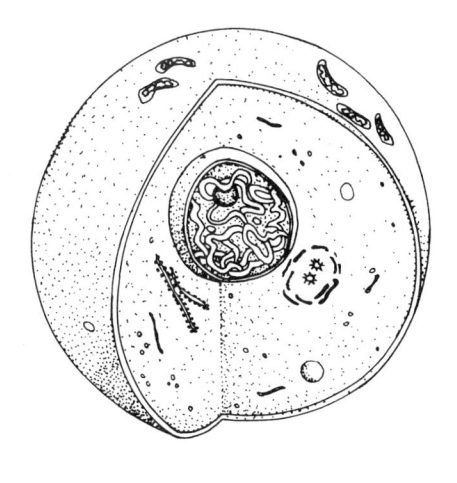

Figure 8-2: Cells are three dimensional units of life.

organelles include the **golgi apparatus**, responsible for carbohydrate formation, and **ribosomes** which are involved with protein **synthesis** (production).

The nucleus is an important part of every living cell for it is here that reproduction of the cell takes place. It is the nucleus that also directs the cellular activity. Within the nucleus are special protein strands called **chromosomes** which contain the directions for making body proteins. The chromosomial strands are normally paired. The chromosomes can be retrieved from the nucleus of a person's cell and can be paired for study.

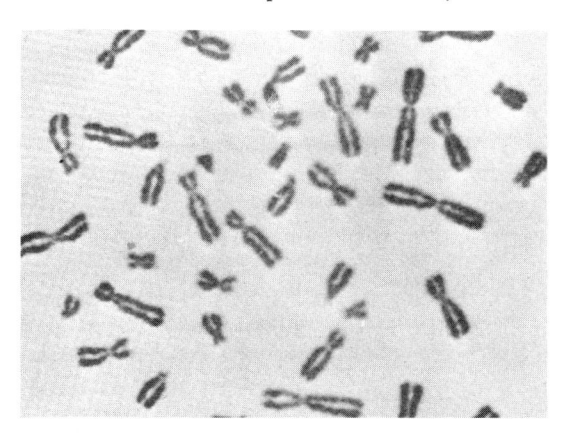

Figure 8-3: Chromosomes as seen under the microscope.

CELLS—BASIC UNITS OF HUMAN STRUCTURE 131 *

Figure 8-4: The phenotype of the mother is also seen in the child (courtesy of The National Foundation March of Dimes).

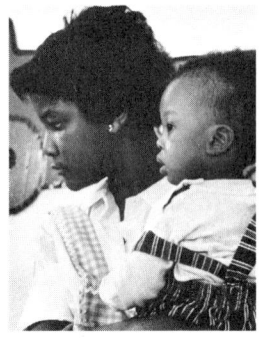

One member of each pair was originally contributed by the mother and one member by the father of the individual. Attached to the chromosomes are tiny bead-like proteins called genes. The genes carry directions for making all the proteins of the body and the proteins determine the characteristics. For example, genes carry the directions for the making of proteins to form brown hair or blue eyes. Brown hair and brown eyes are the obvious characteristics of the hereditary make-up (**phenotype**).

Genes also carry information on how to make the proteins that form normal red blood cells. If the genes are normal their directions will also be normal and the cell protein formed will be normal. If the gene is defective, the directions will be defective and the specific proteins formed will be incorrect. In sickle cell anemia, a defective gene results in the formation of an abnormal protein in the red blood cells. These red cells assume an odd, sickle-like shape and produce a form of **anemia**. Sickle cell anemia is a serious genetic disease. That is, it is inherited.

Figure 8-5: Comparison of normal and sickled red blood cells. *(courtesy of The National Foundation March of Dimes).*

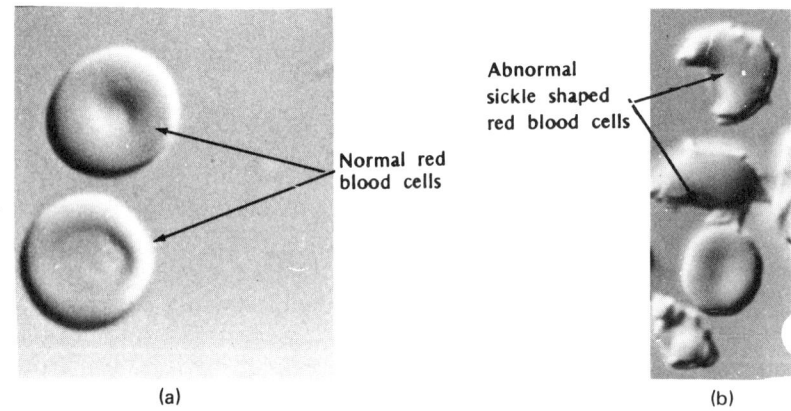

The genetic make-up of an individual is called the **genotype**. The two genes which control a given characteristic such as hair color, body structure, or eye color are called **alleles**. Alleles may be the same or different. If the alleles for a specific characteristic are the same, the person is said to be **homozygous** (having like genes). An individual who has unlike genes for a specific trait is **heterozygous**.

It is easy to understand that if two genes control the color of the eyes and both genes carry directions for brown eyes, the individual's brown eyes express his genetic make-up. If, however, a person inherits a gene for blue eyes from his father and a gene of black eyes from his mother, resulting black-colored eyes do not reveal all his genetic make-up. Genes such as the genes for black eyes need only one gene for expression. They are called **dominant** genes. When a dominant gene from one parent is paired with a recessive gene from the other, the dominant demonstrates its presence. Some genes need two like genes for expression. Blue eyes are an example. Genes for blue eyes must come from both parents. These genes are called **recessive**.

The study of the genes is called genetics. Genetics is a rapidly growing field of knowledge. Much new information is being learned about the effect of genes on newborn abnormalities. A person who is homozygous for a defective recessive gene will express the abnormality. Sickle cell anemia is a homozygous recessive disorder.

Another such disorder is phenylketonuria (**PKU**). There the defective genetic code results in an inability to metabolize certain proteins properly and, if untreated, results in **mental retardation** (lack of mental development).

A person will not demonstrate a defect for a trait if he is heterozygous (one dominant, one recessive gene) and the defect is in the recessive gene. He will, however, be a carrier with the possibility of transferring the defect to his children. Genetic counseling helps identify carriers and alerts parents to the possible consequences for a future generation.

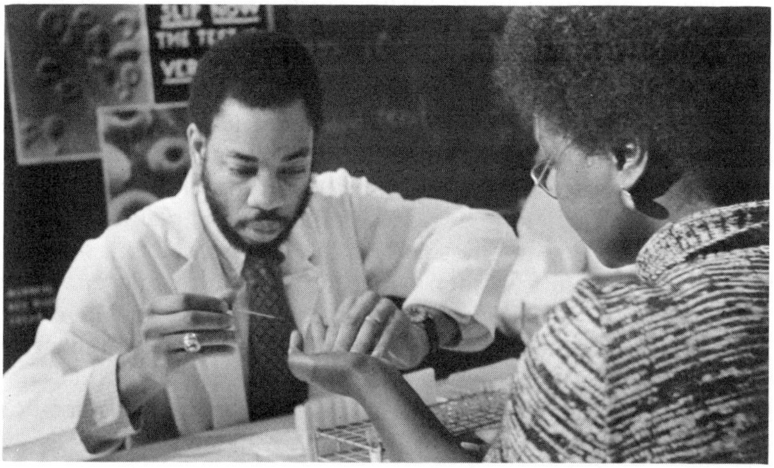

Figure 8-6: Blood is being drawn prior to genetic counseling *(courtesy of The National Foundation March of Dimes).*

EMBRYOLOGY

All the cells in the human body have a common origin. They all derive from one original cell, the **fertilized ovum**. The fertilized ovum is formed by the union of the **gametes** (reproductive sex cells). The **sperm** or male gamete fuses with the **ovum** or female gamete. This process is called **fertilization**. It is during fertilization that genetic material is combined and the genotype of the individual formed. That is to say, it is during this time that genetic defects are established in the new individual and genetic disorders such as PKU and sickle cell anemia begin.

Figure 8-7: (a) Fertilization occurs as the sperm fuses with the ovum; (b) fertilization and implantation: 1) sperm deposited in vagina; 2) union of sperm and ovum in tube; 3) implantation of fertilized ovum in endometrium *(courtesy of Ethicon, Inc.)*.

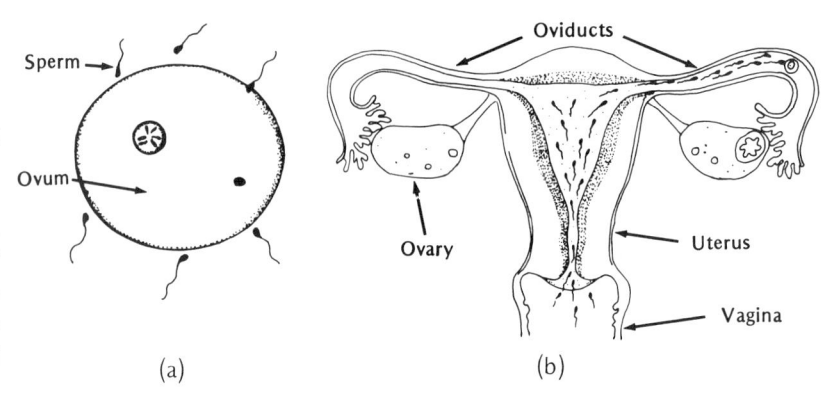

The sperm and the ova, together, form the new individual called, in this early phase, the **zygote**. The single-celled zygote develops through a series of cell divisions and then multiplications (**mitosis**) over a nine-month period into an individual human capable of independent life. The nine-month period of pregnancy development of a baby is called the period of **gestation**. The pregnancy reaches **term** (limits) when the baby is matured and ready to be delivered.

The normal period of gestation is divided into three periods (**trimesters**), each three months in length. Fertilization takes place usually in the **Fallopian tube** or **oviduct**. The zygote, undergoing progressive change, moves along the tube to the womb (**uterus**) where it becomes embedded (**implanted**) in the uterine wall. Some of the tissue of the uterine wall and some of the developing embryo then combine to form the **placenta**, the organ which is the source of nutrients and oxygen for the baby. The baby is attached to the placenta (called the afterbirth later) by the **umbilical cord** and is surrounded by amniotic fluid contained in a thin membraneous bag called the **amniotic sack** or **membrane**. There it remains housed and protected until **delivery** (passage out of the body).

During the first trimester all the body's basic structures are formed in the **embryo** (term applied during the first trimester) but independent life is not possible. The term **abortion** is used to express a pregnancy lost before the end of the third month. After that period a lost pregnancy is termed a **miscarriage**.

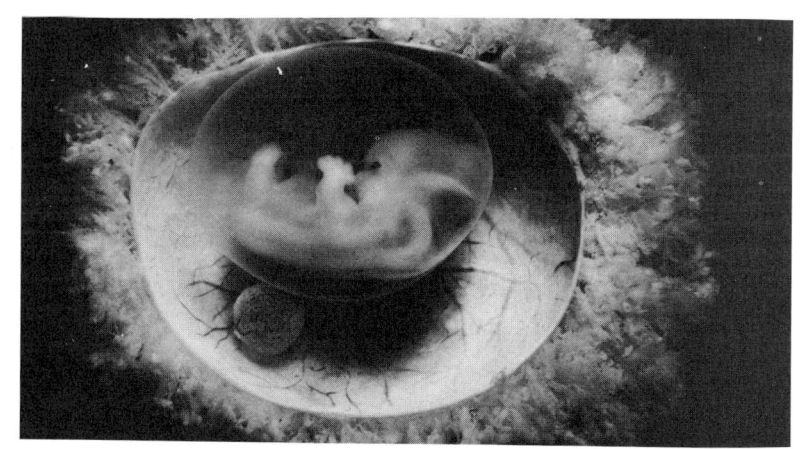

Figure 8-8: Embryo during first trimester of pregnancy *(courtesy of The National Foundation March of Dimes).*

During the **second trimester** (months 4-6) and **third trimester** (months 7-9) the baby is called a **fetus**. The basic structures formed in the embryo are further developed and matured. The closer to term or maturity the baby is when delivered, the better the chances for survival, of course.

In the third trimester the fetal structures mature and the baby gains weight until at term it weighs about 7 to 8 pounds and is approximately 20 inches long. The normal pregnancy is also measured as 40 weeks, or 10 **lunar** (moon) months or 280 days.

Premature (before maturity) babies, often termed **preemies**, are those born early with a low birth weight. Preemies require specialized supportive care in an intensive neonatal nursery.

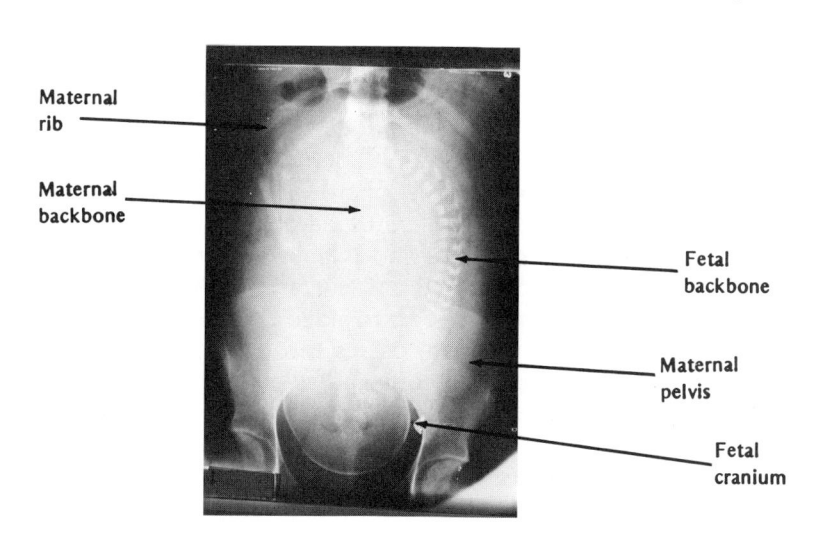

Figure 8-9: X-ray shows the pregnant female at term. Try to identify the fetal backbone and cranium, and the maternal pelvis.

EMBRYOLOGY 135

Figure 8-10: Premies require specialized supportive care in an intensive neonatal nursery.

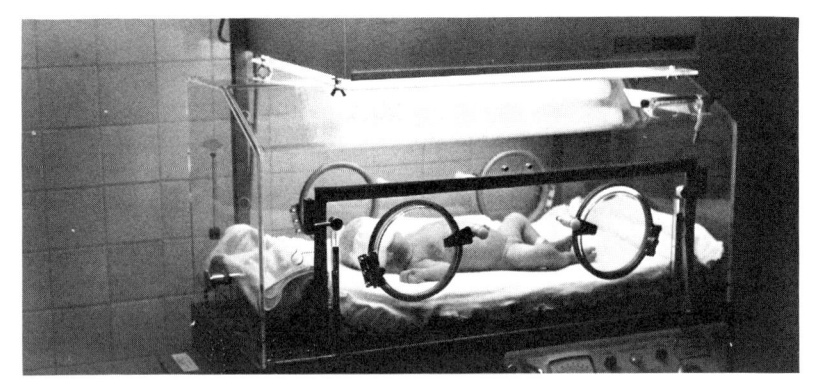

OBSTETRICS

The term **gravida** is used to denote a pregnant woman. The number of pregnancies is indicated by the word followed by a number. For example, a woman pregnant for the fourth time is a gravida IV. The woman who is pregnant for the first time and delivers her first living child is known as a gravida I, and as a **primipara** (para I). If the gravida I does not deliver a **viable** (able to live) child she is known as a **nullipara** (no living child). A person who is pregnant for the third time but has lost one baby before birth would be designated as gravida III, para I until the birth of the living child. She would then become gravida III, para II.

When the end of gestation is reached, the pregnant woman is referred to as being **parturient** (giving birth). The birth process begins when the woman goes into labor. **Labor** is the process by which the mother's body expels the fetus from the womb to the outside.

There are three stages of labor. In the first, the lower part of the womb softens and **dilates** (enlarges the opening). The baby then drops lower in the pelvic cavity and is ready to move through the **birth canal** (area bounded by the vagina and the bones of the pelvis). Frequently, at the beginning of labor, the amniotic sack ruptures (breaks open) and its fluid (water) gushes forth. In the second stage of labor, the baby actually moves through the birth canal and is delivered to the outside. Then the umbilical cord is tied and cut and the baby is ready for independent life. During the third stage of labor the placenta separates from the uterine wall, passes through the birth canal, and is also delivered with the cord and other membranes. That is why the placenta is now called the afterbirth. The placenta, cord, and membranes are together called the **secundines**.

Not all pregnancies follow such an easy, normal course. Sometimes an ovum may be fertilized and implanted outside

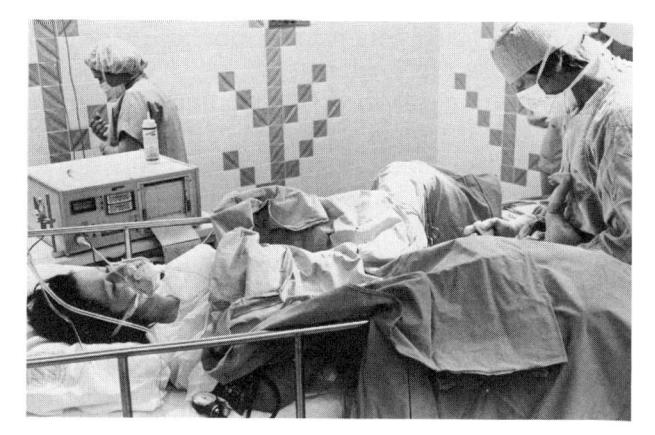

Figure 8-11:
This parturient woman has just completed the second stage of labor by delivering the baby.

the uterus. That is an **ectopic** pregnancy and cannot be carried to term. Or labor may be unusually long and the birth difficult (**dystocia**). In some cases of dystocia, the problem is that the fetal head is too large to pass through the maternal pelvis. This condition is known as **cephalo-pelvic** (head-pelvis) disproportion. If the disproportion is sufficiently great, it may be necessary to deliver the child by performing surgery called a **cesarean section** (hysterotomy).

Normally the placenta is attached high up on the uterine wall and is delivered after the birth of the baby. A placenta implanted low in the wall (**placenta previa**) is likely to separate prematurely. Premature separation of the placenta threatens the life of the infant because the infant's source of oxygen has been cut off. The condition presents danger to the mother from excess loss of blood.

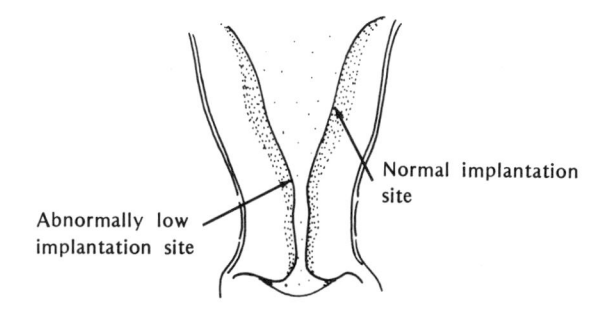

Figure 8-12:
In placenta previa the placenta is implanted abnormally low *(courtesy of Ethicon, Inc.).*

Other problems such as breech birth, or prolapsed cord may complicate the delivery process. In most cases the baby is delivered head first (**cephalic presentation**). Presentation of any other fetal part such as the buttock is called a **breech** presentation. Breech births are usually more difficult to deliver and may require a cesarean section.

The umbilical cord is composed of blood vessels and supporting tissue which act as a lifeline from the placenta to the baby. The placenta and cord are normally delivered together in the third stage of labor. Sometimes the cord **prolapses** (drops down out of place) into the birth canal during the first stage of labor. As the baby begins to move through the canal, considerable pressure is exerted against the prolapsed cord, compressing the blood vessels and shutting off the fetal supply of oxygen. Like placenta previa and breech birth, a prolapsed cord increases the risk to both mother and infant.

In the short time of the **prenatal period** (before birth) many changes are taking place. In those nine months, a single-celled zygote reproduces itself millions of times by the complex process called mitosis. In addition, some of the cells begin to change (**differentiate**) becoming more and more specialized. Some of the cells will eventually **secrete** (produce) different body fluids. Some, like white blood cells, will play the protective role of phagocytosis and others will be specialized in other ways. All the ultimate millions of cells will have developed from the single cell, the fertilized ovum.

Some cells in the body remain in their original site to form tissues and body structures. Some cells function in a somewhat independent manner, moving through the body fluids to distant sites. White blood cells are an example of this kind of cell that can move to distant sites. Most cells that are alike are bound together in the body to synchronize their activity, forming tissues.

Tissues are groups of cells performing a similar function. A tissue is made up of special cells: **intercellular** (between the cells) materials which hold the cells together and **interstitial** (intercellular) fluid.

Figure 8-13:
A tissue is groups of cells performing a special function.

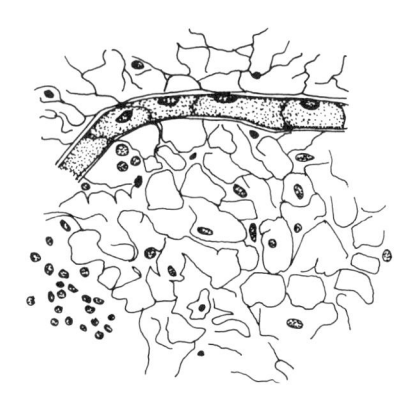

*138 *HUMAN DEVELOPMENT*

The study of tissues is called **histology**. There are four basic tissue groups: epithelial, connective, nervous and muscular.

Epithelial tissues have cells closely packed together. Their special function is secretion, excretion and protection. Epithelial tissues form the **membranes** (sheets of tissues) that line the internal body cavities and those which open to the outside. They also form a covering for the body (**skin**). Other membranes secrete **mucus** (thick sticky fluid). They are called **mucous membranes**. They line cavities which open to the outside such as the nose and mouth. Another type of membrane secretes **serous fluid** (thin watery fluid). Serous membrane lines cavities which do not open to the outside, such as the dorsal and ventral cavities.

The **diaphragm** is the dome-shaped muscle that divides the ventral cavity into a thoracic and an abdominal cavity. The serous membranes further divide these two large cavities into smaller sections or cavities. For example, the **peritoneum** divides the abdominal portion of the anterior cavity into a **peritoneal cavity** surrounded by peritoneum, a **pelvic cavity** bounded by the pelvic bones, and a **retroperitoneal space** (behind the peritoneum). The **thoracic** (chest) cavity is divided by the **pleura** (membrane around the lungs) and the **pericardium** (membrane around the heart) into four spaces; the right and left pleural space, the pericardial space, and the **mediastinum** space (behind the heart).

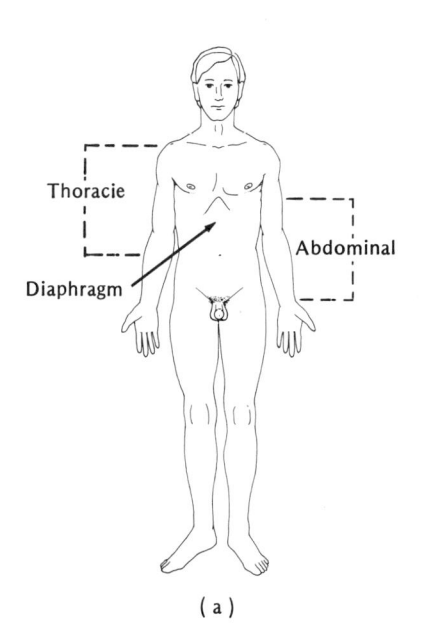

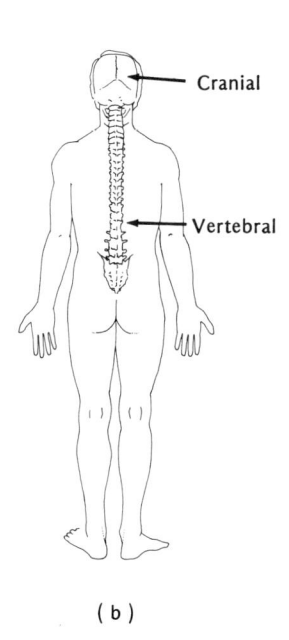

Figure 8-14: (a) Anterior view of body cavities; (b) posterior view of body cavities; (c) anterior view of membranous cavities; (d) posterior view of membranous cavities *(courtesy of Picker Corp.)*.

OBSTETRICS 139 *

(c)   (d)

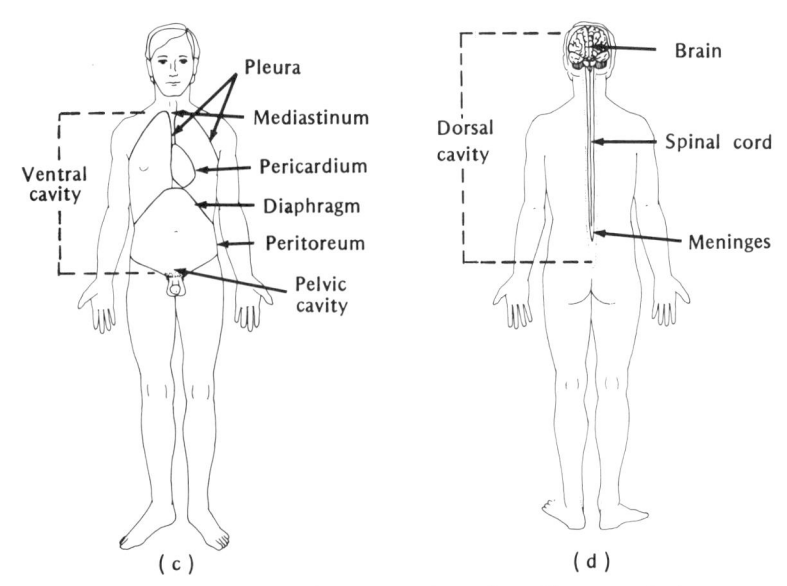

The peritoneum, pleura, and pericardium each have two layers; one that lines the cavity called the **parietal** (pertaining to wall) layer, and the other called the **visceral** (covering the organs). A small amount of serous fluid is found between the two layers. The dorsal cavity is lined by the three-layered **meninges** (serous membrane). The outer layer of meninges is the **dura mater** (tough mother). The middle layer is the **arachnoid mater** (cobweb mother). The inner layer which clings tightly to the organs is called the **pia mater** (soft mother).

There is a relatively large space between the arachnoid mater and pia mater (**subarachnoid space**) in which a special fluid circulates, called **cerebrospinal fluid**. The cerebrospinal fluid cushions the delicate brain and spinal cord much the same as the embryo is cushioned by amniotic fluid. Look at the chart and diagram to see which organs are located in which space.

Synovial epithelial membranes line the cavities of moveable joints and produce a lubricating liquid called **synovial fluid**.

The second type of tissue is called **connective tissue** (ct). As its name implies, it serves to connect other tissues. Some tissues included in this category are **elastic connective** tissues, which is stretchy, **fibrous** connective tissue which is very firm and **reticular** connective tissue which is very delicate. Blood, bone (**osseous**), and fat (**adipose**) tissues all belong to this connective tissue class.

The third type of tissue is **nervous tissue**. It is highly differentiated to be responsive to **stimuli** (excitement) and to conduct

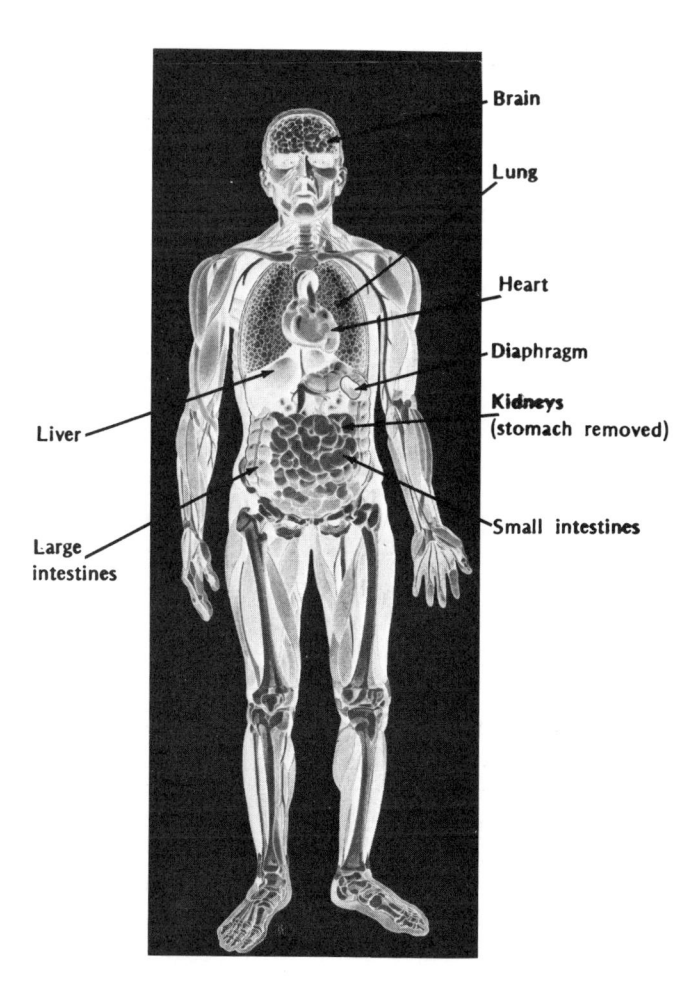

Figure 8-15: Organs of the body *(courtesy of Picker Corp.)*.

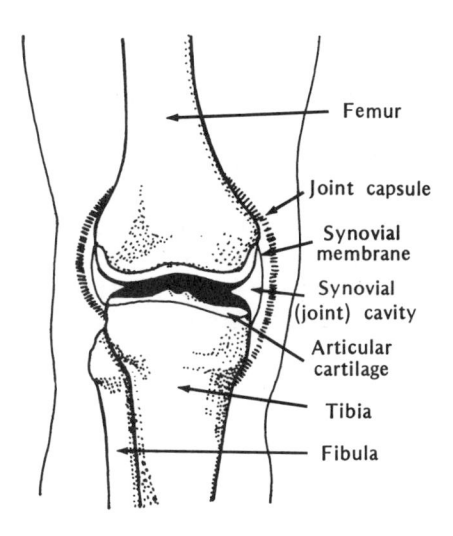

Figure 8-16: The knee joint (articulation): the construction of a movable joint prevents bone ends from scraping against each other. Anterior view, kneecap removed: 1) femur; 2) joint capsule; 3) synovial membrane; 4) synovial (joint) cavity; 5) articular cartilage; 6) tibia; 7) fibula *(courtesy of Ethicon, Inc.)*.

the **nerve impulse** (an electrical wave). This tissue forms the brain and spinal cord and nerves of the body.

The fourth type of tissue is muscular tissue. There are three kinds: the **cardiac** which forms the walls of the heart; the **smooth** or **involuntary** (or **visceral**) which forms the skeletal muscles and the walls of organs; and the **voluntary** or **striated** which forms the bulk of the body and serves in movement.

Figure 8-17: Microscopic appearance of striated (skeletal) muscle *(courtesy of Ethicon, Inc.)*

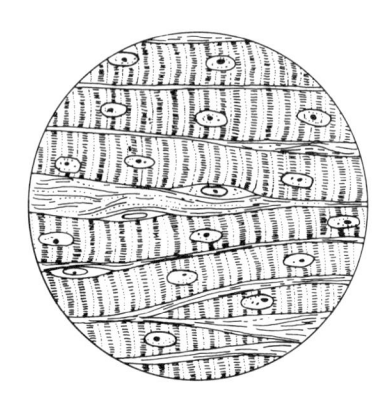

In the embryo, these tissues differentiate and combine to form organs (**viscera**). **Organs** (tissues grouped together for a specific function) are located throughout the body. They are composed of several tissue types. Each organ is specialized for a particular role in the body. For example, the heart keeps blood moving and the kidney secretes **urine** (a liquid waste).

Certain bodily organs function in an interrelated way to carry out some major physiologic process, such as producing urine and then **excreting** (eliminating) it from the body. A series or organs related in this way forms a **system**.

There are nine basic systems. All are **vital** (life necessary) to a healthy person. One of the systems is the urinary system. It produces and excretes urinary fluid and includes several organs: the kidneys, the ureters, the bladder and the urethra. The kidneys do not secrete urine, however, without the aid of the blood vessels which bring waste products in the blood to them. Each system contributes to the effective functioning of the entire body. Since the body systems are so interdependent, any pathology in one puts stress on all others.

SUMMARY

The human organism is a highly complex, beautifully organized structure composed of tissues, organs and systems which originally all evolved from a single fertilized cell. Housed in the female uterus until birth, the fertilized cell gradually develops into a baby capable of independent life upon delivery. Many medical and scientific terms learned in this chapter pertain to the organization of the human body, its development after conception, and the birth process.

PRACTICE & REVIEW

...n and define the new special terms you have been using. Remember, ...arned how to pronounce them at the beginning of this chapter.

...eles _____

...tercellular _____

...aphragm _____

...fferentiate _____

...terstitial _____

...troperitoneal _____

...terozygous _____

...eninges _____

...sarean section _____

...achnoid mater _____

...double-check the meaning of the terms above by studying the brief ...ions given in the Glossary-Index at the back of this text.

...ourself quickly before going on to learn other medical and professional terms. Use these ...eview exercises to practice for your new work in health services. Your teacher will also help ...ommending various other Study Activities.

OBSTETRICS 143 *

A. In the diagrams reproduced on this page, label the structures listed below:

1. diaphragm
2. cranial cavity
3. vertebral cavity
4. thoracic cavity
5. abdominal cavity
6. lungs
7. heart
8. brain
9. liver
10. small intestines

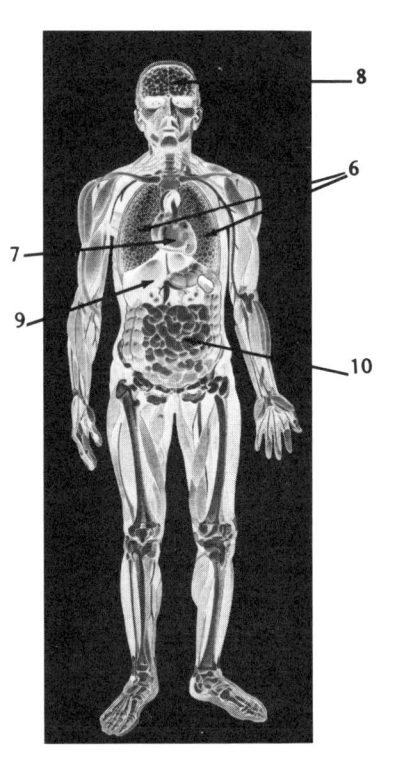

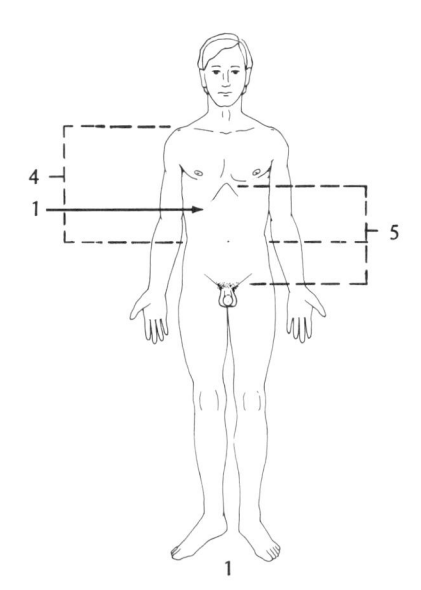

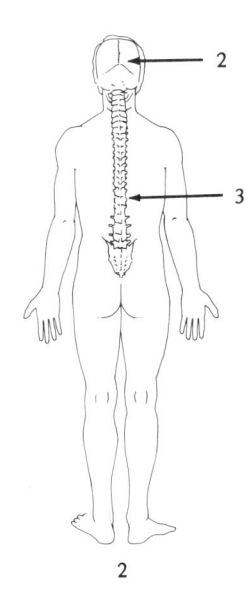

*144 *HUMAN DEVELOPMENT*

B. In the following sentences underline the words that are new in this chapter:

1. <u>Adipose tissue</u> is another name for fat.
2. The delivery of the baby is through the <u>birth canal</u>.
3. In <u>heterozygous</u> individuals, one <u>allele</u> is <u>dominant</u>, giving rise to an individual whose <u>phenotype</u> and <u>genotype</u> are different.
4. <u>Placenta previa</u>, <u>prolapsed cord</u>, and <u>cephalo-pelvic disproportion</u> are all conditions that might require <u>cesarean section</u>.
5. The <u>mitochondrion</u>, the <u>golgi apparatus</u>, and the <u>ribosomes</u> are cellular <u>organelles</u>.
6. <u>Ligaments</u> and <u>tendons</u> are composed of fibrous connective tissue.
7. The <u>umbilical cord</u> connects the <u>fetus</u> to the <u>placenta</u> which is attached to the wall of the uterus.
8. The male <u>sperm</u> and female <u>ovum</u> are the <u>gametes</u>.
9. Nervous tissue responds to <u>stimuli</u> and conducts a <u>nerve impulse</u>.
10. <u>Mucous membranes</u> secrete <u>mucus</u>.

C. Match the word on the right with the best statement on the left:

___ 1. A liquid waste	a. cytoplasm
___ 2. The study of tissues	b. urine
___ 3. The oviducts	c. peritoneum
___ 4. Another name for the womb	d. pleura
___ 5. A double-walled membrane covering the lungs	e. histology
___	f. system
___ 6. A group of organs carrying out a specific function	g. cytology
___	h. uterus
___ 7. Pertaining to the organs	i. viable
___ 8. Able to live	j. visceral
___ 9. Pertaining to bone	k. Fallopian tubes
___ 10. Study of the cell	l. osseous

After studying Chapter 9

The Integumentary System

You should be able to:

* Pronounce and define each of its new medical words and phrases and use the new technical jargon.

* Identify the structures in the integumentary system.

* Name three abnormal conditions of the integumentary system.

MEDICAL WORDS

PRONOUNCE THESE TEN NEW WORDS WITH YOUR TEACHER:

alopecia (al″o-pe′she-ah)
conjunctivitis (kon-junk″ti-vi′tis)
contractures (kon-trak′tūrs)
excoriation (eks-kor-e-ā-shun)
erythema (er″ĭ-thema)

pyretogenous (pi″rĕ-toj′ĕ-nus)
sudoriferous (soo″do-rif′er-us)
ecchymosis (ek″ĭ-mo′sis)
malaise (mal-āz′)
laceration (las″ĕ-ra′shun)

The **integumentary system** is composed of the skin and its **appendages** (accessories). Appendages include the nails, glands, hair, and breasts.

The role this system plays in the body is a vital one. It protects the body by forming mechanical barriers to disease. Some of the glandular secretions are bacteriostatic, and this is also protective since it keeps bacterial populations low. The integumentary system also plays a role in the synthesis of vitamin D, aids in maintaining a constant temperature, and helps monitor the external environment.

The skin is sometimes referred to as an organ because it contains several types of tissues. Some of the appendages, such as glands, are deeply embedded in the total structure and hence are considered a part of the whole **integument** (skin).

The skin covers the entire body and its study is called **dermatology**. The appearance of the skin reveals a great deal about the general health of the individual, and the skin is an excellent indicator of many pathologic conditions.

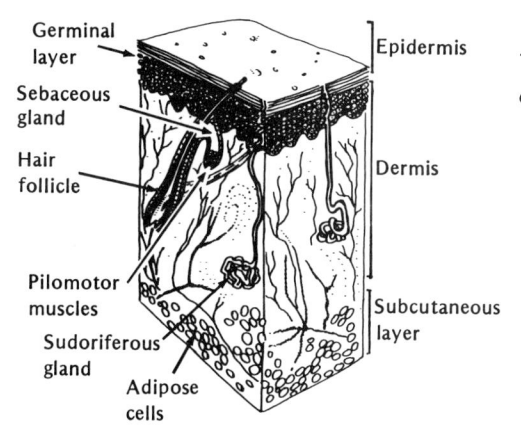

Figure 9-1: The skin *(courtesy of Ethicon, Inc.)*.

STRUCTURE OF THE SKIN

There are two functionally separate but anatomically fixed layers to the skin; the epidermis and dermis.

The **epidermis** is the outer layer of skin and is constantly being **shed** (lost). This part of the skin is many layers of cells thick. The bottom-most layer of epidermis is called the **germinal layer** (reproductive layer). As new cells are produced in this layer, they are pushed upward to the surface and flattened and eventually shed. The tissue forming the epidermis is **squamous** (scale-like) epithelium. The epidermis contains no blood vessels and therefore cells in this part of the skin receive less nourishment. **Melanin** granules (pigment) are found in this skin layer as well as in the hair and eyes. Melanin gives color to the skin. The more melanin, the darker the pigmentation.

Nails

Nails are horny skin appendages found on the distal, dorsal surfaces of fingers and toes. As part of the epidermis, they help protect the sensitive fingertips and toes.

The Dermis

The **dermis** (**corium** or true skin) lies beneath the epidermis and is solidly attached to it. The dermis is well supplied with nerves and blood vessels. It is here that appendages such as glands, hair follicles, and sense organs are located. These structures are all held in place by an extensive network of connective tissue.

Glands are specialized organs which secrete specific substances. Three types of glands are located in the dermis. The **sebaceous glands** secrete **sebum** (an oily substance) and open into the hair shaft. The sebum keeps the hair lubricated and less brittle. The sebum normally reaches the skin in small amounts, lubricating the outer layer of epidermis.

Sudoriferous glands are also found in the dermis but they have **ducts** (tubes) which lead directly to the surface of the skin.

Because they pour their secretions through ducts, they are called ducted or **exocrine** (secreting externally) **glands**. Other glands in the body which do not open to the outside but, instead, pour their secretions into the bloodstream are called **ductless** or **endocrine** (internally secreting) **glands**.

Sudoriferous glands secrete **sweat** (perspiration). Sweat is a salty fluid and is poured onto the surface of the skin. There it evaporates into the atmosphere, thus serving to cool the body. Sweat also contains some antibacterial substances which help to control the skin flora. There are approximately two million sudoriferous glands in the skin of the body. They provide a very effective mechanism for maintaining the **homeostasis** (constancy) of body temperature. Cystic fibrosis is an inherited disease characterized by excessively thick mucus and abnormal secretions of saliva and sweat. Analysis of perspiration can help to establish a diagnosis of cystic fibrosis.

Figure 9-2: Cystic Fibrosis Analyzer *(courtesy of Sherwood Medical Industries)*.

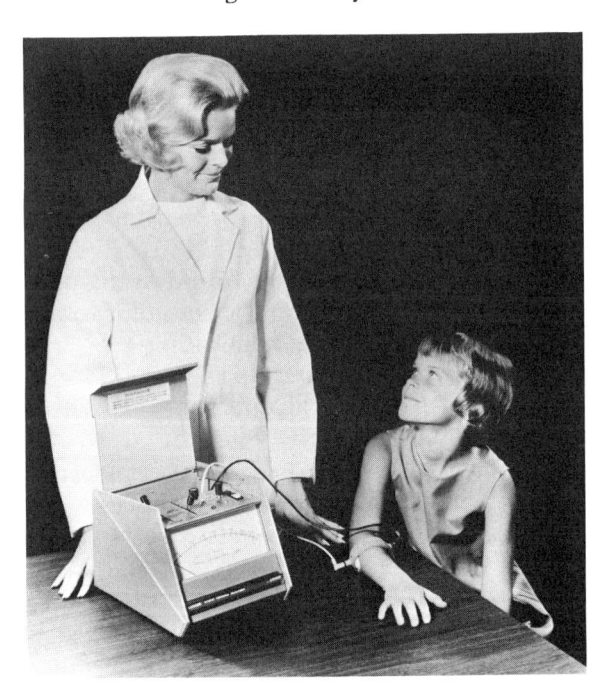

Ceruminous glands are located in the skin which lines the external ear canal (external **auditory meatus**). They secrete a waxy substance, **cerumen**. This secretion traps materials before they get deep into the ear and cause problems. Occasionally cerumen becomes hardened, interferes with hearing, and must be removed.

* 148   *THE INTEGUMENTARY SYSTEM*

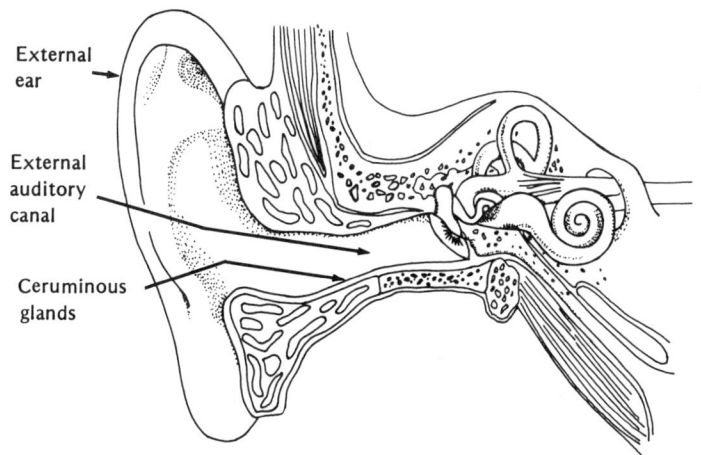

Figure 9-3: Location of ceruminous glands *(courtesy of Picker Corp.)*.

External ear
External auditory canal
Ceruminous glands

Hairs

Hairs are slender thread-like structures which develop from hair follicles in the dermis and project out through the epidermis. The cells of the hair are modified epidermis. Hair is distributed all over the body except for the soles of the feet and palms of the hands. Men tend to have a heavier distribution of hair than women and therefore are more **pilose** (hairy). Men also tend to lose their hair (**alopecia**) earlier than women. In lower animals, hairs serve a protective function by providing protective warmth. Various kinds of clothing do some of this for humans.

Small **pilomotor** (hair movement) muscles are attached to the hairs. When the pilomotor muscles **contract** (shorten) the hairs assume a straighter posture and there is a small elevation of the skin, called a "goose bump."

The Sense Organs

The sense organs are specialized nerve endings which respond to **sensations** (impressions) of touch, heat, cold, pain and pressure. Messages are carried by the nerves to the brain area (**sensorium**) which perceives sensations and keeps us aware of changes in the external environment.

The Subcutaneous Tissue

The subcutaneous tissue, though not actually part of the skin, is a layer of fatty connective tissue which firmly anchors the skin to the underlying muscle and **fascia** (fibrous connective or binding tissue). The fascia hold internal structures together. The subcutaneous tissue is highly vascular and serves as an insulating area to prevent undue heat loss over the entire body.

Body Temperature

The skin is of great importance in maintaining a constant and favorable body temperature. The body may be likened to a giant chemical factory whose chemical enzymes only function under strict temperature conditions or limits. These enzymes

STRUCTURE OF THE SKIN 149 *

Figure 9-4: Compare the Farenheit and Centigrade temperature readings on the thermometer.

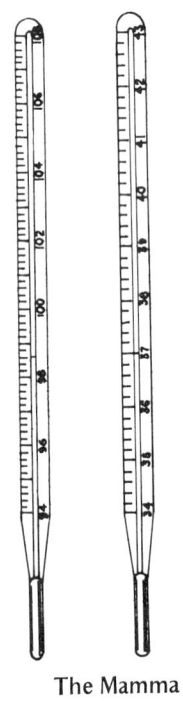

The Mamma

can only operate within relatively narrow limits: if the temperature is raised too high (**hyperthermia**) or drops too low (**hypothermia**), the body cannot survive.

Temperature (heat level) is measured mechanically with an instrument or tube called a thermometer. Two scales of temperature measurement are used in medicine. The **calibrations** (gradations) are usually marked on the tube in the **Fahrenheit scale (F)**, but they may also be in the **Celsius (C)** scale. Celsius readings are those figured with the centigrade system developed by Anders Celsius, a Swedish astronomer. Although there is a formula for converting temperature readings from one scale to the other, most health facilities utilize either the Celsius or the Fahrenheit system for all their measurements. Gabriel Fahrenheit was a famous German physicist.

Important equivalents on these two scales are:

Fahrenheit (F°)	Celsius (C°)	Effect
32°	0°	Water freezes
98.6°	37°	Average body temperature
212°	100°	Water boils

An elevation in body temperature is called fever or **pyrexia**. Many patients become **pyretic** (feverish) when invaded by **pyretogenous** microbes (fever producing) such as the **pneumococcus** or **meningococcus**.

The **mamma** or breasts are present on the anterior chest wall of both men and women. But normally full **mammoplasia** (breast development) of the mammary glands occurs only in women; the term "breast" is used primarily about females.

The **mammary glands** are modified sweat glands that secrete milk for the newborn. The process of secreting milk is known as **lactation**. Lactation begins about 3 days postpartum. The size and activity of the breasts are under the control of **hormones** (secretions of endocrine glands). A pigmented area, the **areolar**, is found at the end of each breast. At the center of the areolar is the **nipple**, through which the milk flows. The **lactiferous** (milk conveying) ducts of the breast empty into the nipples.

Neoplastic changes in the breast tissues are very common. Both benign and malignant neoplasms can develop. Only a tissue biopsy can afford a definitive diagnosis. Surgical procedures to remove the **morbid** (diseased) tissue include a **simple mastectomy** (removal of the breast tissue only) and a **radical mastec-**

*150 *THE INTEGUMENTARY SYSTEM*

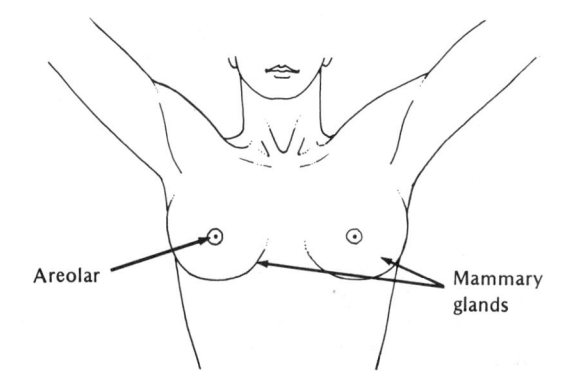

Figure 9-5: The mamma *(courtesy of Picker Corp.)*.

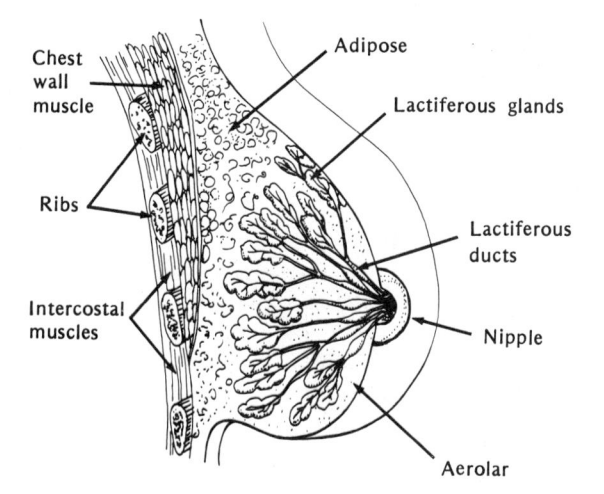

Figure 9-6: The process of secreting milk is called lactation.

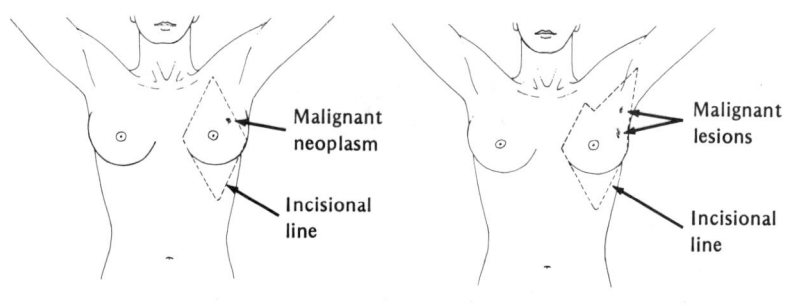

Figure 9-7: (left) Simple mastectomy *(courtesy of Picker Corp.)*.

Figure 9-8: (right) Radical mastectomy *(courtesy of Picker Corp.)*.

tomy. In a radical mastectomy the entire breast, the underlying muscle, and **axillary** (pertaining to the armpit) lymph nodes are removed.

Most breast tumors can be found early by women who regularly examine their own breasts. Early discovery, before there is an opportunity for metastasis, greatly improves the

STRUCTURE OF THE SKIN 151 *

prognosis for complete recovery. Suspicious **masses** (lumps or irregularities) can be further investigated by **mammography**. Mammography is an X-ray photographic technique used to visualize breast abnormalities. **Thermography** (heat record), is a technique that identifies actively growing tissues by recording the heat they produce.

Figure 9-9: Mammography is a special X-ray technique used to examine the breasts *(courtesy of General Electric Co.).*

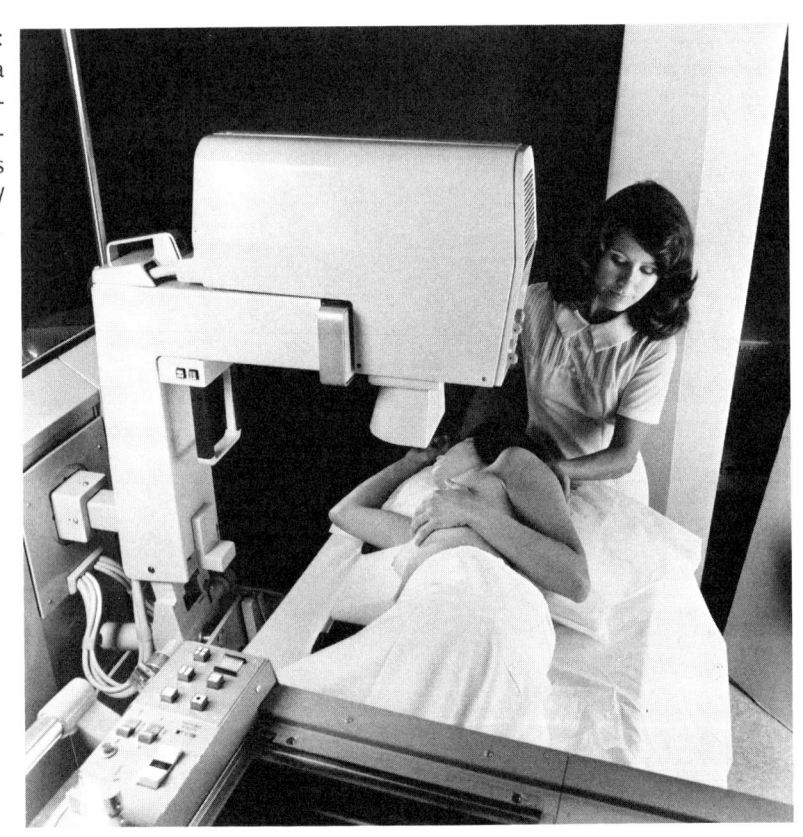

Skin Lesions

The skin reveals information not only about its specific condition, but about the general health of the body as a whole. Trauma to the skin results in visible lesions. General systemic conditions such as pyrexia, **dehydration** (water loss), **hypoxia**, communicable disease, and allergies are also demonstrated in skin changes. In addition, specific dermatological conditions are diagnosed by the altered character of the skin.

Trauma damages the tissues of the skin. Look at Table 9-1 to see some of the descriptive terms of **cutaneous** (skin) lesions.

Table 9-1

Kind of Lesion	Description of Skin
laceration	cut or break in the skin
excoriation	scratches
abrasion	rubbed or scraped area
contusion	bruise
ecchymosis	flattened black and blue due to bleeding into the tissues
keloid	tumor-like growth of scar tissue
ulcer	open sore or crater
decubitus	ulceration due to pressure
fissure	narrow slit or cleft
crust	scab

Many communicable diseases give rise to characteristic skin eruptions (lesions) called **exanthema** (rashes). The exanthema are usually associated with other **constitutional** (systemic or general body) symptoms. Constitutional symptoms which accompany childhood communicable diseases include pyrexia, cough, **coryza** (nasal discharge), headache, general **malaise** (general feeling of ill health) and **conjunctivitis** (inflammation of the conjunctiva). Look at the next table to learn some of the descriptive terms used with rashes.

Table 9-2

Kind of Rash	Description of Skin
erythema	redness of the skin
macule	a discolored, non-elevated spot
papule	small, rounded, solid elevation
vesicle	a blister
pustule	a small elevation filled with pus

Skin-Color Variations

The color of the skin indicates much about the general health of an individual. Someone described as robust, with a

STRUCTURE OF THE SKIN 153

ruddy complexion, immediately conjures up the vision of a healthy individual. On the other hand, a person described as wan and pale gives the opposite impression. Look at the following descriptive terms in Table 9-3 and try to visualize the appearance of each patient.

Table 9-3

Skin Condition	Discoloration or Change	Possible Problem
cyanosis	bluish/dusty	lack of oxygen
jaundice	yellow	liver disease
pallor	absence of color	hemorrhage
rubor	red	inflammation
flushed	red	pyrexia
bronzing	yellowish, brownish	disorder associated with Addison's disease

Allergies

Allergies or hypersensitivities are frequently associated with **pruritis** (itching) and various skin eruptions. Erythemas, **maculopapular** rashes, vesticular eruptions, and crusting are all very common.

Allergies are unusual reactions to certain substances known as **allergens**. Allergens are usually harmless but they can cause certain hypersensitive people to form a special kind of antibody in the tissues. When the allergen enters the body the first time (**sensitizing contact**), the body reacts by developing the special antibodies. The person is unaware that the antibody-forming activity is taking place. Subsequent contact with the allergens brings on a reaction between the allergen and antibody which results in the release of certain chemicals, such as **histamine**, in the body. The allergic reactions are in response to such liberated chemicals.

Allergic reactions frequently affect the respirations, digestions, and skin of the allergic individual. Sometimes the response is so severe it is life threatening such as in **anaphylactic shock**, an extreme hypersensitivity reaction. There are some terms related to allergies in Table 9-4.

Table 9-4

Allergic Reactions	Skin Description
dermatitis	inflamed skin
urticaria	slightly elevated, reddened patches called hives
wheals	local areas of edema and itching
wheeze	whistling, respiratory sound
eczema	skin rash that itches, blisters, oozes, and scales
scales	thin flakes of epithelial cells

Some of the more common allergies include **dermatitides** (collective skin inflammations) of various kinds, eczemas, **hay fever** (allergic response with sneezing, itching eyes, runny nose), and **asthma** (condition with difficult breathing).

Burns

Remember that the protective layers of skin cover the entire body. So it is the skin which receives the initial and most severe damage if the human body is subjected to excessive fire or other external heat. The severity of a burn is classified according to the amount of tissue damage, as either first, second, or third degree.

Table 9-5

Severity of Burn	Signs and Symptoms	Tissue Involved
first degree	erythema	epidermis damaged
second degree	vessicle formation	epidermis destroyed, dermis damaged
third degree	damage to deeper layers, destruction of superficial layers	epidermis, dermis destroyed, subcutaneous and below damaged or destroyed

In a **first degree burn**, the most minimal in tissue damage, the epidermal tissue is traumatized but not destroyed. The area heals rather readily and there is no permanent damage. In **second degree burns**, the epidermis is destroyed and vessicles form, separating the epidermal cells from the dermis. Again

STRUCTURE OF THE SKIN 155 *

Figure 9-10:
(a) First degree burn traumatizes the epidermis;
(b) second degree burn with an accumulation of fluid separating epidermis and dermis, forming a blister;
(c) third degree burns destroy epidermis, dermis, and underlying structures.

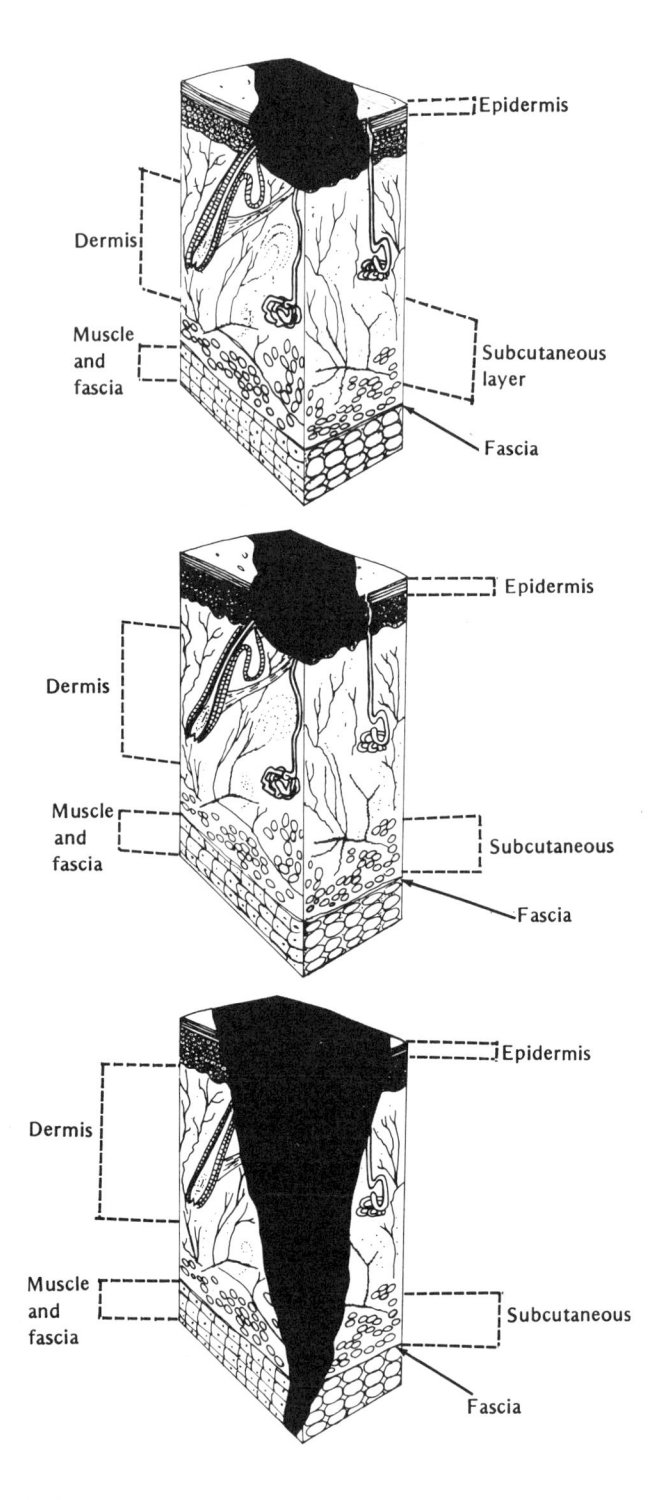

*156 *THE INTEGUMENTARY SYSTEM*

healing is relatively uneventful with no **residual** (lasting) effect. In third degree burns, both the epidermis and dermis are destroyed and underlying tissues are traumatized and may have irreversible damage as well. This is the most serious form of burn that can occur. It also may result in disfigurement and **deformity** (distortion).

When large tissue areas are destroyed, the tissues may be unable to repair the original tissues with tissues of the same type. Usually, however, the area is replaced during healing with a strong fibrous, connective tissue called **scar**. The scar fills in the area and maintains the integrity of the body, but it cannot carry out the functions of the original tissue that formed the area. Scars tend to contract and become smaller as they develop, forming contractures and bringing the edges of the area closer together. **Contractures** (abnormal shortenings) result in distortion of normal body contours. When they are between moveable parts, there is a loss of mobility.

Scars may enlarge and become sharply raised above the level of the normal skin surface. These are **keloids** (tumor-like fibrous growths). People vary in their tendency to form keloid tissues. Some form them more readily than others.

The mortality rate for extensive third degree burns is relatively high due to loss of fluids and **electrolytes** (salts) from the body, and due to infections, since the protective defensive skin covering is lost. Pain from burns is intense and many larger hospitals have **intensive burn units** (IBU) to provide the specialized care these patients need.

CASE STUDY

Fourteen-year old Robert Leslie received a chemistry set for his birthday. His father cautioned him about its use and suggested that Robert wait to use it until the weekend when his father would be home. Robert agreed that was the best plan and put the set into the closet.

The next morning, Robert's friend, Wayne, came over. Before long the two boys were in the garage with the chemistry set. An explosion followed and both boys were burned. Wayne received first and second degree burns on his chest and arms. Robert was less fortunate. He was severely burned about the head and left arm with second and third degree burns.

He required intensive care in the IBU of the medical center for several months. In the period immediately following the injury and for some time after, Robert's condition was critical, due to fluid and electrolyte imbalance and the ever-pending threat of infection.

He has now returned home but faces long years of treatment and reconstructive surgery as attempts are made to restore the use of his left hand.

Figure 9-11: Third degree burns may require extensive restorative therapy *(courtesy of Upjohn, Homemakers Home and Health Case Services, Inc.).*

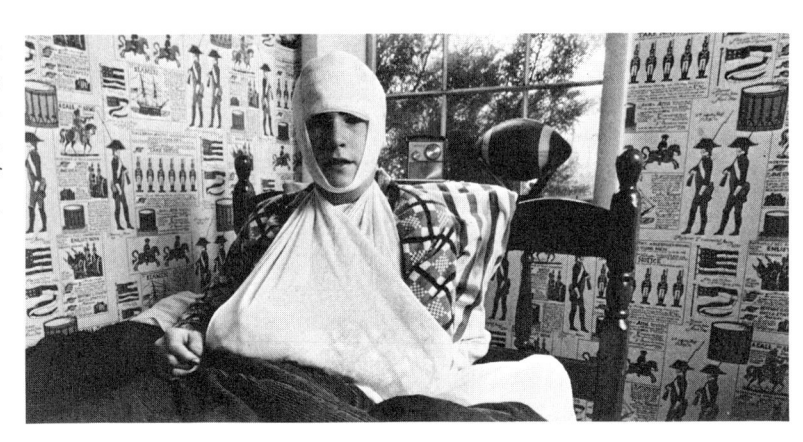

SUMMARY

The integumentary system, composed of the skin and its appendages, is subject to its own pathology. It also reflects the state of health of the body as a whole.

PRACTICE & REVIEW

Explain and define the new special terms you have been using. Remember, you learned how to pronounce them at the beginning of this chapter.

1. alopecia _____

2. conjunctivitis _____

3. contractures _____

4. excoriation _____

5. erythema _____

6. pyretogenous _____

7. sudoriferous _____

8. ecchymosis _____

9. malaise _____

10. laceration _____

Now, double-check the meaning of the terms on page 158 by studying the brief definitions given in the Glossary-Index at the back of this text.

Test yourself quickly before going on to learn other medical and professional terms. Use these short review exercises to practice for your new work in health services. Your teacher will also help by recommending various other Study Activities.

A. Match the words on the right with the best statement on the left.

    ____ 1. Another word for perspiration   a. alopecia
    ____ 2. Pressure sore   b. axillary
    ____ 3. General feeling of ill health   c. fascia
    ____ 4. Fibrous connective tissue which binds other tissues in the body   d. sweat
                                         e. urticaria
    ____ 5. Hairy   f. ecchymosis
    ____ 6. Narrow slit or cleft   g. allergies
    ____ 7. Nasal discharge   h. caryza
    ____ 8. Sensitivities to allergens   i. decubities
    ____ 9. Flattened black and blue area due to bleeding in the tissues   j. fissure
                                         k. pilose
    ____ 10. Characterized by hives   l. malaise

B. Label the diagram reproduced on this page with the terms below:

1. dermis
2. epidermis
3. sebaceous
4. subcutaneous fat
5. sudoriferous gland
6. hair follicle
7. nerve ending
8. pilomotor muscle

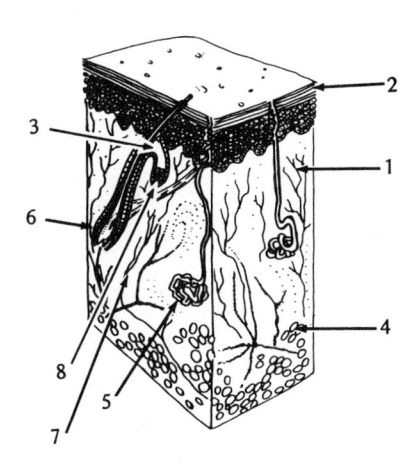

STRUCTURE OF THE SKIN

After studying Chapter 10
The Respiratory System
You should be able to:

* *Pronounce and define each of its new medical words and phrases and use the new technical jargon.*

* *Identify the anatomical structures of the respiratory system.*

* *Name five abnormal conditions of the respiratory system.*

MEDICAL WORDS   PRONOUNCE THESE TEN NEW WORDS WITH YOUR TEACHER:

atelectasis (at″e-lak′tah-sĭs)
choana (ko-a′nah)
copious (ko′pĭ-us)
dysphonia (dĭs-fo′ne-ah)
emphysema (em″fĭ-se′mah)
hyperpnea (hi″perp-ne′ah)
intralaryngeal (in″tr-lar-ing′eal)
parenchyma (pah-reng′kĭ-mah)
pneumorrhagia (nu″mora′je-ah)
spirometer (spi-rom″ĕ-ter)

Each living cell must be provided with a constant supply of **oxygen** (O_2) (an odorless, colorless gas) as well as a method to rid itself of its byproduct, **carbon dioxide** (CO_2) (gaseous waste). Oxygen is used by the cell to provide energy, and carbon dioxide is the useless residue produced during this metabolic process.

$$\text{nutrients} + O_2 = \text{energy} + \text{water} + CO_2$$

CELLULAR RESPIRATION   The activity shown in the equation above describes a chemical reaction and is known as **cellular respiration**. **Hypoxia** (oxygen deficiency in the tissues) is a very serious condition and **anoxia** (no oxygen) is severe hypoxia and incompatible with life.

The respiratory system brings into the body the oxygen needed for cellular energy-making and removes carbon dioxide from the body. This body system which conducts **respiration** is located at the superior end of the body while some of the cells requiring its service are at far distant points, like those in the fingers and toes. The system of blood vessels and the blood convey the O_2 to the cells and the CO_2 away. Two gaseous exchange points are necessary: one point is between the **alveolus** (terminal part of the respiratory system) and the blood vessels, and another point between the blood vessels and the cells.

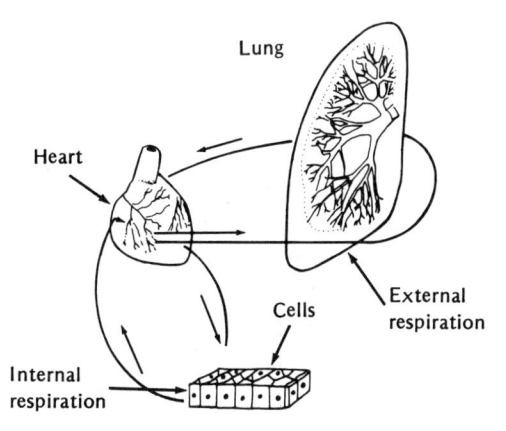

Figure 10-1: Points of gaseous exchange.

External respiration is the exchange of gases between the alveoli and the blood. **Internal respiration** is the exchange of gases between the blood and tissue cells. The air in the alveolus is separated from the blood in the vessels by a thin partition known as the **blood gas barrier**.

The oxygen moves into the bloodstream and the carbon dioxide moves from the bloodstream into the alveolus by the process of diffusion. **Diffusion** is the movement across a membrane resulting from a greater concentration of gas on one side than the other. When a person inspires, the concentration of O_2 moving in the alveolus is greater than in the concentration of oxygen in the blood, so the O_2 moves across the membrane into the bloodstream. At the same time the CO_2 levels in the blood are higher than in the CO_2 levels in the alveolus, so CO_2 diffuses across the membrane to the alveolus.

Gas Transport in the Blood

Only a small amount of the major blood gases, oxygen and carbon dioxide, are carried dissolved in the liquid portion of the blood. Most of the oxygen transported in the red blood cells is combined with the protein, **hemoglobin**. Combined with hemoglobin, the oxygen is transported as **oxyhemoglobin**. The carbon dioxide is carried in three chemical **compounds** (combinations).

THE RESPIRATORY TRACT

The respiratory tract extends from the nose to the alveolus and is lined with ciliated mucous membrane. It is divided into

THE RESPIRATORY TRACT 161 *

Figure 10-2: The respiratory system and related structures *(courtesy of Picker Corp.)*.

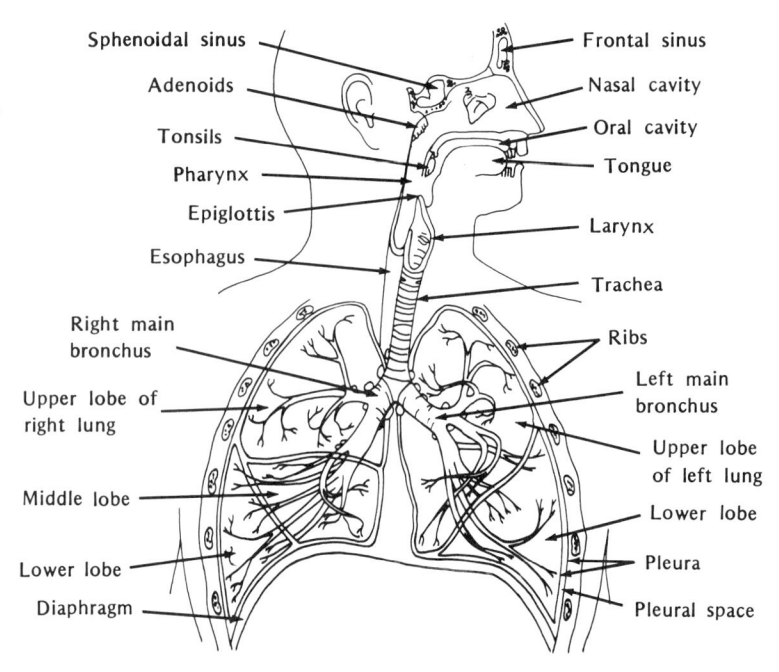

the upper respiratory system (**URS**) and lower respiratory system (**LRS**). The upper respiratory system begins in the head and extends into the mediastinum. It includes the nose, pharynx, larynx, trachea, bronchi and bronchioles. The lower respiratory tract is composed of the lungs and their double coverings, the pleura. The lung substance is made up of millions of tiny alveolar air sacs and the alveolar ducts which connect the alveolus and the **terminal** (final) bronchioles. The lungs have a spongy consistency. They are found in the pleural cavities within the thorax.

The Nose

The external nose projects from the face. The internal **rhinal** (pertaining to the nose) cavity is divided into two **nasal** (pertaining to nose) cavities divided by a **septum** (partition) made up of **cartilage** (firm, flexible connective tissue). The **palate** separates the nasal cavities from the oral cavity. Two openings, the external **nares**, lead from the outside into the nasal cavity. Tiny hairs, the **vibrissae**, guard these external nares from foreign particles. Two openings, the posterior nares or **choanae** (choana, singular) lead from the posterior nasal cavity to the upper portion of the nasopharynx or upper throat. Tears from the eyes drain into the nasal chambers through the **naso lacrimal ducts** (nose tears). The mucous membrane which begins here and lines the tract is a special membrane. Its tiny mucus

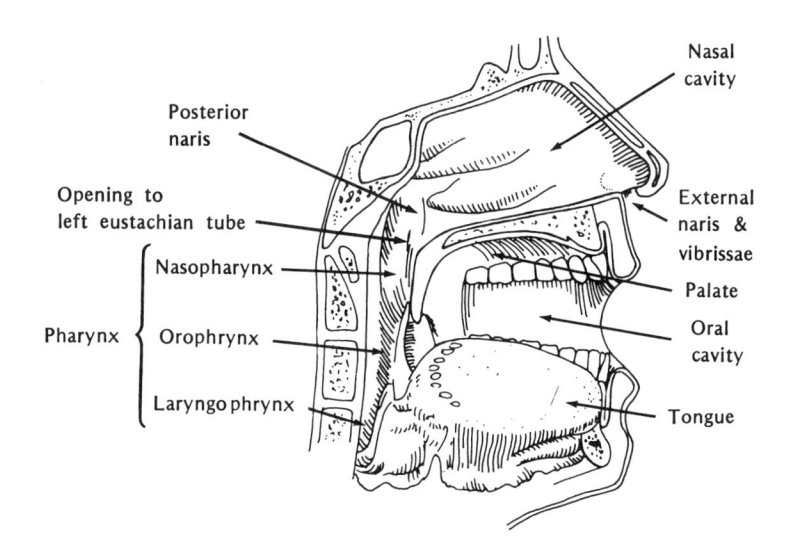

Figure 10-3: Structures of the nose and pharynx *(courtesy of Picker Corp.)*.

producing cells are column shaped (**columnar**) with microscopic cilia. The sticky mucus traps the foreign particles and the constantly beating cilia move it to the outside. The lining of the nose is highly **vascular** (has many blood vessels). So the incoming air is moistened and filtered by the mucous membrane and warmed by the heat of the blood before reaching the lower tract. Tiny **olfactory** (sense of smell) nerve endings are located in the nose. The sense of smell is lost (**anosmia**) when the membranes become swollen (**edematous**) as in an upper respiratory infection (URI). Nose bleeds (**epistaxis**) are associated with some pathologies of the respiratory tract as well as other systemic abnormalities.

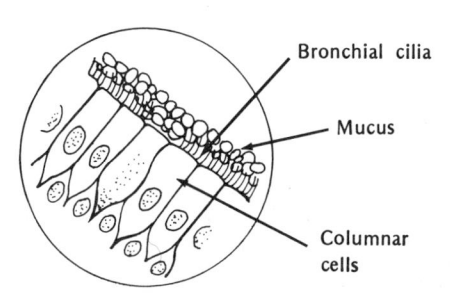

Figure 10-4: Columnar cells of respiratory epithelium *(courtesy of the American Lung Association)*.

The Paranasal Sinuses

Four pairs of paranasal (beside the nose) **sinuses** (cavities) are found in the bones of the skull: the **maxillary** sinus in the maxillae or cheek bones; the **frontal** sinus in the forehead or frontal bone; the **ethmoidal** sinuses in the ethmoid bone; and the **sphenoidal** sinuses. These sphenoidal sinuses are located in

Figure 10-5: The paranasal sinuses *(courtesy of Picker Corp.).*

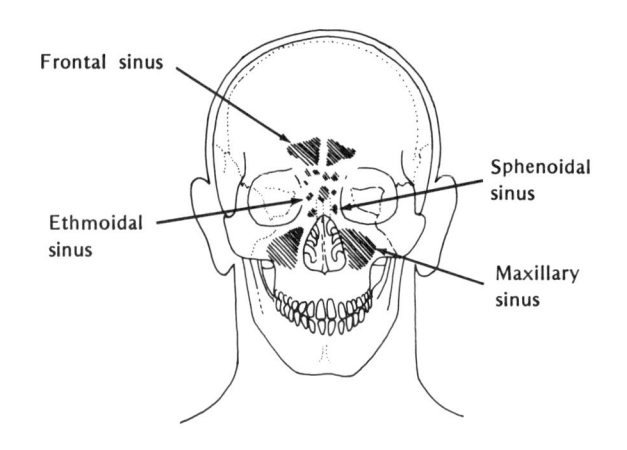

the sphenoid bone which forms the inferior and lateral sides of the internal skull.

The sinuses are also lined with mucous membrane. They make the head light and act as a **resonance** (sound intensifying quality) chamber for the voice.

The Pharynx

The nasal cavity and the **oral** (mouth) cavity both open into the throat or pharynx. The **pharynx** (throat) is a short tube dividing into the **nasopharynx** which communicates with the nasal cavity, the **oropharynx** which communicates with the mouth, and the **laryngopharynx** which leads into the larynx and esophagus. The **eustachian** tubes are openings in the nasopharynx which lead into the middle ear. The **adenoids** (pharyngeal tonsils), masses of lymphoid tissue, are found in this area.

A second pair of lymphoid masses, the **palatine tonsils**, are found on either side of the posterior oral cavity as it opens into the oropharynx. These tissues are part of the normal body defense system and serve to filter out harmful organisms. At times they themselves become the center (**focus**) of infection when invading microorganisms overwhelm them. Then they may have to be surgically removed. The adenoids and tonsils are sometimes removed in the surgical procedures, **tonsillectomy** and **adenoidectomy** (T & A). A small tab of mucous membrane-covered muscle hangs between the oral cavity and the oropharynx, called the **uvula**. The pharynx serves as a dual passageway for nutrients and gases. Through it nutrients pass into the esophagus which leads to the stomach, while gaseous air enters the larynx and flows into the trachea.

The Larynx

The **larynx** (voice box) is the next section of the upper respiratory tract. It communicates above with the pharynx while

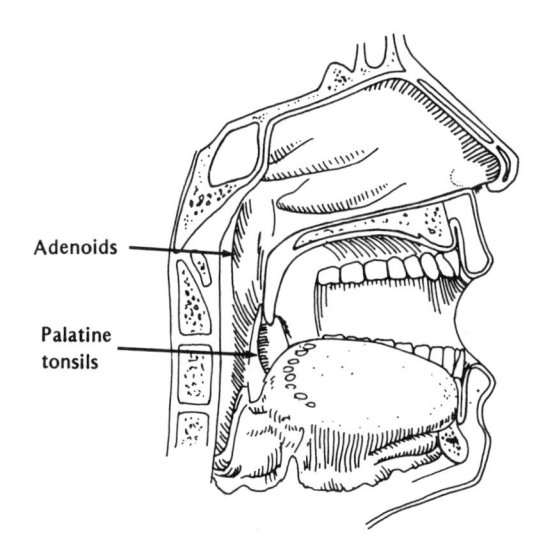

Figure 10-6: Adenoids and tonsils *(courtesy of Picker Corp.)*.

below it is continuous with the trachea. The larynx is made up of a number of pieces of cartilage and is lined with mucous membrane. The largest of these is a shield-shaped cartilage, the **thyroid cartilage**. In adult men the thyroid cartilage is more pronounced than in women. It is called the "Adam's apple."

There are folds of tissue called the **vocal cords** within the larynx (**intralaryngeal**). An opening in the center, the **glottis**, is enlarged or reduced and vocal cords tensed or relaxed in **phonation** (voice production). The tongue, lips, sinuses and pharynx also aid in phonation. **Dysphonia** (difficulty in speaking) is a symptom of laryngitis.

The **epiglottis** (a laryngeal cartilage) protects the glottis so that foreign materials do not enter the lower respiratory tract. The trachea is a tube about four and a half inches long (11.5 cm) and about one inch in diameter (2.54 cm). It is made up of C-shaped cartilaginous rings and smooth muscle lined with mucous membrane and extends into the mediastinum. The trachea serves as a passageway for the air. At its distal end it **bifurcates** (branches into two) to form the right and left bronchi.

The Bronchi

The right bronchus and the left bronchus enter the right and left lungs respectively at their medial surface in an indented area of the lung substance called the **hilum**. Like the trachea, the walls of the main bronchi have cartilage and smooth muscle for support and are lined with mucous membrane. The left main bronchus is shorter and less **vertical** (straight up and down) than the right because of the position of the heart. Each bronchus divides within the lung forming a **parenchyma** (essential organ

The Lungs parts) of bronchioles, terminal ducts and alveoli, supplied with blood vessels.

The two lungs in the body are each enveloped within their own pleural covering. The right lung has three divisions (**lobes**) and the left lung has two. The superior pointed end of the lung, the **apex**, extends just above the **clavicle** (collar bone). The **base** or inferior border of each lung rests on the diaphragm. The parietal pleura is attached to the thoracic wall. The visceral pleura is tightly **adherent** (attached) to the lung surfaces. Only a small **potential** (possible) space exists between the two membranes. This space is the **intrapleural cavity** and is filled with serous fluid.

RESPIRATION

Respiration (breathing) moves air into and out of the lungs. Respiration consists of two phases: **inspiration** (inhalation) allows air to move through the upper respiratory passageways into the lungs; **expiration** (exhalation) forces air back out of the lungs through the same passageways to the outside. The strength of the respiratory effort determines the **volume** (amount of gases measured in ml) that will be moved. The deeper the respiration, the greater the volume of gases passing into and out of the **respiratory tree** (tract).

The Mechanics of Respiration

Respiration is controlled by nerve impulses originating in the respiratory center of the brain. The respiratory center is located in the **pons** and **medulla** which are parts of the lower brain. The nerve impulses from the respiratory center stimulate the respiratory muscles to contract or shorten.

The diaphragm and intercostal muscles are the major respiratory muscles. As they change their shape, the thoracic cage also changes shape, thus increasing the space within it. This allows air to flow into the enlarged space. In other words, the lungs move with the thorax so as to enlarge the **intrapulmonic space** (intralung). Discontinuance of the nerve stimulation allows the muscles to return to their normal, relaxed shape and position. The space within the thorax and lungs is decreased and air moves out. Remember that the entire volume of air or gases in the lungs is not completely exchanged in each respiration.

The volume of air moved in and out of the lungs during inspiration and expiration can be measured with a **spirometer** (volume measuring instrument). Variances from the **norm** (fixed standard) are significant in making diagnosis of respiratory pathology. Look at Table 10-1 to learn the types of volumes and norms for respiratory activity.

Table 10-1

	Respiratory Activity	Air Volume Moved
vital capacity	the greatest amount exhaled after the deepest possible inspiration	4800 ml
tidal	volume of air which flows in and out with each normal respiratory movement	500 ml
complemental	the amount of air that can be drawn into the lungs above tidal volume	3100 ml
supplemental	the amount of air that can be forced out of the lungs after a normal inspiration	1200 ml

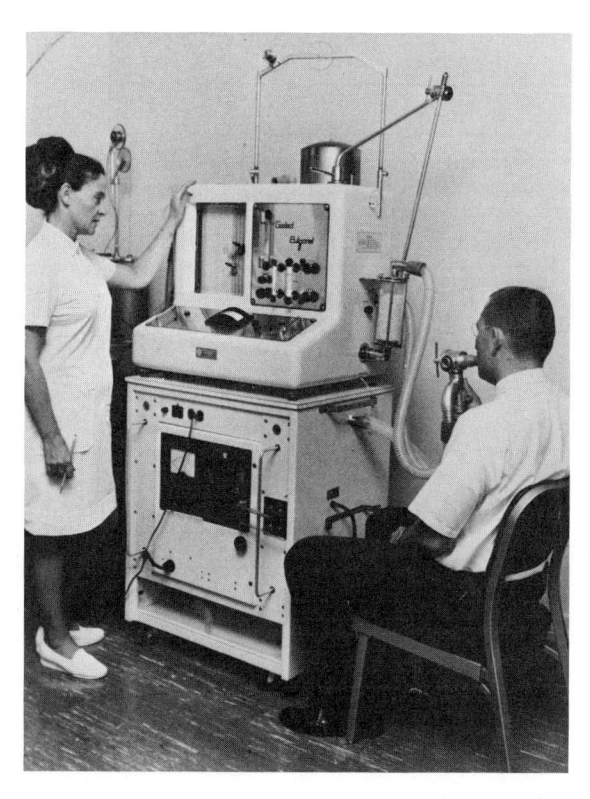

Figure 10-7: The spirometer measures volumes.

RESPIRATION

A certain volume of air cannot be forced out of the lungs once they have been expanded. This volume is known as **minimal air**. The medicolegal pathologist makes use of this information in determining if a neonate was born dead or alive. If the baby had taken even one breath, a **vital** (living) sign, there will be a minimal volume of air trapped in the alveoli. A piece of lung with minimal air floats in water; a piece of lung tissue without minimal air sinks, giving indication of the fetal status at birth.

Respiratory Rate and Rhythm

Most healthy people breathe between 14 and 20 times per minute. The respiratory **rate** (frequency) is altered by many factors such as sleep, exercise, eating, emotions and illness. These same factors alter the **rhythm** (regularity) and **character** (quality) of the respiratory pattern. Look at Table 10-2 to learn some of the terms used to describe respiratory patterns.

Table 10-2

Term	Respiratory Pattern
eupnea	normal rate and rhythm
hyperpnea	increased rate and depth of respiration
tachypnea	rapid, shallow respirations
rales	moist breathing sounds associated with respiratory pathology
apnea	respirations temporarily cease
dyspnea	difficult, painful respiration
stertor	snoring type of respirations
orthopnea	ability to breathe in an upright position only
Cheynes-stokes	periodic deep rhythmic respirations followed by shallow respirations or apnea
hiccough or singultus	involuntary respirations due to spasms of the diaphragm

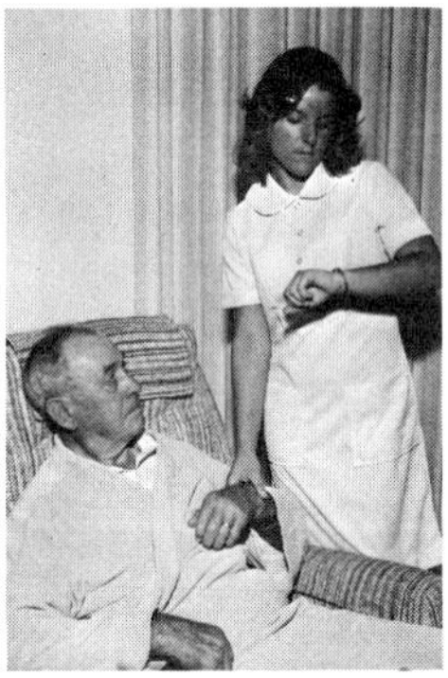

Figure 10-8: The health assistant checks the respiratory rate, rhythm, and character.

Pathology

Any portion of the respiratory tract can become inflamed either by irritants that have been inhaled or by microbes. As a result of the inflammatory process, the tissues either increase their activity or become less functional. For example, rhinitis results in **rhinorrhea** (excessive nasal mucous discharge) following increased activity of the mucous cells. In laryngitis, **aphonia** (loss of voice) is a characteristic symptom.

Usually the suffix "itis" attached to the name of the anatomical part will reveal the location of inflammation. For example, a diagnosis of "bronchitis" indicates that the inflamed area is the bronchus. Two exceptions to this rule are **pleurisy** (inflamed pleura) and **pneumonia** (acute inflammation or infection of the lung).

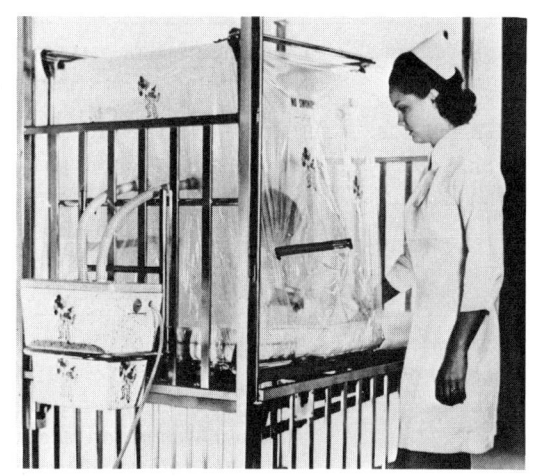

Figure 10-9: This child with bronchitis is receiving oxygen by tent *(courtesy of Continental Hospital Industries).*

The prefix **pneumo** (lung or gas) combines in a number of ways to form commonly used terms. Look at Table 10-3 for a few of the more common terms.

Table 10-3

Term	Meaning
pneumometry	measurement of inspired and expired air
pneumothorax	gas or air in the pleural sac (intrapleural space)
pneumonectomy	removal of a lung
pneumorrhagia	hemorrhage from the lungs
pneumonotomy	incision into the lung

Some of the more serious conditions affecting the respiratory tract include, chronic bronchitis, atelectasis, tuberculosis, pneumococcal pneumonia, empyema and emphysema.

RESPIRATION 169

Table 10-4

Pathology	Description of Respiratory Disease
chronic bronchitis	long term inflammation and infection of the bronchi associated with dyspnea and **phlegm** (heavy mucus) production; the heavy phlegm production **obstructs** (blocks) the passageways; frequently associated with heavy smoking or exposure to other irritants; untreated, the prognosis is guarded.
atelectasis	collapse of all or part of a lung; possible etiology, pneumothorax, or chronic obstruction pulmonary disease (**COPD**) such as chronic bronchitis.
pulmonary tuberculosis	an ancient infectious and communicable disease; the etiologic agent is the *mycobacterium tuberculosis*; early diagnosis improves the prognosis for **arresting** and holding in check (containing) the disease process.
pneumococcal pneumonia	inflammation of the lung due to invasion by the pneumococcus microbe; people between the ages of 15 & 40 are most susceptible; more men than women become infected; the alveoli become filled with fluid and gaseous exchange rate is hampered.
empyema or *pyothorax*	pus accumulates in the intrapleural space; the pus is due to an inefective process; the accumulation of pus causes intrapleural pressure which may force the pleural membranes apart bringing about atelectasis; **thoracentesis** (drainage of the chest) may be performed to relieve the pressure; antibiotics are given to combat the infection.

CASE STUDY

Herman Orville, age 67, a married man and the father of four, was admitted on November 22, in acute respiratory distress to the Intensive Respiratory Care Unit of Raymond Memorial Hospital. His diagnosis was emphysema. The physician orders included:

1. regular diet
2. IPPB C̄ *N.S.* Q.I.D.
3. O$_2$ @ 3 L/min via mask prn.
4. bedrest—BRP.

Emphysema is a progressive degenerative chronic disease in which the terminal bronchioles become obstructed. It is the sequalae of any **C.O.P.D.** In Mr. Orville's case, the C.O.P.D. had been an allergic asthma of many years duration. He had been under medical therapy for many years prior to the present admission. His C.C. on admission was dyspnea. Observation revealed tachypnea, moderate cyanosis and **expectoration** (ejection) of **copious** (excessive) **sputum** (mucus from the lungs). Any **exertion** (physical effort) exacerbated the dyspnea.

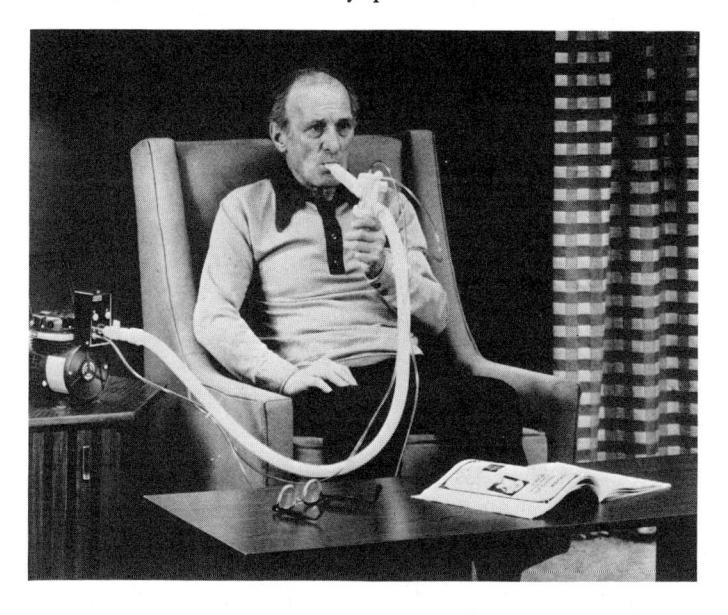

Figure 10-10: The breathing assistor permits the COPD patient to remain at home *(courtesy of Mine Safety Appliances Company).*

The physician ordered bed rest to limit exertion except for bathroom privileges. Oxygen was ordered to alleviate the hypoxia. **I.P.P.B.** (intermittent positive pressure breathing) a technique for improving **ventilation** (process of supplying with fresh air) of the lungs was ordered to be given four times a day. The **N.S.** (normal salt) solution was ordered to help liquify and loosen the phlegm which obstructs the airways.

Kept on this therapeutic regime, Mr. Orville showed gradual improvement and finally was able to be discharged to his home. He was instructed to report to the Respiratory Rehabilitation Department so he could be followed on an out-patient basis.

SUMMARY   *The respiratory system has the vital role of providing an avenue for oxygen intake and carbon dioxide elimination. Since it is open to the outside, it is subject to damage from irritants and infectious microbes. The normal body defenses may be overwhelmed and chronic pulmonary disease may be the result. Many people today suffer from COPD, a major health problem.*

PRACTICE & REVIEW   *Explain and define the new special terms you have been using. Remember, you learned how to pronounce them at the beginning of this chapter.*

1. atelectasis _____
2. choanal _____
3. copious _____
4. dysphonia _____
5. emphysema _____
6. hyperpnea _____
7. intralaryngeal _____
8. parenchyma _____
9. pneumorrhagia _____
10. spirometer _____

Now, double-check the meaning of the terms above by studying the brief definitions given in the Glossary-Index at the back of this text.

Test yourself quickly before going on to learn other medical and professional terms. Use these short review exercises to practice for your new work in health services. Your teacher will also help by recommending various other Study Activities.

    A. Using the diagram provided, label the numbered structures:

1. nasal cavity
2. pharynx
3. larynx
4. trachea
5. right mainstem bronchus
6. left mainstem bronchus
7. left lung
8. diaphragm
9. epiglottis
10. ribs

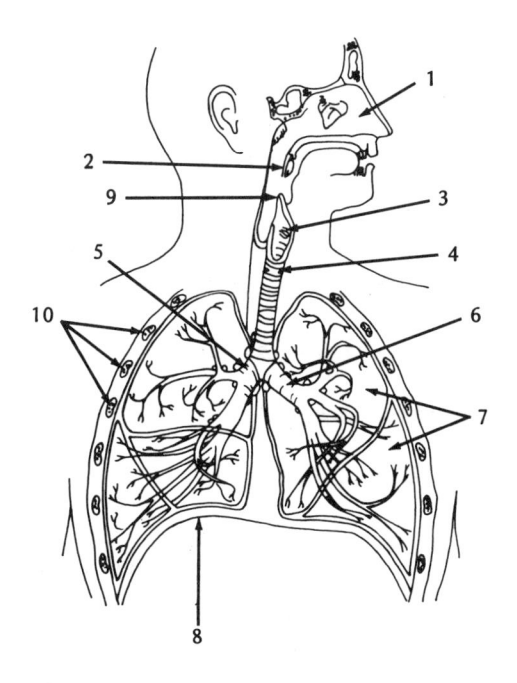

B. Complete the following sentences with the best word from the list below:

palate	obstruct	diffusion	lobes
pneumothorax	septum	volume	vital capacity
olfactory	larynx	hypoxia	pharynx

1. Thick, tenacious phlegm can block or _____ the air passageways.
2. Oxygen moves across the blood gas barrier by the process of _____.
3. The lungs are divided into segments called _____.
4. The _____ separates the nasal cavities from the oral cavity.
5. The structure which serves as a common passageway for food and air is the _____.
6. The _____ nerve endings transmit the sense of smell to the sensorium.
7. The nasal cavity is separated into a right and left side by the nasal _____.
8. The vocal cords are found in the _____.
9. The greatest amount of air exhaled after the deepest possible inspiration is called the _____ capacity.
10. The spirometer measures the amount or _____ of air moved in and out of the lungs.

RESPIRATION 173 *

After studying Chapter 11

The Musculoskeletal System

You should be able to:

* *Pronounce and define each of its new medical words and phrases and use the new technical jargon.*

* *Describe the formation of bones.*

* *Name seven bone markings.*

* *Identify five bones and muscles.*

MEDICAL WORDS   PRONOUNCE THESE TEN NEW WORDS WITH YOUR TEACHER:

amphiarthrotic (am′fe-ar-thrak′tĭk)
arthrochalasis (ar″thro-kal′ah-sĭs)
epiphysis (ĕ-pĭf′ĭ-sĭs)
hematopoiesis (hem″ah-to-poi-e′sis)
ischium (is′ke-um)
myelogenous (mĭ″-ĕ-loj′ĕ-nus)
myosclerosis (mĭ″ĕ-lo-sklĕ-ro′sis)
osteodynia (os″te-o-din′e-ah)
sternocleidomastoid (ster″no-kli″do-mas′toid)
synergistic (sĭn″er-jĭst′ik)

The musculoskeletal system is comprised of the muscles and bones and the joints, tendons and ligaments which hold these structures together.

The bones and **skeletal muscles** (attached to skeleton) give structure and form to the body, protecting the delicate organs within the body and its membranous cavities. Together with the tendons, ligaments and joints, the bones and skeletal muscles enable the body to move. The bones act as levers to which the skeletal muscles are attached by tendons. Movement occurs at the joints as the skeletal muscles shorten, pulling their points of attachment to the bones closer together. The shortening of the muscles changes the angle between the bones.

All adult human bone has an inner cavity that is filled with a soft, organic tissue called bone marrow. Some of this soft material produces blood cells (**hematopoiesis**), which circulate in the blood stream, while the rest of it becomes fat.

There are three types of muscle tissue. The skeletal muscles, which function in movement, the cardiac muscle that

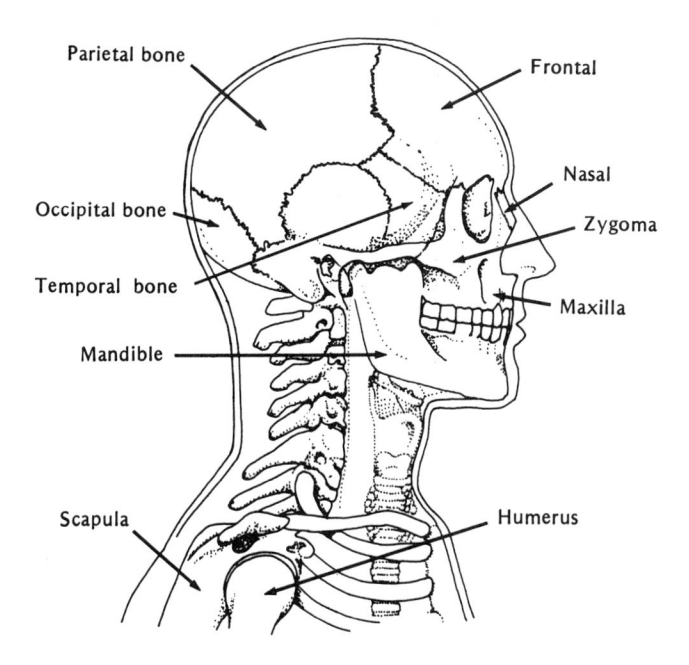

Figure 11-1: Bones of the cranium *(courtesy of Picker Corp.)*.

forms the heart wall, and the smooth muscle that forms the walls of the viscera.

THE BONES

There are 206 bones of the body. You can see most of these bones easily when you look at a skeleton. A few, however, like the internal skull and face bones, are more difficult to see unless the skull is **disarticulated** (separated).

The bones of the body may be studied by dividing the skeleton into an appendicular and axial skeleton. The *axial* skeleton includes the skull (**cranium**), backbone (**vertebrae**), *ribs* and breastbone (**sternum**).

The **appendicular** skeleton includes the **pelvic girdle** which supports the lower limbs, the **shoulder girdle** which supports the upper limbs, and the arms and legs (**extremities** or limbs). The hip bones forming either side of the pelvic girdle are a fusion of three bones: the **ilium**, **ishium**, and **pubis**. Called the **ossa coxae**, they articulate with the **sacrum** posteriorly to complete this bony girdle which encircles the pelvis. The pubic bones are articulated at the midline with a band of connecting cartilage called the **symphysis pubis**. The **shoulder girdle** is composed of the shoulder blades (**scapulae**) and collar bones (**clavicles**).

Figure 11-2: (a) The human skeleton *(courtesy of Picker Corp.)*; (b) lateral view of skeleton *(courtesy of Picker Corp.)*.

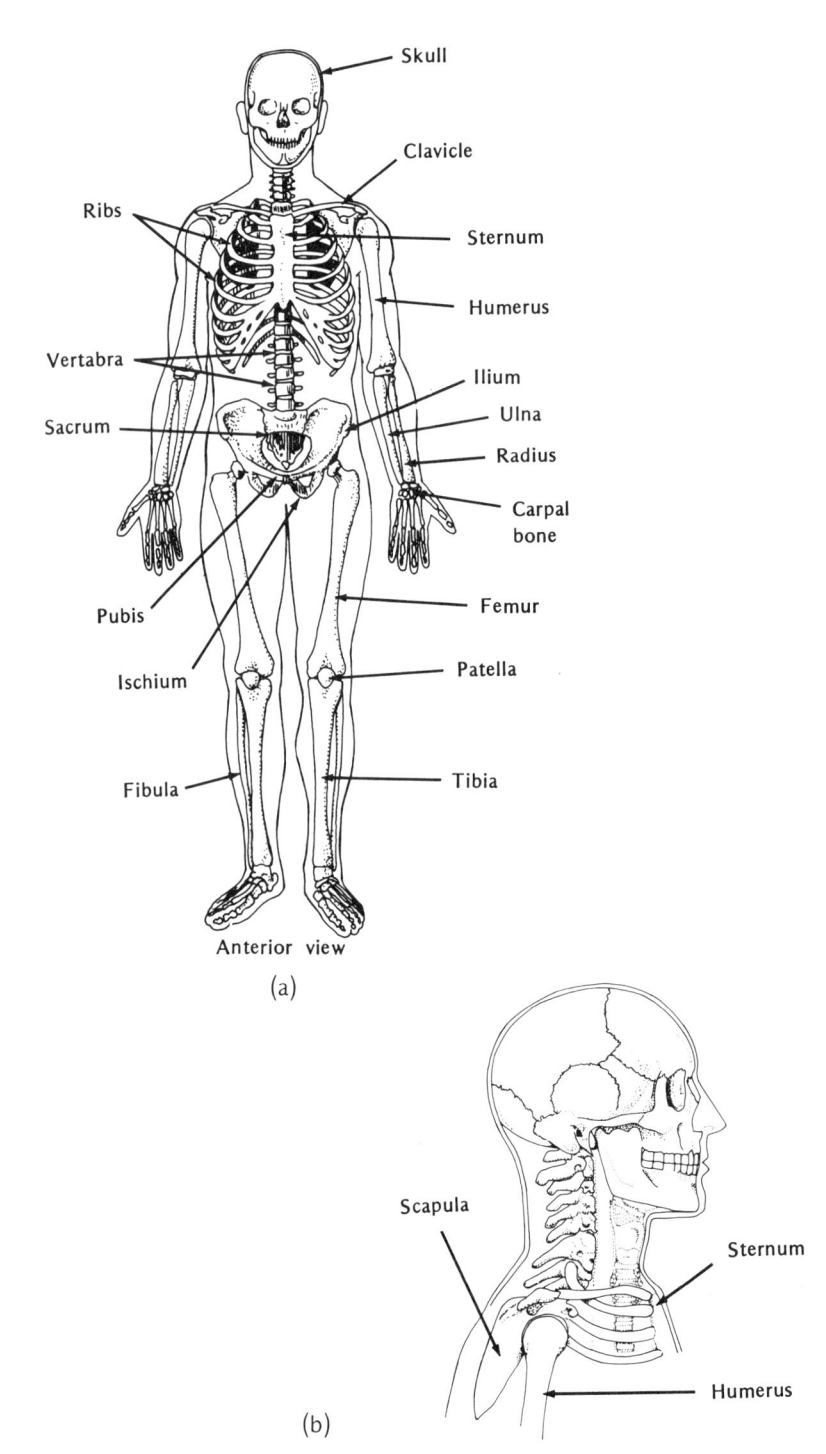

(a) Anterior view

(b)

176 *THE MUSCULOSKELETAL SYSTEM*

Look carefully at the diagrams of the skeleton to learn the names and locations of the major bones. Notice that if an imaginary line is drawn at midline, the bones on one side are duplicates of those found on the opposite side.

The general shape identifies four types of bones in the body: flat ones, like the scapula; short ones, like the carpals; long ones, like the femur; and the irregular ones, like the vertebrae. Notice the **femur** (thighbone), and then the **patella** (knee cap), and then the **carpal** bones which form the wrist. Then examine the vertebrae that form the backbone (**spine**). As you can see, these bones are not alike. You could easily distinguish one bone from the other because they represent the four different kinds. Each has its own **markings** or characteristics.

There are a large number of distinctive bone markings. There are, however, two general groupings by contours. Some have visible projections, others have visible depressions. For example, the term **fossa** means a basin-like depression. It is used to describe a hollowed-out area on the scapula called the **glenoid fossa** and one on the temporal bone into which the **mandible** (lower jaw bone) fits. The mandible fits into the **mandibular fossa** of the temporal bone.

Other markings, like **trochanter**, are used only when describing a specific bone. For example, the greater trochanter is a large, roughened prominence found only on the femur. Still other important markings apply to several bones with similar projections or ridges or knobs.

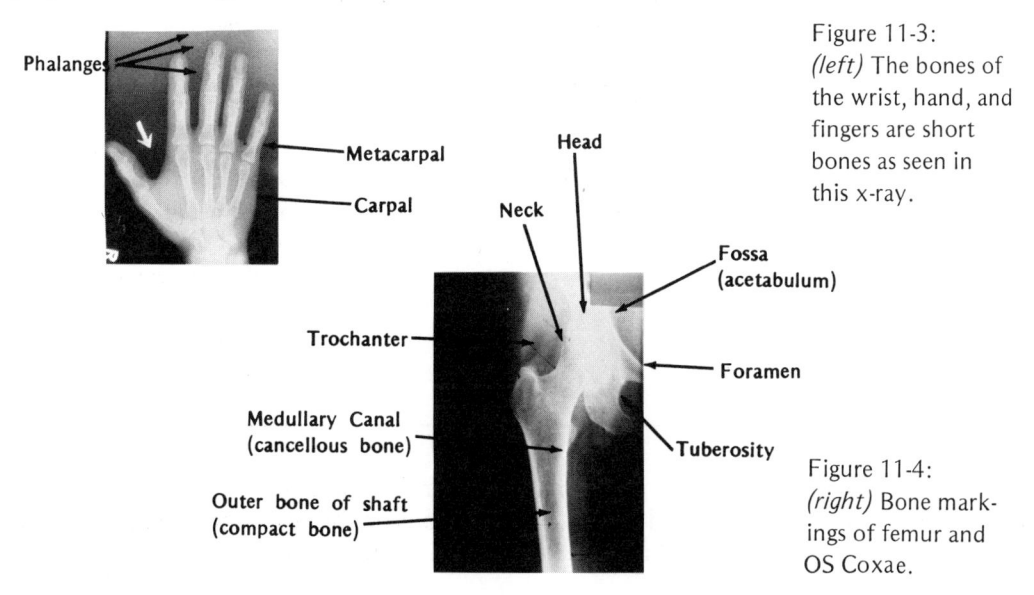

Figure 11-3: *(left)* The bones of the wrist, hand, and fingers are short bones as seen in this x-ray.

Figure 11-4: *(right)* Bone markings of femur and OS Coxae.

THE BONES 177 *

Table 11-1

Markings (Projections)	Description	Examples of Bones
head	rounded projection supported on a constricted neck	humerus/femur
process	prominence	styloid process radius xiphoid process of sternum
condyle	rounded eminence which is knuckle-like	occipital bone, femur
tuberosity	large rounded irregular projection	ischium, tibia
crest	prominent border or ridge	ilium, fetal maxilla

Table 11-2

Markings (Depressions)	Description	Examples of Bones
sinus	cavity	frontal/maxillary
facet	flat, shallow surface	ribs, vertebrae
foramen	large opening	occiput, ossa coxae
meatus	canal	temporal bone
sutures	line of cranial bone unions	*coronal suture* between the frontal & parietal bones *squamosal suture* between the parietal & temporal bones *lambdoidal suture* between the parietal & occipital bones

Histology   Bones are composed of two types of osseous tissue: **compact** or hard bone and **cancellous** or spongy bone. Compact bone is solid and relatively heavy. Cancellous bone is lightweight.

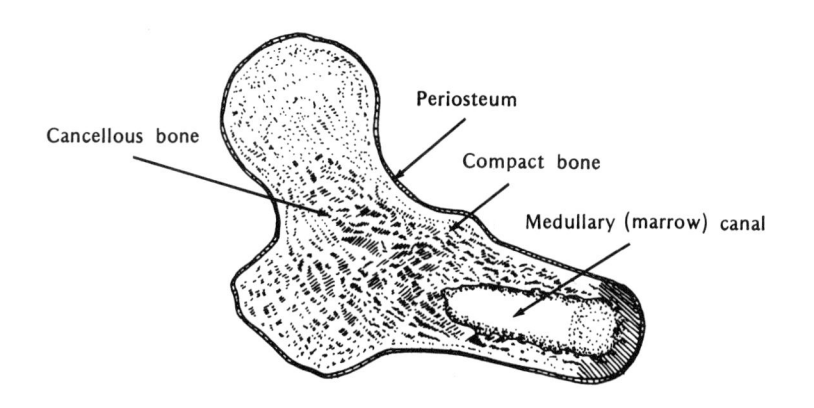

Figure 11-5: Compact and cancellour bone *(courtesy of Ethicon, Inc.)*.

Compact bone forms the outside bone and gives strength to the structure. Despite its solid appearance, microscopic soft bone cells (**osteocytes**) form the living cellular portion of the bone.

The spongy cancellous bone is found inside the hard compact bone in areas not subject to great stress. Red bone marrow in cancellous bones is the site of **hemacyte** (blood cell) production. The cranial bones are formed of two layers of compact bone with a layer of cancellous bone between them. The layer of cancellous bone is called the **diploe**.

In children, menatopoiesis (blood-forming activity) is carried on in the **myelogenous** (bone marrow) tissue of all cancellous bone. In adults, only specific cancellous bone carries out this same hemopoietic activity. In adults it occurs in the cancellous bone at the proximal ends of the humerus and femur, in the bodies of the vertebrae, and in the cranial diploe, ribs, ossa coxae, and sternum.

Bone Formation

Bone is formed of osseous tissue which is formed in one of two different ways; from membranes (**membranous**) or from cartilage (**cartilaginous**). The long bones, such as the femur, are developed as osteocytes that gradually replace the cartilage cells of the cartilaginous skeleton that is formed in the fetus. The process of replacing **chondrocytes** (cartilage cells) with osteocytes is called **ossification** (conversion to bone).

The bones of a newborn's skull are formed from membranes of fibrous connective tissue. These fibrous connective tissue cells are gradually replaced by bone cells. But these bones are not completely ossified or converted to bone at birth. This

Figure 11-6: The femur: note the parts of the long bone.

"incompleteness" allows the head to **mold** (shape) so it can pass through the birth canal.

At birth, the unossified membranous areas of the skull are called **fontanels**. The **anterior fontanel** is between the frontal and two parietal bones and is roughly diamond-shaped. The **posterior fontanel** is found between the parietal bones and the occipital bone and is roughly triangle-shaped.

The **periosteum** (membrane around bone) covering the compact bone serves as a point of attachment for tendons and ligaments. Bones grow in circumference from the cells of this tissue. The **endosteum** (bone lining) is a membrane that lines the medullary canal. In adults, the **medullary canal** (center cavity) of long bones is filled with fat. The shaft of the bone is called the **diaphysis**; each end the **epiphysis**.

A line of cartilage called the **epiphyseal cartilage** is found between diaphyses and epiphyses. This tissue is gradually ossified in a child so that it increases the length of the body's bones.

The prefix **osteo-** means bone. It is used in a large number of word combinations. Review the terms you already know and learn some new ones. Analyze and learn the new words and word combinations in Table 11-3.

Table 11-3

ostalgia (osteodynia)	pain in the bone
osteoarthritis	inflammation of bones and joints
ostectomy	excision of a bone
osteitis	inflammation of a bone
osteotomy	surgical cutting of a bone
osteectopia	displacement of bone
ostempyesis	bone tumor
osteoclasis	surgical fracture of a bone
osteometry	measurement of bones
osteotome	a bone cutting knife
osteopathology	disease of the bone
osteoporosis	metabolic bone disease
osteoma	bone tumor
osteomalacia	softening of bones
osteomyelitis	pyogenic bone infection

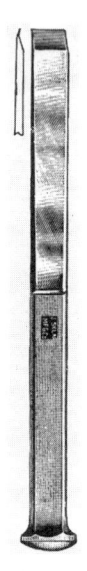

Figure 11-7: "Osteotome" *(courtesy of American Hospital Supply Corp.).*

Bones join or **articulate** at certain points where they meet. It is at these joinings or **joints** that movement takes place. Movement at a joint changes the relationship of the bones articulating at that point. The same type of movement is not possible at all joints, and at some points of articulation there is no mobility at all. The articular ends of the bones are covered by a smooth connective tissue composed of **hyaline cartilage**. There it is called **articular cartilage**.

There are three types of joints; immovable, slightly movable, and fully movable. Joints at which there is no movement are **synarthrotic** (immovable). The suture joints of the cranial part of the **skull** (cranium and face) are examples of synarthrotic joints.

JOINTS

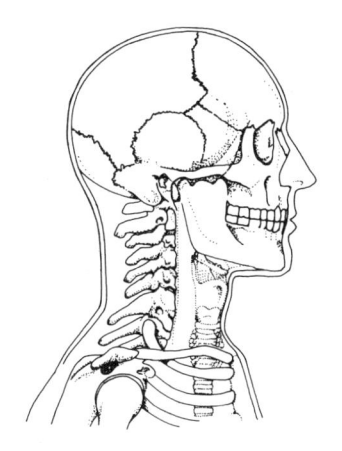

Figure 11-8: Suture joints of skull (synarthrotic joints).

Amphiarthrotic joints are slightly movable joints. The sacroiliac joint (between sacrum and ilium) is an example of an amphiarthrotic joint. A freely movable joint is called **diarthrotic**. Diarthrotic joints are also called **synovial joints** because a capsule around the diarthrotic joint is lined with synovial membrane.

Several different types of diarthrotic movements are possible. Keep in mind that movement at the joints changes the relationship and angle between the bones. Several important terms are used to describe the changes in the bony relationships.

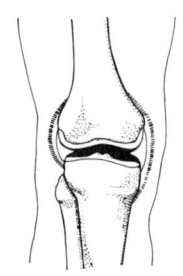

Joint Movements

Figure 11-9: The knee joint (articulation—knee cap removed); the construction of a movable joint prevents bone ends from scraping against each other *(courtesy of Ethicon, Inc.)*.

A diarthrotic joint is protected by a joint capsule. The joint is held together by ligaments and the synovial lining of the capsule secretes just enough synovial fluid to keep the joint lubricated to prevent friction. **Ligaments** are tough fibrous connective bands which hold bones together at the joints.

Figure 11-10: (a) Flexion decreases the angle between bones; (b) extension increases the angle between bones; (c) abduction means moving away from the midline; (d) adduction means moving toward the midline.

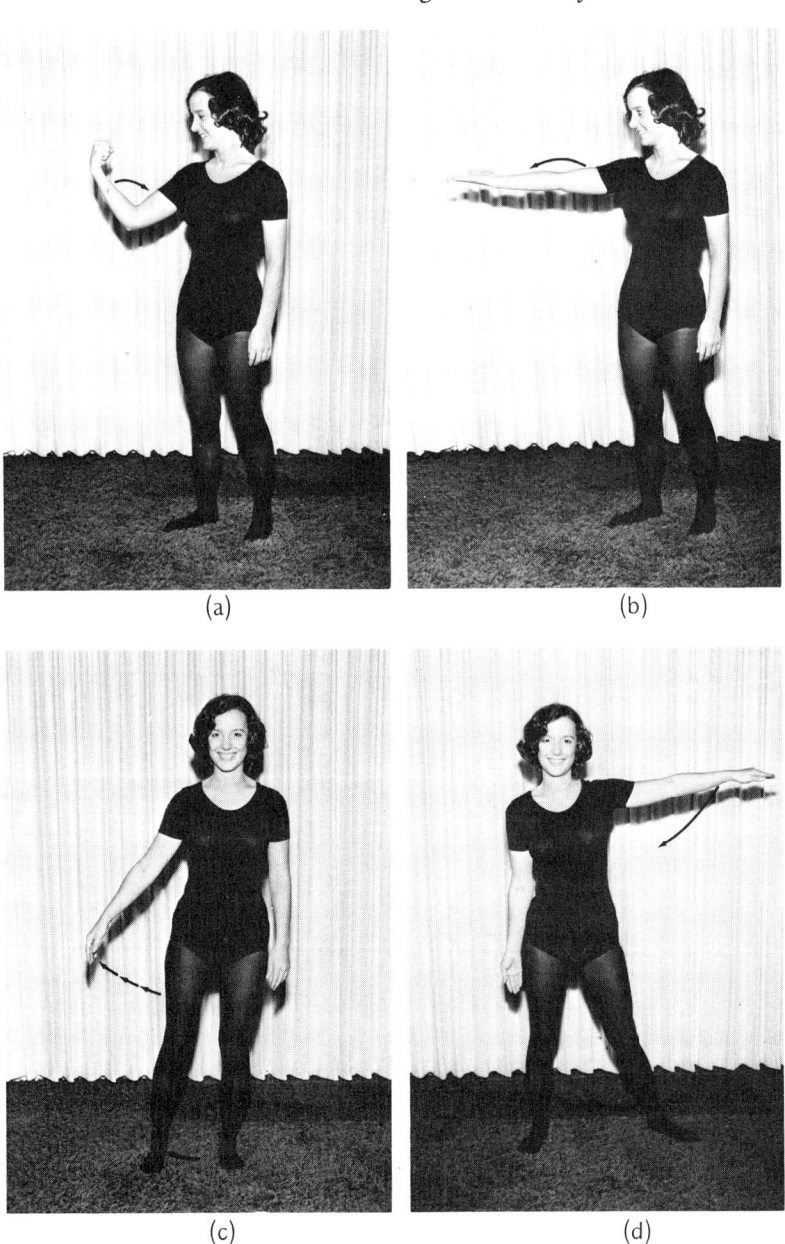

(a) (b)

(c) (d)

*182 *THE MUSCULOSKELETAL SYSTEM*

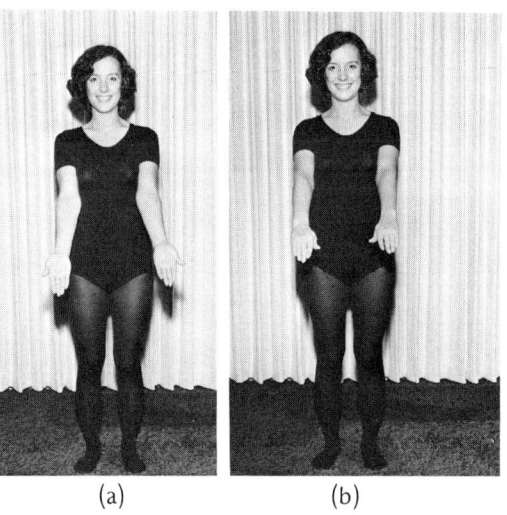

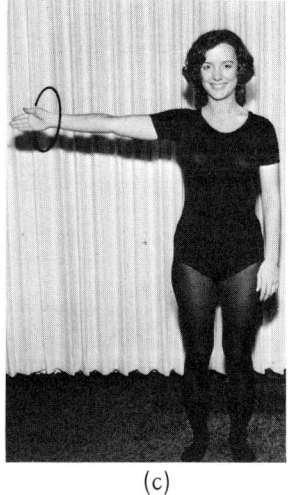

Figure 11-11:
(a) Supination means palms up with the radius and ulna parallel;
(b) pronation means palm down with the radius crossed over the ulna;
(c) rotation means moving a part around a central axis.

Table 11-4

Movement	Description	Example of Joint
flexion	decreased angle	bending arm at the elbow decreases the angle between humerus and ulnar and radius
extension	increased angle	straightening the arm at the elbow increases the angle between humerus and ulnar and radius
abduction	movement away from midline	moving the arm or part to the side away from the body
adduction	movement away from midline	moving the arm or part back toward midline of body
supination	palm of hand up	ulna and radius are parallel as they are in anatomic position
pronation	palm of hand down	the radius is crossed over the ulna
rotation	revolving motion	the whole arm is pivoted at the shoulder without changing the position of the bones

The prefix meaning joint is **arthro-**. Here are some of the words which are formed by combining the prefix with different endings.

Analyze and learn the new terms in Table 11-5.

Table 11-5

arthrectomy	excision of a joint
arthralgia or *arthrodynia*	pain in a joint
arthrotomy	incision of a joint
arthrocele	joint swelling
arthritis	inflammation of a joint
arthrodesis	surgical fusion of a joint
arthroempyesis	suppuration in a joint
arthroclasia	joint manipulation
arthrophyte	abnormal growth in a joint cavity
arthrochalasis	abnormal relaxation of a joint

Figure 11-12: Rectus femoris muscle, it's origin and insertion *(courtesy of Ethicon, Inc.)*.

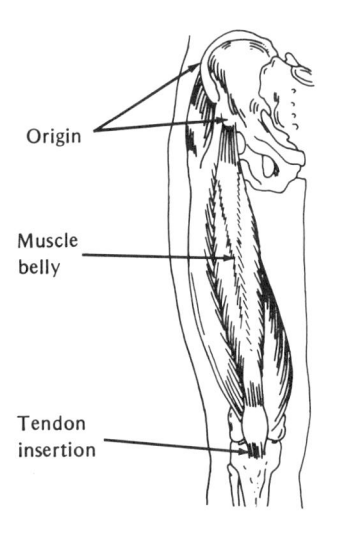

SKELETAL MUSCLES

The skeletal muscles are **striated** or striped, and are also called **voluntary** because they shorten or contract on command of the human will. These muscles have three parts: origin, body, and insertion. The **origin** or starting point of the muscle is the place where it is attached to a bone. Its **body** is the central part or belly of the muscle. Tendons stretch or extend across one or more joints to attach or insert the muscle to the bone on the other side. That point of attachment is called its **insertion**. Tendons are fibrous bands of connective tissue that attach skeletal muscles to the bones. When stimulated, skeletal muscles contract, pulling the point of insertion toward the point of origin, thus changing the joint position. When these muscles are not deliberately contracted they are partially relaxed. In other words, they do not exert a strong pull over the joint at all times. But they do, however, maintain a steady state of partial contraction. This is called **tonus**. Muscles without tone or tonus are soft or flabby (**flaccid**).

Muscles usually act in groups. One muscle is usually the major muscle in an action. It is called the **prime mover**. The other muscles in the group are **synergistic** (enhancing another's action) to the prime mover. Muscles with an opposing action are called **antagonists**.

Muscles derive their names in several ways. There are many skeletal muscles, and it is easiest to learn their names in groups. Some muscles are named for the bones to which they are attached or are near. The **sternocleidomastoid** muscle and **sacrospinalis** muscle are named in this way. The sternocleidomastoid muscle is found attached to the sternum, clavicle, and **mastoid process** of the temporal bone. The sacrospinalis begins at the sacrum and travels up the spinal column to insert on the occipital bone of the skull.

Names of Muscles

Some muscles are named by the action they perform. For example, contractions of the **flexors** on the anterior part of the forearm flex the fingers, and contractions of the **extensors** on the posterior arm extend the fingers.

Some muscles are named for a special characteristic such as the **triceps brachii** which has three heads or points of origin and is located on the posterior upper arm. The triceps brachii extends the elbow joint. The **biceps brachii** (two heads or points of origin) found on the anterior upper arm flexes the elbow joint. It is antagonistic to the triceps.

Study Figure 11-13 to learn the names of the major muscles and their general location.

The prefix **myo-** means muscle. Here are some of its combined forms to analyze and learn:

Figure 11-13: Muscles of the body *(courtesy of Ethicon, Inc.)*; anterior view; posterior view.

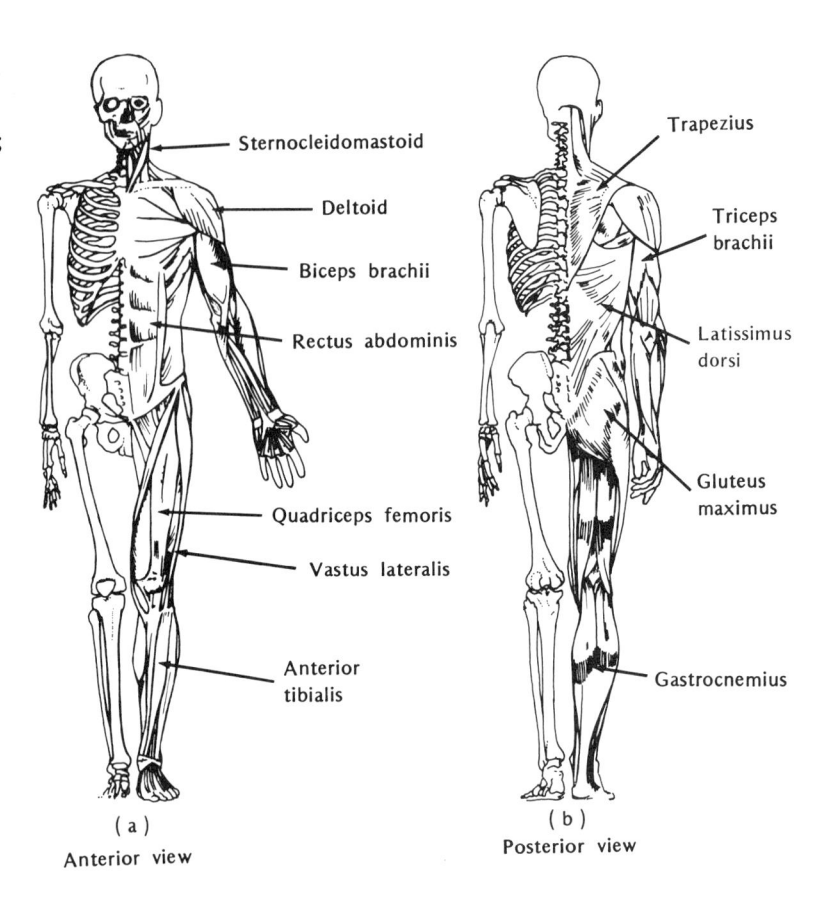

(a) Anterior view

- Sternocleidomastoid
- Deltoid
- Biceps brachii
- Rectus abdominis
- Quadriceps femoris
- Vastus lateralis
- Anterior tibialis

(b) Posterior view

- Trapezius
- Triceps brachii
- Latissimus dorsi
- Gluteus maximus
- Gastrocnemius

Table 11-6

myology	study of muscles
myomalacia	softening of muscles
myopathy	diseases of muscles
myosclerosis	hardening of a muscle
myospasm	involuntary muscular contraction

MUSCULOSKELETAL PATHOLOGY

Pathology of either muscles or bones or joints affects the functional ability of the whole musculoskeletal system. Loss of some degree of mobility is one of the major problems associated with such illness. Consider, for example, what the team leader of an orthopedic unit in a small general hospital had to do to plan care for these new patients:

1. A. Holtz, 14 yrs. old, with multiple fractures (fx);
2. S. Hartley, 8 yrs. old, with scoliosis;
3. B. Eckert, 48 yrs. old, with rheumatoid arthritis;
4. T. Lizel, 19 yrs. old, with myesthenia gravis; and
5. P. Smith, 35 yrs. old, with muscular dystrophy.

In planning for their care, the team leader reviewed the pathology involved. See page 188-90 for their case histories.

Bone Fractures

Bones are hard tissues and when they are subject to stress or severe trauma they break (**fracture**). There are several kinds of fractures but each results in loss of mobility of the part fractured and some damage to the surrounding musculature. See the summary in Table 11-7.

Table 11-7

Types of Fractures	Description of Breakage
simple	bones remain in proper position (**alignment**) but are broken through
compound	part of broken bone protrudes through the skin
comminuted	the broken bone is splintered
greenstick	bone only partly broken, not all the way through
compression	bone fragments are pressed together, as in vertebral fractures
compacted	bone fragments firmly driven into one another

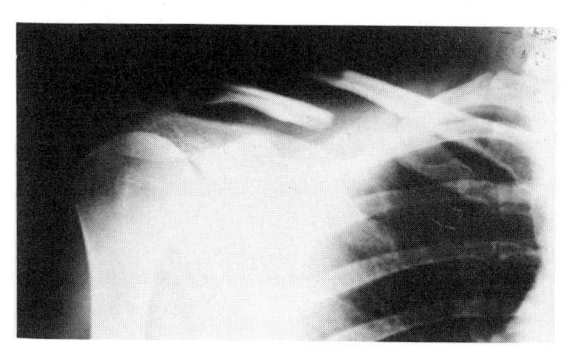

Figure 11-14: Compound fracture of the clavicle.

Figure 11-15: Cominuted fracture.

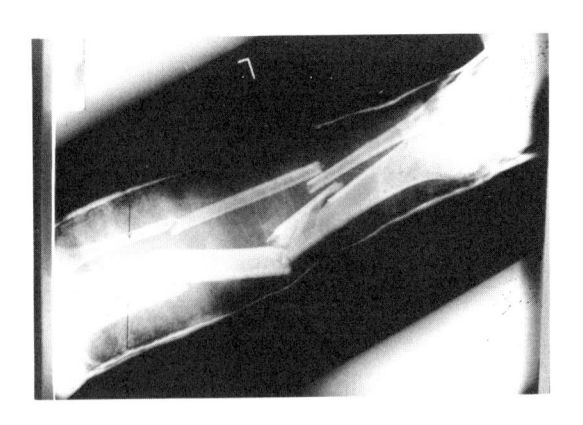

Figure 11-16: Casts are used to immobilize a fracture and maintain alignment *(courtesy of Ely Lily Co.)*.

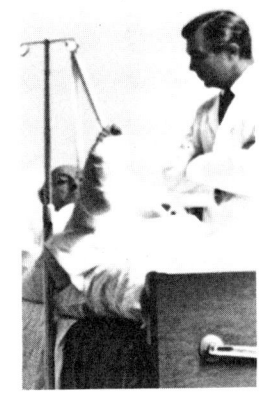

In fracture therapy, **realignment** (repositioning) of the fractured bone is the first stage of treatment. This repositioning is called the **reduction** of the fracture. The second stage of fracture therapy is **immobilization** (keeping immovable) until reossification is completed. Reductions are either closed or open. In a **closed reduction** the orthopedist uses his hands to **manipulate** the bones until they are realigned. Then he/she immobilizes the part, usually with a **cast** (rigid covering) or splint. An **open reduction** is a surgical procedure. An **incision** (surgical opening) is made over the fracture site and some form of mechanical aid such as bone nails, screws or pins are used to hold or **fix** the fractured bone. This type of immobilization is called an internal **fixation**. The incision is then closed and held in place with **sutures** until healing takes place. Frequently **traction** (pulling apart) is used both before and after an open reduction to prevent severe prolonged muscle spasm (**tetany**). The steady pull of traction keeps the injured muscle from contracting too strongly. Traction is also a major immobilization technique.

CASE 1

Andy Holtz miscalculated the distance to the pier while water skiing. His admission diagnosis was a compound fracture of the right humerus and a simple fracture of the right ulva, compression fracture of the skull and multiple contusions and abrasions. An open reduction was performed on his arm and internal fixation was done, using a pin in the humerus. The simple fracture of the ulna in the lower half of his arm was reduced by manipulation and fixed with a cast. He is now recovering (**recuperating**) nicely. The prognosis for complete recovery is excellent.

THE MUSCULOSKELETAL SYSTEM

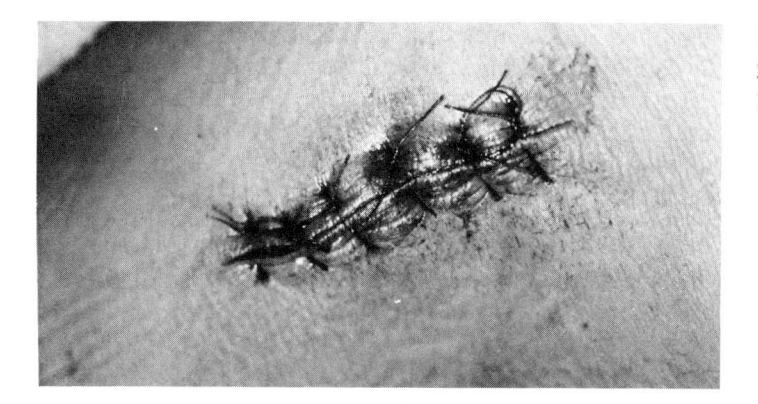

Figure 11-17: Sutures support the incision until healed.

Spinal Deformities

The vertebral column normally is straight when viewed posteriorly. From a lateral view, there are normally four slight curves. They are: the cervical, thoracic, lumbar and sacral curves. An abnormally pronounced thoracic curve is called **kyphosis**, commonly known as hunchback. A pronounced lumbar curve is called **lordosis** or sway back and a lateral curvature of the normally straight spine is called **scoliosis**.

CASE 2

Sammy Hartley was born with a congenital scoliosis and bilateral clubfeet (**talipes**). The latter have already been corrected. He does, however, still walk with a slight **limp** (lameness). Now having been admitted to the orthopedic unit, he is being **worked up** (readied) for surgery to straighten his spine and correct the abnormal curvature.

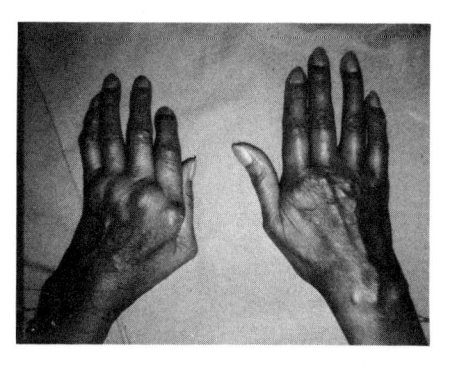

Figure 11-18: Note the deformity caused by rheumatoid arthritis.

There are two major forms of arthritis: rheumatoid arthritis and osteoarthritis. **Rheumatoid arthritis** affects the synovial membrane of the diarthrotic joints so that an acute inflammation of the joint occurs. The condition affects more women than men and usually strikes younger persons. It is characterized by periods of remission and exacerbation. It is the most crippling form of arthritis. **Osteoarthritis**, another form of arthritis, results in damage to the articular cartilage of weight bearing joints such as the hips and knees. It is a progressive condition and usually affects older persons.

CASE 3

Mrs. Eckert first experienced arthralgia several years ago. Her right knee and finger joints showed signs of inflammation and a diagnosis of rheumatoid arthritis was made. Her current episode has exacerbated the condition and she is so immobilized that hospitalization is required.

Myasthenia gravis is a chronic disease characterized by muscular weakness. The problem appears to be related to some defect at the points where nerves contact the skeletal muscles at neuromuscular junctions so that the body's command to contract is ineffective. **Muscular dystrophy** is characterized by muscular **atrophy** (wasting away). The etiology of this disease is unknown, except that the severe loss of muscle protein is somehow caused by faulty nutrition.

CASES 4 & 5

Both Tom Lizel and Patricia Smith are suffering from serious muscular pathologies. However, Tom's myasthenia gravis is responding to medication. He will be discharged from the hospital soon. Mrs. Smith requires almost complete care because she has gradually become disabled from muscular dystrophy. Not all forms of this disease are crippling, but hers is. For this patient, the prognosis is guarded.

* * *

In one way or another each of these five patients has mobility limited to some degree for at least a period of time. So the nurses on duty in the orthopedic unit realize that special consideration has to be given to this fact when providing care to the patients.

SUMMARY

The musculoskeletal system is composed of the muscles, bones and joints. Besides holding the body upright it is involved in the formation of certain blood elements and in protecting the more delicate body structures. One of the most significant other functions of the musculoskeletal system is to make the body mobile. Pathology of the system almost always results in some limitation to that mobility.

Explain and define the new special terms you have been using. Remember, you learned how to pronounce them at the beginning of this chapter.

PRACTICE REVIEW

1. amphiarthrotic _____
2. arthrochalasis _____
3. epiphysis _____
4. hematopoiesis _____
5. ischium _____
6. myelogenous _____
7. myosclerosis _____
8. osteodynia _____
9. sternocleidomastoid _____
10. synergistic _____

Now, double-check the meaning of the terms above by studying the brief definitions given in the Glossary-Index at the back of this text.

Test yourself quickly before going on to learn other medical and professional terms. Use these short review exercises to practice for your new work in health services. Your teacher will also help by recommending various other Study Activities.

A. Various bone markings are listed here. Write the name of each beside the best description in the five statements below:

    crest   meatus   foramen   process
    sinus   suture   head   facet

1. Rounded projection supported by a constructed neck. _____
2. Line of bone unions in the skull. _____
3. Cavity. _____
4. Large opening. _____
5. Prominent border or ridge. _____

B. Match the words on the right with the best statement on the left:
1. Projections and depressions which are characteristic of a bone
2. Bones of the cranium and face
3. Another name for the shoulder bone
4. Another name for the knee cap
5. Means the study of muscle
6. Freely movable joints
7. Lateral curvature of the spine
8. Name applied to voluntary muscles
9. Decreasing the angle between two bones
10. Another name for pain in a joint

a. lordosis
b. scoliosis
c. arthroclosis
d. arthrodynia
e. markings
f. myology
g. skull
h. patella
i. scapulae
j. diarthrotic
k. striated
l. talipes
m. flexion

C. Read these ten statements, then choose from the list the term that best completes each one:
1. A person who is recovering from an illness is said to be _____ .
2. The proper name for the condition commonly called hunchback is _____ .
3. Immovable joints are called _____ joints.
4. The term meaning turned to bone is _____ .
5. The membrane which lines long bones is called the _____ .
6. The places where bones meet and movement takes place are called _____ .
7. Skeletal muscles are attached to bones by _____ .
8. Immobilization of fractured bones by use of nails, screws, and pins is called an internal _____ .
9. The major muscle responsible for a specific movement is called the _____ .
10. Another name for joint pain is _____ .

arthralgia	joints	ossified	ligaments
synarthrotic	recuperating	prime mover	arthrodesia
endosteum	tendons	fixation	kyphosis

D. There are several kinds of bone fractures. Name those being described in the spaces below:
1. Part of the bone protrudes through the skin. _____
2. Bone only partly broken through. _____
3. Bone fragments pressed together. _____
4. The bone is splintered. _____
5. Bone fragments driven into one another. _____

After studying Chapter 12
The Cardiovascular System
You should be able to:

* *Pronounce and define each of its new medical words and phrases and use the new technical jargon.*

* *Identify the structures of the heart.*

* *Describe the flow of blood through the circulatory system.*

PRONOUNCE THESE TEN NEW WORDS WITH YOUR TEACHER: MEDICAL WORDS

arrhythmias (ah-rith′me-ahs)   lymphadenitis (lim-fad″ē ni′tis)
cardiomegaly (kar″de-o-meg′ah-le)   megakaryocytes (meg″ ah-kar′e-o sīts″)
extracoporeal (ĕk″strah-kor-po′rē-al)   phlebitis (fel-bi′tis)
infarction (in-fark′shun)   sphygmomanometer (sfig′mo-mah-nom′e-ter)
granulocytes (gan′u-lo-sīts″)   vasculature (vas′ku-lah-tūr″)

The **cardiovascular** (heart-vessel) **system** is a continuous, closed network of interrelated tubes conveying a body fluid called **blood**. The pumping heart propels the blood throughout the body by means of this tube system. The blood carries needed products to the cells and waste products away for disposal.

The cardiovascular system includes the body fluids, the heart, and **vasculature** (systematic structure of tubes and vessels). This body system is subject to so much stress and pathology that its diseases rank first in U.S. morbidity rates. Among them, heart disease is one of the major health problems when measured in terms of **incidence** (number of cases) of mortality and disability.

Fluids are the medium for exchange of nutrients and waste   THE BODY FLUIDS
products within the body. Their movement is the mechanism by which important substances are carried from their source of production to their point of use or discharge. Phagocytes, for example, use the body fluids to travel to the areas of the body

needing protection from infectious organisms and other foreign agents.

Body fluids are derived from and ultimately return to the cardiovascular system. The body fluids include: the blood which flows in the blood vessels; the **interstitial** or tissue fluid which bathes the cells; the **lymph** which is found in the lymphatic vessels; and the **intracellular** fluid which is found within the cells.

The fluids of the body are located in three compartments separated by **semipermeable** (selective fluid passage) membranes and they move back and forth between them. The walls of the blood vessels are the boundaries of the **intravascular** compartment. The cell walls encompass the intracellular compartment. The interstitial compartment is found between the walls of the vessels and the walls of the cells.

The movement of substances from one compartment to another is dependent upon a number of factors. Gases such as O_2 and CO_2 move by a process of diffusion. When these gases and certain substances in solution cross through a semipermeable membrane, the process is called **dialysis**.

Dialysis occurs because pressure differences on either side of the membrane force gases and selected substances from the side of greater pressure to the side of lesser pressure. Other materials, such as nutrients, also move through the membrane by dialysis and by two other processes as well.

The two other processes are filtration and osmosis. In **filtration**, materials move because of the weight of the column of fluid behind them. This is the principle process for moving substances out of the intravascular compartment. The blood pressure supplies the driving or filtering force.

Osmosis is water-drawing power. This process pulls water and dissolved substances through a semipermeable membrane. The presence of proteins aids in creating this osmotic pull. Osmosis and dialysis are the principal modes of fluid movement from the intravascular and interstitial compartments.

By tracing the pathway of a nutrient such as the carbohydrate, **glucose**, we can see how the forces cooperate. Carried in the intravascular compartment, the glucose passes by filtration and dialysis into the interstitial compartment. It then moves by dialysis and osmosis into the intracellular compartment where it is utilized in cellular respiration. **Edema** (swelling) means that excess fluid remains behind in the interstitial spaces.

The Lymph Fluid

Not all of the intersitial fluid returns directly to the bloodstream. Some of it is drained off into the lymphatic vasculature.

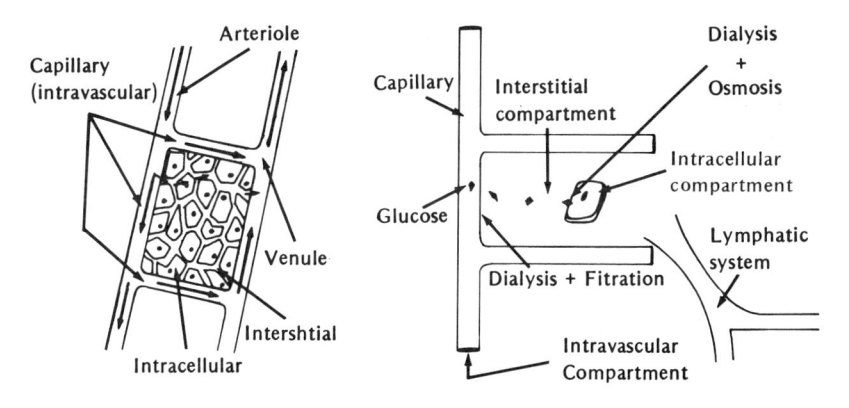

Figure 12-1 *(left)* Fluid Compartments.

Figure 12-2: *(right)* Materials move from one fluid compartment to another by the processes of dialysis, filtration, and osmosis.

The watery interstitial fluid that drains into the lymphatic system is known as lymph. As lymph it is drained through a system of lymph vessels and lymph nodes. Finally, it drains back into the blood vessels, once more becoming part of the blood.

The **lymph nodes** (known also as glands) are small masses of lymphoid tissue found throughout the lymph channels. They arc particularly numerous in the axillary, cervical, and groin areas. Large numbers of **lymphocytes**, or special phagocytic white blood cells, are located in the nodes and serve to remove injurious substances from the lymph before it returns to the general circulation. At times, however, infectious microbes which have invaded body tissues drain into the lymph ducts and overwhelm the lymphocytes. Then the lymphocytes are unable to destroy the microbes through phagocytosis and various illnesses result.

Average Blood Volume

The volume of blood in the adult human body averages between 4,000 ml to 6,000 ml or between about 8½ to 12 pints—according to size and weight. It is a sticky, salty, red fluid composed of solid elements and a liquid containing many dissolved substances.

Solid Elements in Blood

The solid elements, or cells, are basically of three kinds: erythrocytes (RBC), leukocytes (WBC), and thrombocytes (**platelets**). The erthrocytes are the most numerous. They contain the red pigment, hemoglobin. The average RBC count is 5,000,000 per cubic mm of blood. Erthrocytes are produced in the bone marrow. Shortly before they are released into the bloodstream, they lose their nuclei. They circulate for about four months and then, worn out, are destroyed by the cells of the liver, bone and spleen.

Erthrocytes are the prime carriers of oxygen in the body. They pick up their load of O_2 at the lungs and carry it to the

THE BODY FLUIDS

Figure 12-3: Erythrocytes are round. Note the absence of the nucleus, leaving an indentation *(courtesy of The National Foundation March of Dimes).*

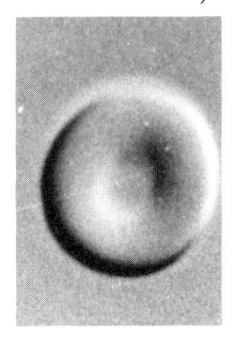

cells throughout the body. Insufficient O_2 in the blood is called **hypoxemia** and is often caused by hemoglobin imbalances. Sometimes, pathology of the blood-producing cells of the bone results in **polycythemia** (excess RBC). Either too few erythrocytes or too little hemoglobin results in **anemia**. Polycythemia and anemia are blood **dyscrasias** (abnormalities). In cases of **hemorrhage** (escape of blood), so much blood can be lost that life is threatened. Normally the blood's clotting mechanism is a protective body defense to guard against hemorrhage.

The thrombocytes are also produced in the **marrow** (soft bone tissue). They are not whole cells but are broken-off pieces of the very large cells called **megakaryocytes**. There are from 200,000 to 400,000 of these microscopic colorless fragments in each cubic millimeter (mm^3) of blood. They prevent undue loss of blood by starting the clotting process when blood vessels are ruptured. A substance, **thromboplastin**, found within the thrombocytes combines with an inactive substance, **prothrombin**, found in the liquid portion of the blood. Thromboplastin and prothrombin form a new substance **thrombin**. Thrombin then combines with still another protein found in the liquid portion of blood called **fibrinogen** to form the insoluble **fibrin**. The fibrin forms tiny solid strands which trap the rest of the blood components forming a **thrombus** (clot). Reread the section on thrombocytes and see how many times the prefix thrombo- has been used in the terminology to relate to clot or clot formation.

Figure 12-4: Blood clotting mechanism prevents excessive blood loss.

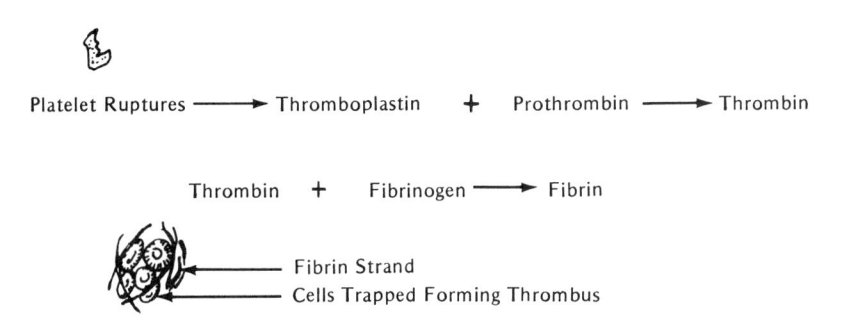

Platelet Ruptures ⟶ Thromboplastin + Prothrombin ⟶ Thrombin

Thrombin + Fibrinogen ⟶ Fibrin

— Fibrin Strand
— Cells Trapped Forming Thrombus

Leukocytes are not all alike. But they all fulfill a protective role in the body both in the formation of antibodies and by their power for phagocytosis. Some of the leukocytes have **granules** (particles) in their cytoplasm which can be stained and some do not. On this basis, the leukocytes can be classified as **granulocytes** (cells with granules) and **agranulocytes** (cells without granules).

Figure 12-5: Leukocytes.

Eosinophil Neutrophil

Lymphocyte

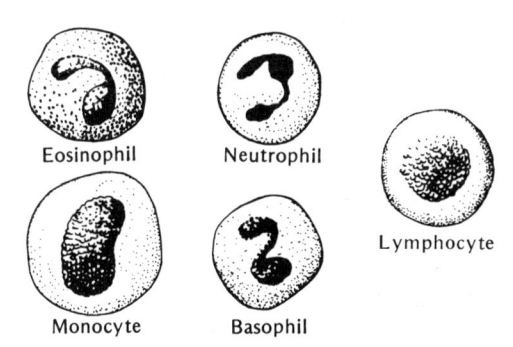

Monocyte Basophil

The granulocytes are identified according to their degree of affinity for a particular stain. For example, those called **basophils** (basic loving) have an affinity for basic stains which are easily taken up by the granules in the cytoplasm. Two other granulocytes are the **eosinophils** (eosin stain-loving) and the **neutrophils** (neutral stain-loving). The neutrophils, which are the most numerous, are known as **polymorphonuclear leukocytes** (WBC with nuclei of many shapes) or simply as "**polys**." The granulocytic WBC are produced in the bone marrow.

The agranulocytes, the **monocytes**, and lymphocytes lack granules and are not produced by the bone marrow. These cells are produced in special lymphoid tissue throughout the body. Look at Table 12-1 to see the relative quantities and qualities of the various cells in the blood.

Table 12-1

Kind of Leukocyte	Percent in Average WBC Count	Production Site	Identifying Characteristic
neutrophils	55-65	bone	takes neutral stain
basophils	0-1	bone	takes basic stain
eosinophils	1-4	bone	takes eosin stain
monocytes	25-40	lymphoid tissue	no granules
lymphocyte	3-7	lymphoid tissue	no granules

Liquid Portion of Blood

The **plasma** (liquid portion of blood) is a pale, yellow fluid. It comprises 55% of the total blood volume and is a solution in which many cellular substances are in suspension. It holds proteins, such as fibrinogen and prothrombin, salts, such as **sodium** chloride (NaCl), nutrients, such as glucose, and waste products such as **urea**.

The solid elements of blood, such as the RBC (red blood cells) and platelets, remain in the intravascular compartment. But other substances in solution and the WBC (white blood cells) move into the interstitial compartment. The white blood cells are able to change their shape and squeeze out of the blood vessels.

The composition of fluids in the three compartments is variable, depending on the tissue needs. Remember, the fluids are normally in continuous movement: from the bloodstream to the interstitial compartment, into the cells, back to the bloodstream, from the interstitial fluid through the vascular wall, or back to the blood by way of the lymph system. **Ischemia** (lack of blood to an area) results in hypoxia. Pypoxia, unrelieved, leads to anoxia. Anoxia, unrelieved, leads to **infarction** (death of the tissues).

The prefix, hemo or **hemato**, meaning blood, is used with a large number of medical terms. Look at the list below to review some of the more common ones:

hematology	study of blood
hemacyte	blood cell
hemoglobin	oxygen carrying pigment of blood
hemolymph	blood and lymph
hemolysis	rupturing of RBC

THE HEART

The heart is a four-chambered, hollow pump which propels the blood through the system of blood vessels. The heart is located in the pericardial sac in the anterior mediastinum.

The walls of the heart are muscular tissue (**myocardium**) with very special characteristics. This tissue, unlike other muscle tissue, can shorten or contract without nervous stimulation. This **intrinsic** (of internal origin) ability to contract is found only in this very special tissue. **Extrinsic** (external) nervous stimulation does alter the rate and rhythm of the contractions. The heart is lined with smooth epithelial tissue (**endothelium**) which is continuous with the lining of the blood vessels. It is divided into a right and left side by a septum. The upper chambers are the right and left **atrium** and the lower chambers are the right and left **ventricles**. The section called the **interventricu-**

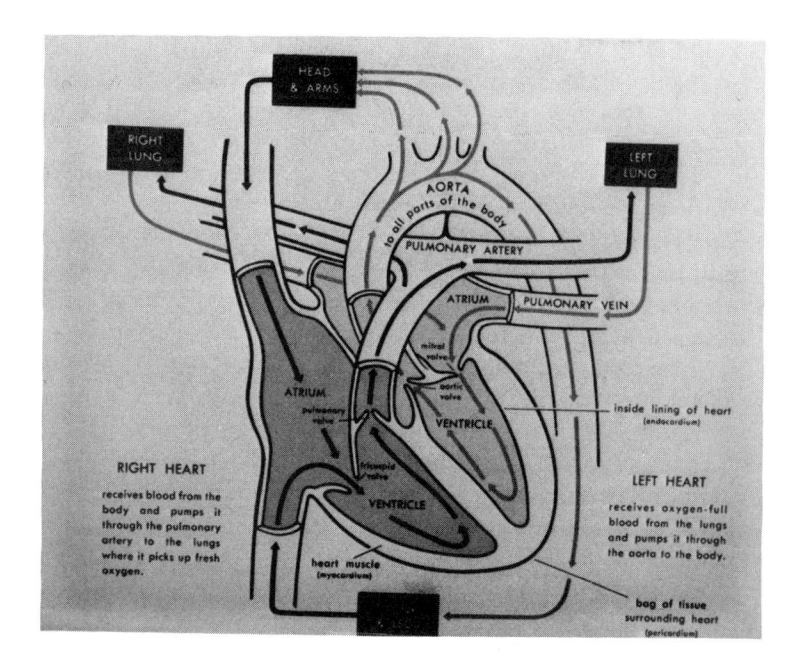

Figure 12-6: The heart is a four chambered pump (courtesy of The American Heart Association).

lar (between the ventricles) septum is much thicker than the one called the **interatrial** (between the two atria) septum. A small depression in the interatrial septum is called the **fossa ovale** (oval depression). It is the visible evidence that before birth the blood flowed from the right atrium to the left atrium through the **foramen** (opening) **ovale cordis**. Shortly after birth that fetal foramen closes, thus changing the direction of the major blood flow in the heart. Only a slight ditch or depression remains in the septum after the closing.

Valves (folds which temporarily close a passageway) separate the upper atrium from the lower ventricle on each side. The **tricuspid** valves (three cups or flaps) are found on the right side and the **metral** or **bicuspid** valves (two cups or flaps) are found on the left.

Large blood vessels enter the two atria and leave the two ventricles. The **superior vena cava** drains blood from the head, neck, and upper extremities. The **inferior vena cava** drains blood from the trunk and lower appendages. Both the superior vena cava (**SVC**) and the inferior vena cava (**IVC**) drain blood into the right atrium. At the same time, blood is returning from the lungs through the four **pulmonary** veins into the left atrium. The blood entering the right atrium is **deoxygenated** (oxygen lost) because it has given up part of its oxygen load to the tissues. The blood returning to the left atrium is well **oxygenated** (loaded with oxygen), since it has just picked up a fresh supply of oxygen in the lungs. These vessels are all **veins**, since they are returning blood to the heart. Blood leaving the heart is carried by blood vessels called **arteries**.

The blood flows from the two atria through the tricuspid and bicuspid valves into the right and left ventricles as the atria slightly contracts. From the right ventricle, blood flows out to the lungs through the **pulmonary artery**. From the left ventricle the blood is pumped into the **aorta** (largest artery) and out through its many branches to the body.

The entrance to the pulmonary artery and the aorta is guarded by a valve called the **semilunar** (half moon) valve. Like the tricuspid and metral valves, these valves prevent back flow of blood. The aortic semilunar valves and the pulmonary semilunar valves are each shaped like three solid half circles—or like the half moon from which they derive their name.

Figure 12-7: Cardiac circulation.

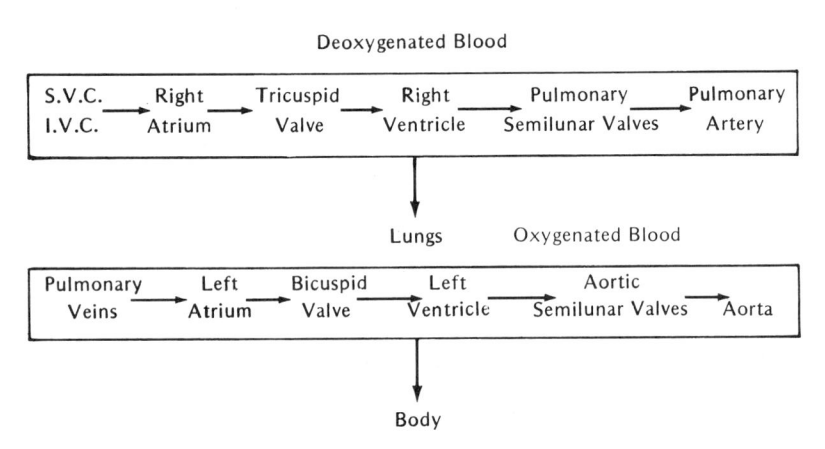

Deoxygenated Blood

S.V.C. / I.V.C. → Right Atrium → Tricuspid Valve → Right Ventricle → Pulmonary Semilunar Valves → Pulmonary Artery

↓

Lungs   Oxygenated Blood

Pulmonary Veins → Left Atrium → Bicuspid Valve → Left Ventricle → Aortic Semilunar Valves → Aorta

↓

Body

The Cardiac Cycle

The blood flows through the heart in a synchronated, rhythmic manner. The atria contract together, forcing the blood through the **atrioventricular valves** which open under pressure. The ventricles receive the blood and as they contract, the semilunar valves are forced open, while the atrioventricular valves close. Once the blood passes through the semilunar openings, these valves close, preventing back flow into the ventricles. Then the ventricles relax, ready to receive more blood from the atria. There is a short pause between the closing of the two sets of valves. The whole cycle normally lasts about eight-tenths of a second, and the valve closings give rise to the characteristic heart sounds of "lubb dubb." The louder, more pronounced sound, "lubb," occurs when the cuspid valves close and "dubb,"

* 200   *THE CARDIOVASCULAR SYSTEM*

the softer, more muffled sound, occurs at the closing of the semilunar valves.

The alternate contraction and relaxation of the atria and ventricles is called the **cardiac cycle**. The cardiac cycle occurs in response to intrinsic stimulation by special nodal tissue, located within the myocardium, and to extrinsic stimulation by nerves connected to the central nervous system. Without extrinsic stimulation, the cardiac cycle would reoccur about 70-80 times per minute. The normal cycle occurs up to 100 times per minute.

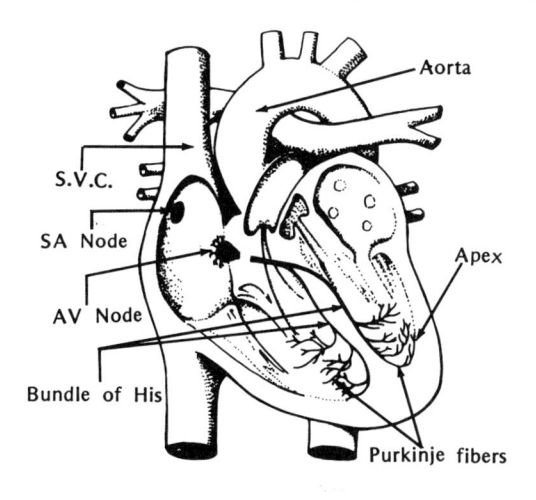

Figure 12-8: Cardiac conduction system.

Special neuromuscular tissue known as **nodal tissue**, directs the intrinsic rhythmicity of the cardiac cycle. This nodal tissue has characteristics of both nervous and muscular tissue. It is composed of the **sinoatrial mass (SA node)**, the **atrioventricular mass (AV node)**, the **bundle of His (interventricular bundle)**, and the **Purkinje fibers** (terminal fibers embedded in the myocardium).

Each part of the nodal tissue masses has its own intrinsic rate for sending out electrical impulses, but since the SA node has the fastest firing rate, it acts as the pace setter and is called the pacemaker. Impulses generated at the SA node, in the right atrium, spread across the atria and the atrial muscular tissue contracts in response. The impulses reach the AV node, also in the right atrium, close to the atrioventricular wall, and cause it to fire. That generates impulses through the bundle of His in the interventricular septum and out to the Purkinje fibers to the ventricular walls. The ventricles respond by contracting, forcing the blood through the semilunar valves. The electrocardiogram or ECG is a recording of this electrical activity.

The Heart's Conduction System

The tightening or pumping action of the ventricles is called ventricular **systole** (contraction) and relaxation or loosening action is known as ventricular **diastole**. Extrinsically, the **accelerator** (speed up) **nerve** stimulates more rapid firing of the SA and AV nodes during periods of physical or emotional stress so the heart beat becomes more rapid (**tachycardia**). After stress has diminished, impulses from another nerve, **the vargus**, slow the heart rate.

If the cardiac contraction rate drops below 60 **bpm** (beats per minute) in the female and 50 bpm in the male, it is known as **bradycardia** (slow heart action). When pathological changes prevent the nodal tissue from fulfilling its pacemaking activity, a condition called **heart block** results. Then an artificial pacemaker may have to be used. An electronic device, it can be implanted in the body (**intracorporeal**) near the heart under the chest muscles. Sometimes such an artificial pacemaker is worn strapped to the outside of the body (**extracorporeal**).

The **pulse** is the wave of pressure exerted against the walls of the arteries in response to ventricular systole. It can be felt as a series of recoils and expansions against the fingers if a person palpates an artery after lightly compressing it.

Figure 12-9: Intracorporeal pacemaker *(courtesy of Medtronic, Inc.)*.

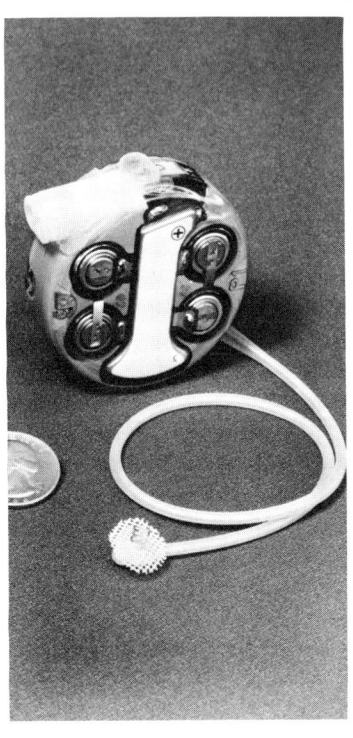

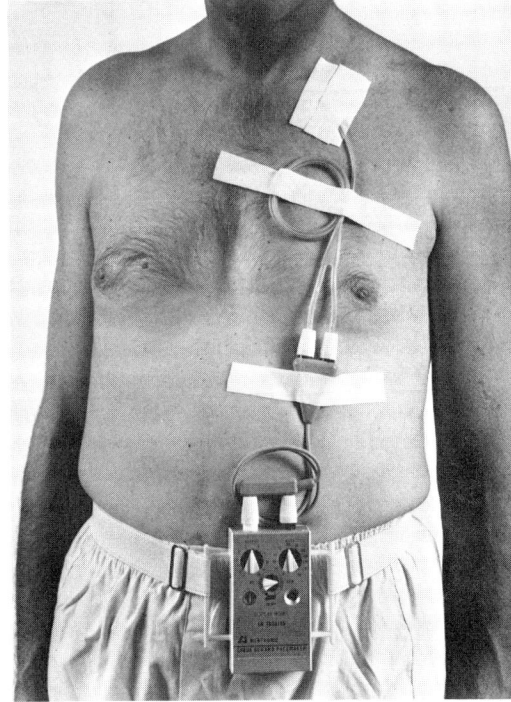

Figure 12-10: Extracorporeal pacemaker *(courtesy of Medtronic, Inc.)*.

The pulse may be felt this way each time the ventricles contract. Normally, the pulse rate is regular. Any cardiac irregularities are called **arrhythmias** and are reflected in the pulse. If the ventricular contraction is weak, it may not be perceived in a patient at the pulse site. That patient, therefore, has a pulse **deficit** (shortage or lack). To be accurately read, the pulse must be taken by placing a stethoscope over the pointed apex of the heart and listening to the closing of the valves to determine ventricular systole.

Blood Pressure

The force the blood exerts against the vascular walls is called the **blood pressure**. It is greatest when the ventricles contract and lowest when they relax. The arterial blood pressure is usually measured with an instrument called the **sphygmomanometer** (pulsation measurer). The most common site to obtain an arterial reading is the upper arm. The recording is made for the highest pressure reading (systolic) and lowest pressure reading (diastolic) and is usually written as B.P. 140 (systolic)/80 (diastolic). The measurement is calculated in millimeters (mm) of mercury pressure.

The average adult's blood pressure is 120/80 mm Hg. The difference between the systolic and diastolic reading is usually about 40 mm of mercury (Hg) pressure. This difference is known as the **pulse pressure**. Low blood pressure (**hypotension**) is an arterial pressure measuring below 100/70 mm Hg. High blood pressure or hypertension is an arterial blood pressure measuring 140/90 or higher. The blood pressure in the major veins can also be measured. Measurement of blood pressure in a large vein such as the inferior vena cava is called **Central Venous Pressure**. It, CVP, is a very significant factor in certain cardiac diseases.

THE VASCULATURE

A vast network of blood vessels serve the tissue needs and supply the pathways for the blood and lymph. Several types of vessels make up the vascular network. **Arteries** lead from the heart, branch out to become just smaller **arterioles** and then **capillaries**. It is at the capillary level that the vital exchanges take place. The capillaries in turn drain into larger vessels (**venules**) and then still larger vessels, veins. The veins drain back into the heart. **Lymphatic capillaries** drain into lymph vessels, into blood carrying veins, and back to the heart. One difference between the two kinds of blood vessels is the direction of fluid flow; another is in their anatomy.

The Arteries

The arteries have three walls or coverings (**tunica**). The innermost or **tunica intima** is ultra-smooth epithelial tissue; the

Figure 12-11: Major arteries and veins. Can you tell how some were named? *(courtesy of Ethicon, Inc.)*.

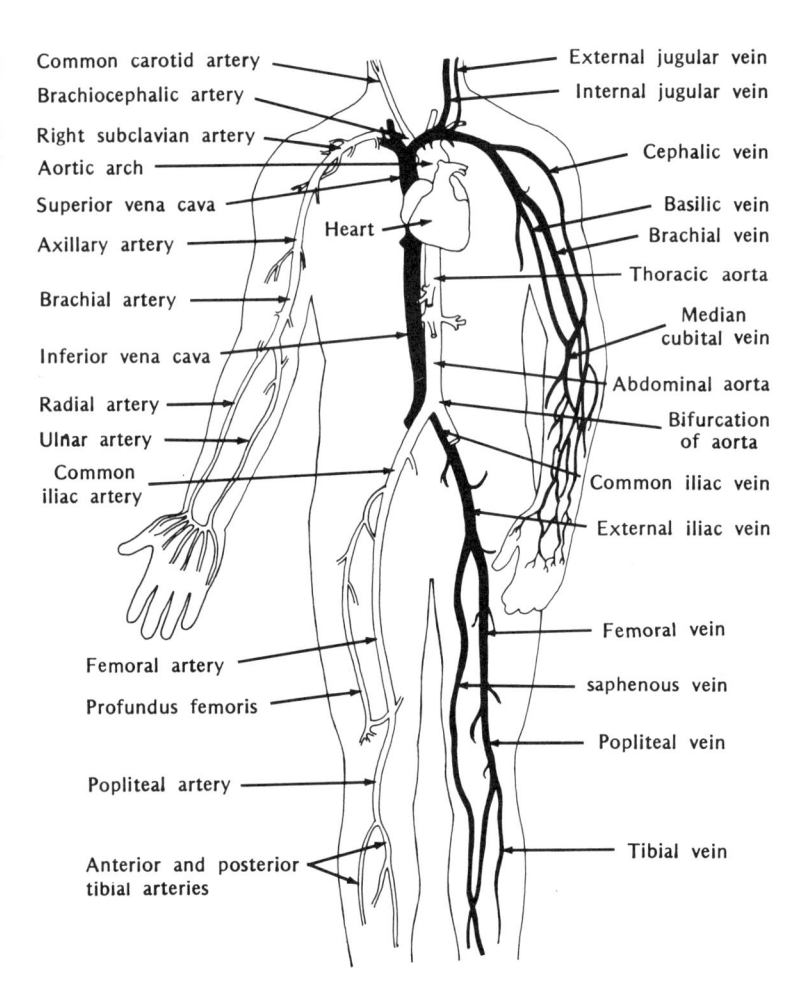

middle muscular layer is the **tunica media**; and the outer layer is the **tunica adventitia** (outer coat). Veins have the same layers but the tunica media is thinner and, within some of the larger veins, the tunica intima forms valves.

Arteries depend on the recoil ability of the thick tunica media and the propelling force of the ventricular systole to keep the blood moving. Gravity also assists most of the largest arteries to carry blood. The veins lack these advantages and aids to blood flow. Since venal blood flows upward mainly, they carry most of the blood against gravity, lack heavy muscular walls, and must depend on the pressure of adjacent muscles and their valves to keep the blood moving forward and up toward the heart.

An inflammation of the veins is called **phlebitis**. A major danger associated with phlebitis is that the inflammatory process roughens the normally smooth vascular lining. And that rough endothelium predisposes to clot formation. A thrombus could **occlude** (block) a blood vessel, but an even greater danger is the possibility that a part of the thrombus will break off and form an **embolus** (moving clot) that could lodge in the lungs (**pulmonary embolism**). A pulmonary embolism prevents adequate **perfusion** (blood flow) of the lungs. Pulmonary embolism has a relatively high mortality rate. It is sometimes necessary to withdraw blood to examine its composition. Withdrawal of blood from a vein is done by **venipuncture**.

The lymphatic vessels are similar to the veins and have valves. Remember the lymph nodes are found along their course. The capillaries have the thinnest walls of all. They are only 0.01 mm in diameter; just big enough to allow the erythrocytes to pass through them one at a time.

Some day you will want to learn the names of all the major blood vessels and all the major circulatory patterns. Three major circulatory patterns or pathways are: the vessels forming the cerebral circulation or the **Circle of Willis**, the collection of vessels draining the digestive tract or the **portal system**, and the vessels of coronary circulation which nourish the myocardium itself. Two branches, the right and left coronary arteries, pass from the aorta, supply the myocardium, and drain into the right atrium through the **coronary sinus**, a vein on the posterior heart.

Blood vessels are frequently named for the bone or body area close to them or to the body area being served. So arteries and veins serving an area frequently have the same name. For example, the ulnar artery and ulnar vein are found close to the ulna bone of the forearm, while the subclavian artery and vein are found beneath the clavicle. Study the lists below to learn the names and general location of the major arteries.

These are examples of blood vessels named for adjacent bones:

Figure 12-12: In a venipuncture, blood is withdrawn from a vein *(courtesy of Sherwood Medical Industries).*

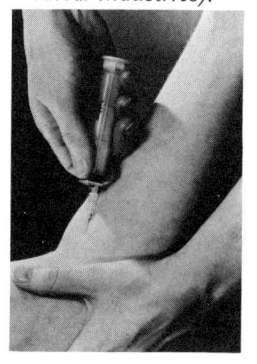

Name
Blood Vessels

	Bone
femoral	femur
iliac	ilium
sacral	sacrum
radial	radius
tibial	tibia

THE VASCULATURE 205

These are examples of blood vessels named for organs served:

	Organ
renal	kidney
ovarian	ovary
splenic	spleen
hepatic	liver
gastric	stomach

These are examples of blood vessels named for body areas:

	Body Area
facial	face
brachial	upper arm
axillary	axilla
lumbar	loin
intercostal	between the ribs

Figure 12-13: Coronary circulation: the main coronary arteries and their many branches come down over the top of the heart carrying oxygenated blood to the myocardium (courtesy of The American Heart Association).

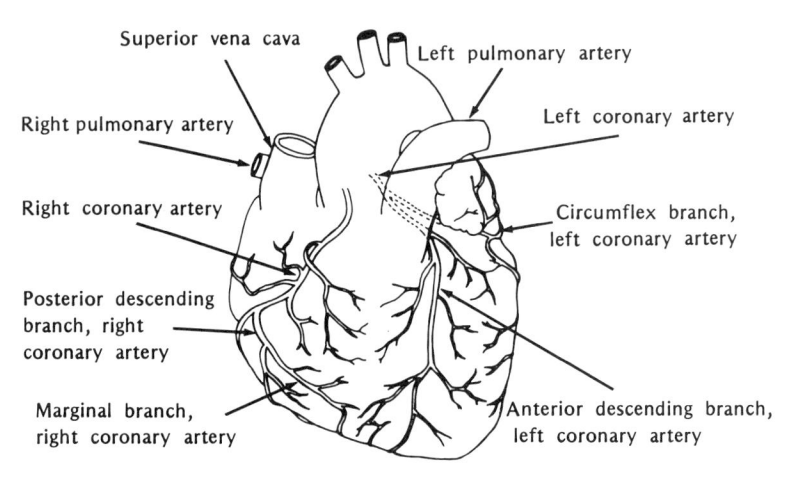

The smaller lymphatic vessels all drain into two large lymphatic vessels. These are the **thoracic duct** which carries lymph from the left side of the body, right trunk and leg into the left subclavian vein and the **right lymphatic duct** which carries lymph from the right side of the head, neck, right arm, and shoulder into the right subclavian vein.

* 206 *THE CARDIOVASCULAR SYSTEM*

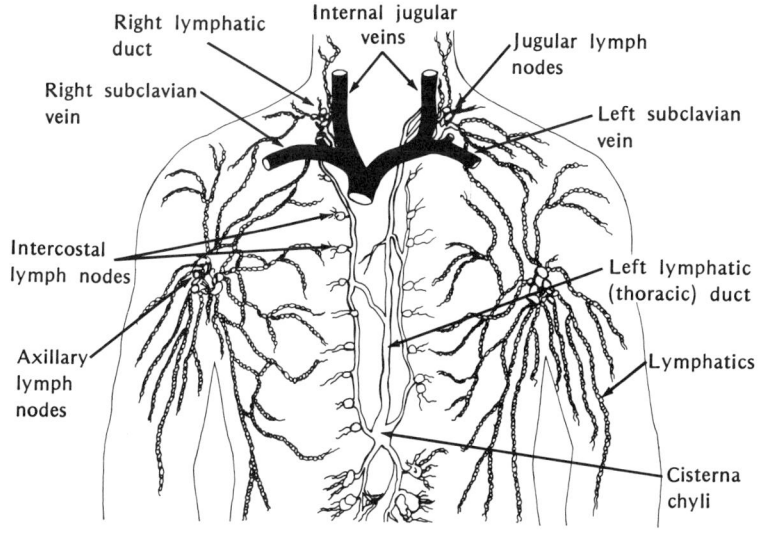

Figure 12-14: Lymph vascular system: tissue fluids gathered all over the body by the lymph system are emptied into the bloodstream at the junction of the internal jugular and subclavian viens, right and left *(courtesy of Ethicon, Inc.).*

Cardio- is a prefix used to describe the heart and is used in multiple combinations. Study the following terms. You will recall some of the combining forms and some will be new.

cardiac arrest	heart stoppage
cardiodynia	pain in heart region
cardiomegaly	hypertrophy of the heart
cardiorrhexis	rupture of the heart
cardiotoxic	poisonous to the heart
cardiopathy	morbid heart condition
cardiogenic	pertaining to the heart
cardiograph	instrument for recording heart movements
cardiologist	heart specialist
cardialgia	painful sensation in the anterior chest or upper abdomen; heartburn

CASE STUDY

Name: Estes, R.
Diagnosis: Myocardial Infarction
History: 48 year-old married man, father of four daughters, counselor for a large investment firm.

The patient had been in apparent good health until 1958 when his physician diagnosed moderate hypertension. His blood pressure was 156/110, p. 92. His blood tests revealed an elevated cholesterol and triglycerate level (composed of cholesterol and triglycerides, fatty substances found in the plasma). At that time, because of his age, sex, history of hypertension, and hematology findings, Mr. Estes was considered at risk for atherosclerosis, which is another name for hardening of the arteries.

The therapeutic regime prescribed for the patient included antihypertensive drugs and a diet low in saturated fats. He was advised to stop smoking, maintain his current adequate weight level, and to make an effort to alter his life style to lower the tension levels. For several years, Mr. Estes lived a successful life in relative health. In 1966, there was a marked deterioration of his condition.

On Thanksgiving Day of that year, after a particularly heavy meal, Mr. Estes complained of cardiodynia and shortness of breath. He was seen in the Emergency Room of City Hospital where his condition was diagnosed as **angina pectoris** (temporary cardiac ischemia) or transitory ischemia attack (**TIA**). His blood pressure had risen and he was admitted as an in-patient to the I.C.C. unit of the hospital for observation and treatment. His physician called in a cardiologist as a consultant to assess the cardiac status.

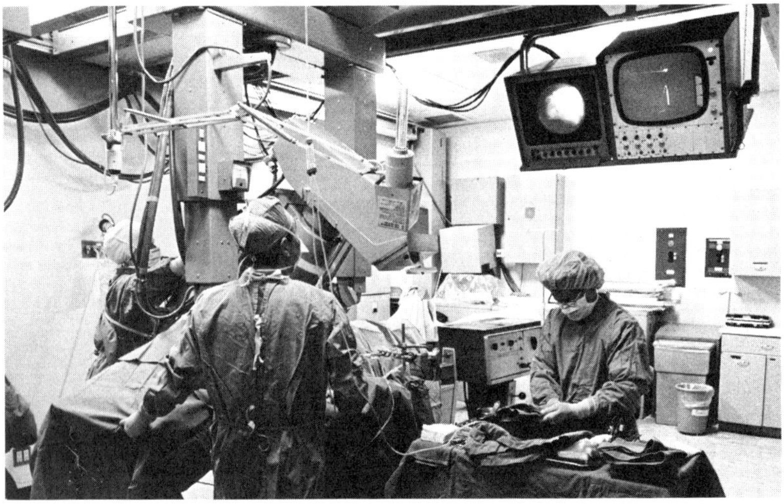

Figure 12-15: Cardiac catheterization: as the catheter is passed into the femoral vein and into the heart, the cardiac surgeon monitors it's progress on the screen overhead.

The cardiologist performed an **arteriogram** (artery X-ray). He also introduced a small catheter through the femoral vein and threaded it up into the heart. (This procedure, called a **cardiac catheterization**, aids in making a diagnosis of cardiac pathology.) In this instance, the diagnostic tests revealed partial occlusion of the right coronary artery and almost complete occlusion of one branch of the left coronary artery.

Bypass surgery was advised for Mr. Estes. This type of surgery creates an alternate route of blood vessels to carry blood around an obstructed area. The surgery was performed successfully the first week of December, 1966. Blood vessels were removed from Mr. Estes' leg and placed in his heart. They were **anastomosed** (interconnected) with the coronary vessels above and below the occluded areas. During convalescence the patient was advised that this bypass surgery would supply his ischemic myocardium with blood and, although dietary control and antihypertensive drugs could help, the advanced atherosclerosis was progressive. His prognosis was considered guarded.

In early 1968, the Emergency Medical Technicians were called to Mr. Estes' home because he was complaining of severe substernal pain, nausea, and shortness of breath. By the time the technicians arrived, Mr. Estes was in cardiac arrest. The paramedics attempted to revive him with cardiopulmonary resuscitation (CPR) but he was **moribund** (dying). Mr. Estes was pronounced Dead on Arrival (**DOA**) when he was brought to the hospital emergency room.

Post Mortem (after death) Diagnosis: Myocardial Infarction.

Contributing Factors: Hypertension and Atherosclerosis.

SUMMARY

The cardiovascular system, composed of the body fluids and vessels, serves as the transportation system for the body. Because it is subject to high levels of stress, pathology of the system is the cause of many major health problems.

PRACTICE & *Explain and define the new special terms you have been using. Remember,*
REVIEW *you learned how to pronounce them at the beginning of this chapter.*

1. arrhythmias _____
2. cardiomegaly _____
3. extracorporeal _____
4. infarction _____
5. granulocytes _____
6. lymphadenitis _____
7. megakaryocytes _____
8. phlebitis _____
9. sphygmomanometer _____
10. vasculature _____

Now, double-check the meaning of the terms above by studying the brief definitions given in the Glossary-Index at the back of this text.

Test yourself quickly before going on to learn other medical and professional terms. Use these short review exercises to practice for your new work in health services. Your teacher will also help by recommending various other Study Activities.

A. In this list the prefix "cardio-" is common to all the terms. Complete them by adding the proper ending after you read the definitions:

1. hypertrophy of the heart   cardio _____
2. rupture of the heart   cardio _____
3. poisonous to the heart   cardio _____
4. morbid heart condition   cardio _____
5. pertaining to the heart   cardio _____

B. In the following ten sentences, circle the number of the false statements. Remember to consider carefully their meaning in relation to the new terms you learned in this chapter:

1. The pointed portion of the heart is called its *apex*.
2. *Phlebitis* means an inflammation of a vein.
3. The *sphygmomanometer* is an instrument used to measure the temperature.
4. The *tricuspid valve* between the right atrium and left atrium has two cusps.

5. An *intracorporeal* pacemaker is strapped to the outside of the body.
6. A person with *cardiac arrest* is suffering from heart stoppage.
7. *Bradycardia* means a greatly increased heart rate.
8. A *pulse deficit* occurs when there is a difference between the cardiac rate and pulse rate.
9. *Basophils* are named because they take a neutral stain.
10. Leukemia, a serious blood condition, is considered a blood *dyscrasia*.

C. Match the words on the right with the best statement on the left:

____ 1. Low blood pressure	a. anemia
____ 2. Heart pain	b. cardiodynia
____ 3. Blood with too few RBC or too little hemoglobin	c. cardialgia
	d. hemorrhage
____ 4. Blood clot	e. aorta
____ 5. The name of the largest artery	f. fossa ovale
____ 6. Means escape of blood	g. hypotension
____ 7. Meaning of internal origin	h. hypertension
____ 8. An oval depression between the atria	i. thrombus
____ 9. Another name for the sinoatrial node	j. heart block
____ 10. Condition due to a failure in the conduction system	k. intrinsic
	l. pacemaker

After studying Chapter 13

The Endocrine System

You should be able to:

* *Pronounce and define each of its new medical words and phrases and use the new technical jargon.*

* *Identify the major structures of the endocrine system.*

* *Name five hormones produced by the endocrine glands.*

MEDICAL WORDS   PRONOUNCE THESE TEN NEW WORDS WITH YOUR TEACHER:

adenohypophysis (ad″ĕ-no-hi-pof′ĭ-sĭs)
diuresis (di′u-re′sis)
glycosuria (gli″ko-su′re-ah)
menses (men′sēz)
polydipsia (pol″e-dip′se-ah)

puberty (pu′ber-te)
suprarenally (soo″prah-re′nah-lĭ)
hypoglycemia (hi″po-gli-se′me-ah)
pancreas (pan′kre-as)
ketosis (ke″to′sis)

ENDOCRINE GLANDS   The endocrine system is composed of a number of glands and cells scattered throughout the body. They interact with one another and with the various tissues of the body to maintain homeostasis.

Endocrine (internally secreting) **glands** are ductless glands. This is one of the characteristics that distinguishes them from exocrine glands, such as the sudoriferous glands of the skin. They have ducts which lead to (exit) the skin surface; the endocrine glands do not. Endocrine glands are highly vascular and depend upon the blood stream to carry their secretions called hormones throughout the body. The endocrine glands pour their secretions directly into the blood stream. This is another difference between exocrine and endocrine glands. Exocrine glands depend on their ducts for dispersion of their secretions but the endocrine glands depend on the circulatory system.

Histology of Endocrine Glands   Histologically, endocrine glands are epithelial cells held together by connective tissue. These secretory cells produce hormones. **Hormones**, chemical substances produced by the endocrine glands, are **synthesized** (produced) by the glandular cells from substances extracted from the blood stream. Hormones act as chemical stimulators which influence the activity of other cells or organs in the body. For example, the **Follicular Stimulating Hormone (FSH)** is produced by the cells of one endocrine gland, the pituitary, and stimulates changes in the tissues of another endocrine gland, the ovary.

Hormones sometimes inhibit an activity in the body although the word hormone literally means "to incite." In general, through hormones the endocrine glands control **metabolism** (cellular chemistry), the rate of growth and development, and the degree of sexual maturity. An organ directly affected by a hormone is called a **target organ** for that hormone. The target organ for FSH is the ovary.

The rising levels of a particular hormone have a depressing effect on the gland producing the hormone. In this way, hormones are maintained at fairly constant levels. The activities that the hormones promote are controlled by the same method. These hormone-producing glands also interact with one another.

Two systems, the nervous system and the endocrine system, are primarily responsible for the maintenance of homeostasis. The nervous system brings about an immediate response in the target organs. The endocrine system brings about a slower but longer lasting response. The two systems act in harmony with one another. How this is accomplished is rather complex. Two endocrine glands, the pituitary and the adrenals, act as **transducers** (organs in which nervous energy becomes chemical energy), or common organs for the two systems. Their dual role assists in the coordination of the two systems.

The endocrine glands are scattered throughout the body. Several, such as the adrenal glands, are duplicates. Study the figure and Table 13-1 to learn the names and locations of some of the endocrine glands. (p. 212.)

Endocrine Location

The pituitary gland is frequently called the master gland because of the wide ranging affect of its numerous hormones. It is about the size of a cherry. The pituitary gland is, however, not an independent organ. It releases the hormones it secretes upon chemical command from the brain. In fact, the pituitary gland or **hypophysis** is made up of two lobes and a central part, each with its own secretions.

The anterior lobe secretes a number of hormones and is known as the **adenohypophysis** (glandular pituitary). The posterior lobe is called the **neurohypophysis** (nervous pituitary). One of the secretions of the neurohypophysis is the antidiuretic

Figure 13-1: The male and female endocrine system. Endocrine glands secrete some hormones vital to life and others which exert profound influence on all man's activities and metabolic processes *(courtesy of Ethicon, Inc.).*

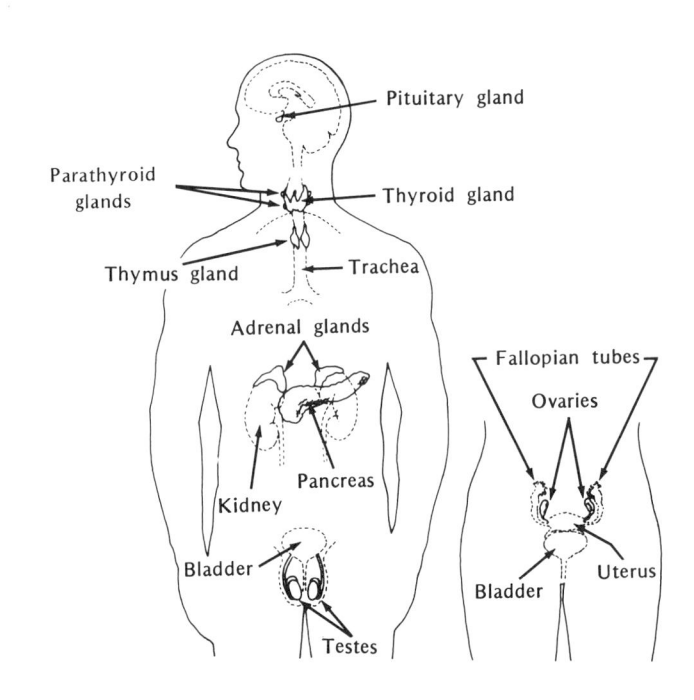

Table 13-1

Endocrine Gland	Anatomical Location
pituitary gland	cranial cavity inferior brain surface
thyroid gland	anterior neck, near the thyroid cartilage
parathyroid glands	embedded in posterior thyroid gland
adrenal gland	retroperitoneal space on top of kidneys
ovaries	female pelvis
testes	scrotal sac
Alpha & Beta cells (Islets of Langerhans)	pancreas

hormone (against **diuresis** or urine secretion). The **antidiuretic hormone** (ADH) is really produced in a portion of the brain called the **hypothalamus** (under the thalamus). ADH is stored in the neurohypophysis and liberated from this site.

The diagram in Figure 13-2 shows some of the relationships of the pituitary gland, the hypothalamus and the thyroid gland. As you can see, many of the hormones are identified by letters. For example, ADH is the antidiuretic hormone, TSH is

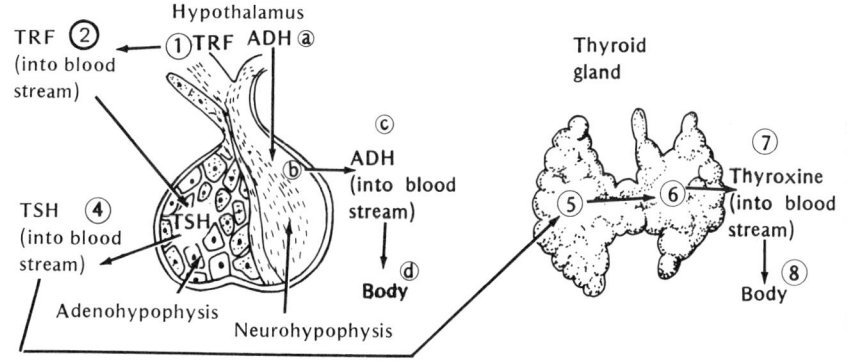

Figure 13-2:
Follow the arrows to see some of the relationships between the hypothalamus, pituitary gland and the thyroid gland and the formation and release of ADH.

the **thyrotropic stimulating hormone**, and TRF is the **thyrotropin releasing factor**.

As you study the diagram you will note that the hypothalamus secretes a hormone, TRF, that is released into the blood stream in response to lowered levels of thyroxine. The TRF is carried to the adenohypophysis where its presence stimulates the cells of the anterior pituitary to secrete the hormone, TSH. The thyrotropic stimulating hormone is secreted into the vasculature and carried to the thyroid gland. The cells of the thyroid gland produce the hormone **thyroxine** which is released into the blood stream. Thyroxine affects the metabolic rate of the body, influencing the amount of oxygen used, the rate nutrients are utilized, the waste products produced, and the rate of growth and maturity achieved.

The **gonads** (the testes) and the ovaries serve a dual function. They produce the gametes and also secrete the hormones responsible for the development of secondary sex characteristics. Those hormones release directly into the bloodstream. The male secondary sex characteristics appear at **puberty**, when the male primary sex organs (the penis, testes, and scrotum) mature and become sexually active.

The testes promote this maturation by releasing the hormone **testosterone**. The male secondary sex characteristics include increased musculature, growth of body hair, especially in the axillary, pubic and facial areas, and the deepening of the voice.

The female secondary sex characteristics also appear at puberty. Two hormones, **estrogen** and **progesterone**, are secreted by the ovaries. The female secondary sex characteristics include growth of hair in the axillary and pubic areas, rounding of body contours, breast development, and the onset of **menses** (menstruation).

The adrenal glands, positioned on top of the kidneys (suprarenally) in the retroperitoneal space, are composed of an

ENDOCRINE GLANDS 215 *

Figure 13-3: Follow the numbers and letters to learn the dual stimulation the adrenal gland receives and to learn how the gland responds.

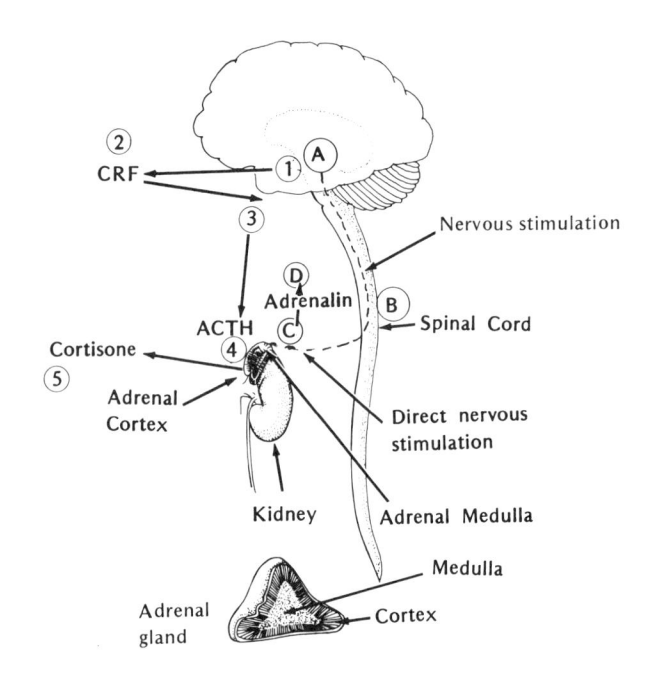

inner portion or **medulla**, and an outer portion or **cortex**. The adrenal medulla develops in the embryo as an extension of the ectoderm so it is formed from tissue similar to nervous tissue. It secretes a group of hormones, one of which, **adrenalin**, augments the nervous system activity.

The cells of the cortex secrete a large number of hormones which influence body metabolism, sexual functioning, and the body's ability to cope with stress. The adrenal medulla gets direct stimulation from the nervous system from which it extends.

The adrenal cortex receives stimulation indirectly from the nervous system. When needed, a **corticotropin releasing factor** (CRF), is sent from the brain to the anterior pituitary gland via the blood stream. In response, ACTH (**adrenocorticotropic hormone**) is released from the anterior pituitary into the blood stream and carried to the adrenal cortex. By this indirect method the adrenal cortex is stimulated to secrete the cortical hormones. There are a large number of these cortical hormones of which **cortisone** is an example.

The **pancreas**, a long, soft gland, is found in the peritoneal cavity. The pancreas is an organ (**viscera**) which produces both endocrine and exocrine secretions. Some of the endocrine cells clustered in the pancreas are called alpha cells. These alpha cells produce the hormone, **glucagon**. Glucagon increases the level of the sugar glucose in the blood stream by causing stored glucose (**glycogen**) to break down into blood glucose. Beta cells are also found in clusters or aggregates in the pancreas. They produce the hormone, **insulin**. Insulin is needed in the body in order for the tissue cells to use glucose as an energy source. Its presence lowers the levels of circulating glucose. These two hormones, insulin and glucagon, are the principal regulators of blood sugar levels.

The parathyroid glands are embedded in the posterior thyroid gland. There are a variable number of these glands; usually around 4-8 parathyroid masses can be found. The parathyroid glands secrete a hormone called **parathyroid hormone** (PTH) which influences the levels of **calcium** (Ca) and **phosphorus** (P). Calcium and phosphorus are elements which form important electrolytes in the body. The electrolytes, or salts, of calcium and phosphorus are important in bone formation, and proper muscle and nerve functioning.

The relationship of the hormones and body activities is very complex. As you continue your medical studies, you will want to learn more about this fascinating subject. Use Table 13-2 to review some of the specific hormones produced by the pituitary and their general affects.

Table 13-2

Pituitary Hormones	*General Function*
Somatotropic Hormone (STH)	stimulates growth
Lactogenic Hormone (Prolactin)	stimulates lactation
Follicular Stimulating Hormone (FSH)	stimulates growth of ovarian follicle
Lutenizing Hormone (LH)	promotes ovulation in the female
Interstitial Cell Stimulating Hormone (ICSH)	stimulates testes in the male to produce sperm
Thyrotropic Stimulating Hormone (TSH)	stimulates thyroid gland
Adrenocortiocotropic Hormone (ACTH)	stimulates adrenal gland
Antidiuretic Hormone (ADH)	stimulates kidneys to retain water

Endocrine Pathology

Pathology involving the endocrine glands results from either overproduction of the hormone (hypersecretion) or underproduction **hyposecretion**. Obviously the hypersecretion of STH in a child is related to that condition called **giantism** which may cause an individual to grow to as much as eight feet in height (approximately 234 centimeters). Hyposecretion of that same hormone in a child results in **dwarfism**. The result is an elfin-like adult—a pituitary dwarf of abnormally small stature.

Many abnormal secretory levels, whether hypersecretion or hyposecretion, are the result of neoplasia. Some neoplasms destroy the normal secretory cells and the gland becomes hyposecretory. Other neoplasia result in the formation of an excess number of secretory cells. Then the gland becomes hypersecretory and puts out excess hormone levels.

To learn the pathologies associated with the endocrine glands, first review what the normal secretions achieve. Then relate hypersecretion with excessive or premature development of those activities, and hyposecretion with inadequate functioning of those tissues normally stimulated.

Take, for example, estrogen and testosterone; the two hormones responsible for development of female and male secondary sex characteristics. Hyposecretion of these two hormones would mean delayed sexual maturity for the girl or boy reaching the normal age of puberty. Hypersecretion would mean that the signs of sexual maturity would appear very early in children. We might, for example, have a five-year old girl menstruating and an eight-year old boy with facial hair and a deep voice.

Look at Table 13-3 to see four pathologies related to the pituitary and thyroid glands.

Diabetes Mellitus

One of the major endocrine pathologies seen today is diabetes mellitus. In this disease, the pathology exists in the cells of the pancreas. The etiology of diabetes mellitus is not fully understood but there is a hyposecretion of insulin which controls blood sugar levels.

This inadequate production of insulin results in **hyperglycemia** (excess blood sugar). Remember, the blood sugar level must be properly controlled since the tissue cells need a constant supply to produce energy. Normally the body's insulin exerts this control in three important ways: first, its presence makes it possible for glucose to pass from the blood through the cell wall into the cell; second, it must also be present for the cells to use the glucose once it enters the cell; third, it promotes the storage of excess glucose as glycogen in the liver. In these three ways, adequate amounts of insulin control and maintain the level of blood glucose normally.

But the hyposecretion of insulin results in a dangerous

Table 13-3

Gland	Hormone	Hypersecretion	Hyposecretion
pituitary	ADH		*Diabetes Insipidus* (normally this hormone prevents excess fluid loss, so inadequate amounts result in excessive urine output; in addition to the abundance of urine produced, essential salts are also lost; a relatively rare but very serious condition)
	STH	*Acromegaly* (abnormal condition resulting from overproduction of the growth hormone after maturity, resulting in excessively large jaws, hands and feet in the adult)	
thyroid	thyroxine	*Exopthalmic Goiter* (overproduction of thyroxine increases the activity of tissues normally stimulated by the thyroid so the *BMR* (*Basal Metabolic Rate*) or rate at which oxygen is consumed increases and the patient experiences tachycardia and hypertension, with weight loss; characteristically the eyes protrude, hence the name *exopthalmic* or out eyes goiter)	*Myxedema* (inadequate production of thyroxin in the adult slows down all metabolic processes and the patient is lethargic or drowsy and functionally sluggish; mentally he becomes dull and his skin becomes very dry; improvement is rapid once drug therapy is started)

ENDOCRINE GLANDS 219

accumulation of glucose in the blood stream because it cannot enter the cells, cannot be utilized by the cells, and cannot be stored. Since the cells cannot utilize needed sugar, they turn to another nutrient, fats. The cells then produce excess acid since they cannot store fats properly. In the process, acid byproducts accumulate in the blood stream. This upsets the homeostasis of the body. If the situation is unrelieved, the patient gradually slips into **acidosis** (an acid state) and loses consciousness and is in a diabetic coma.

Diabetic coma is known as acidosis or **ketosis**, since some of the acid which accumulates in the blood are ketones such as **acetone**. Diabetic coma is the coma of severe diabetic or acidosis or ketoacidosis. Excessive numbers of ketones accumulate in both the body fluids and tissues. These excess sugar and acid substances are carried out of the body with the urine. The amounts of these substances found in the urine are good indicators of the amount accumulating in the blood stream.

The symptoms of diabetes mellitus include loss of weight and fatigue and, since the cells are deprived of their normal nutrition, excessive hunger (**polyphagia**), excessive thirst (**polydipsia**), and excessive urine output (**polyuria**). Frequently, the healing of even minor infections is retarded and excessive sugar can be found in the blood and urine (**glycosuria**).

Treatment consists of monitoring sugar levels and balancing food intake. Sometimes the patient must also take a medical preparation of insulin which must be injected. Insulin must be given in extremely small amounts and is usually injected into the subcutaneous fat layer. Patients who use it must be taught to be constantly on the alert for the signs of hypoglycemia and hyperglycemia.

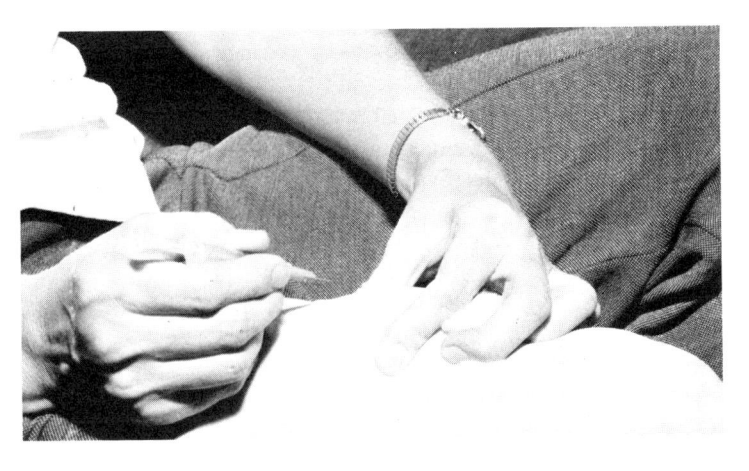

Figure 13-4: Injection of insulin.

Hypoglycemia or low blood sugar is also very serious and can lead to insulin shock. **Insulin shock** occurs either when there is too much insulin or too little sugar in the blood. Anxiety, pallor, sweating and rapid pulse are common symptoms prior to loss of consciousness. Therefore most diabetics carry some easily assimilated sugar to alleviate these conditions and prevent insulin shock which is very dangerous. Both hyperglycemia and hypoglycemia can be fatal if steps are not immediately taken to reinstate the homeostasis. Now read the case history of a person who has diabetes mellitus.

CASE STUDY

Peggy Anderson, age 58, a somewhat obese lady, was first seen by her physician when she appeared complaining of excessive fatigue. She had always been very active and liked to play tennis. But now she found herself exhausted after just one set. She admitted experiencing polyphagia, polydipsia, and polyuria. Weight gain had always been a problem, but, recently she had lost several pounds without conscious effort.

She had a low-grade vaginal infection but did not associate it with her present problem or even think to mention it to her physician until questioned about excoriations noted during the routine vaginal examination. After the general physical, the physician requested a urine specimen which he gave to the office assistant to test. The urine tests for acetone and for sugar revealed a glucosuria and moderate level of acetone. Miss Anderson was admitted to the hospital for additional diagnostic tests, including **Fasting Blood Sugar (FBS)** and **Glucose Tolerance** (G.T.T.) tests. These are two tests of blood glucose levels. Findings in both cases were positive for diabetes mellitus.

The therapeutic regime prescribed for the patient included a diet balanced in fats, protein and carbohydrates. It was designed to control weight reduction. Insulin was ordered to replace the missing hormones. Moderate exercise was sanctioned.

Insulin has to be taken according to a scale. The amount given, or in Miss Anderson's case, taken, would depend upon her ability to utilize sugar in her body. Since excess sugar is "**spilled over**" (excreted) in the urine, Miss Anderson had to learn to perform the same urine testing that the office nurse had done on the initial visit. In this way she would know what doses of insulin she had to take in order to restore the correct balance to her system.

After a period of hospitalization during which the patient's condition was stabilized, she was discharged. She was referred to the Diabetic Clinic to be followed as an out-patient.

SUMMARY

The endocrine system is composed of a series of widely scattered organs and cells which secrete hormones. Hormones are chemicals which influence body activities. There is a great interaction between the endocrine glands and their secretions. One very serious and common endocrine pathology is diabetes mellitus.

PRACTICE & REVIEW

Explain and define the new special terms you have been using. Remember, you learned how to pronounce them at the beginning of this chapter.

1. adenohypophysis _____
2. diuresis _____
3. glycosuria _____
4. menses _____
5. polydipsia _____
6. puberty _____
7. suprarenally _____
8. hypoglycemia _____
9. pancreas _____
10. ketosis _____

Now, double-check the meaning of the terms above by studying the brief definitions given in the Glossary-Index at the back of this text.

Test yourself quickly before going on to learn other medical and professional terms. Use these short review exercises to practice for your new work in health services. Your teacher will also help by recommending various other Study Activities.

A. Complete the ten statements below with the best word from this list:

glucagon polyphagia adrenalin
somatotrophic hypersecretion cortisone
polydipsia glycogen Luteinizing
hyposecretion lactogenic thyroid

1. Sugar is stored in the body in the form of _____.
2. The pancreas produces two hormones, insulin and _____.
3. Excessive hunger often associated with diabetes mellitus is called _____.
4. The letters L.H. are used to denote the _____ hormone.
5. A hormone produced by the medulla of the adrenal gland is called _____.
6. An underproduction of a hormone is called _____.
7. Another name for the growth hormone produced by the pituitary gland is the _____ hormone.
8. Excessive thirst is called _____.
9. The gland located in the anterior neck near the larynx is the _____ gland.
10. Overproduction of a hormone is called _____.

B. Many hormones are identified by letters. Write the proper name beside each of the letter abbreviations for the name of the hormone:

1. STH _____
2. LH _____
3. TH _____
4. ACTH _____
5. ADH _____

C. Match the words on the right with the best statement on the left:

____ 1. Male sex hormone produced by the testes
____ 2. Sugar in the urine
____ 3. Excessive urine output
____ 4. Collective name for the ovaries and testes
____ 5. Hormone produced by the ovaries
____ 6. Another name for the pituitary gland
____ 7. The age of sexual maturity
____ 8. Cellular chemistry
____ 9. Chemicals secreted by the endocrine glands
____ 10. Organ which secretes insulin

a. hormones
b. transducer
c. metabolism
d. puberty
e. polyuria
f. testosterone
g. estrogen
h. hypophysis
i. glycosuria
j. gonads
k. pancreas
l. thyrotropic

ENDOCRINE GLANDS 223 *

After studying Chapter 14

The Nervous System

You should be able to:

* *Pronounce and define each of its new medical words and phrases and use the new technical jargon.*

* *Identify the major structures of the nervous system.*

* *Describe the function of the nervous system.*

MEDICAL WORDS   PRONOUNCE THESE TEN NEW WORDS WITH YOUR TEACHER:

cerebrum (ser'ĕ-brum)
diplopia (di-plo'pe-ah)
encephalosclerosis
  (en-sef"ah-lo-sklĕ-ro'sis)
flaccid (flak'sid)
gustation (gus-ta'shun)

mastication (mas"ti-ka'shun)
myelodiastasis (mi"ĕ-lo-di-as'tah-sis)
neuroma (nu-ro'mah)
proprioceptors (pro"pre-o-sep'tors)
sciatica (si-at'i-kah)

The nervous system is a highly complex network of nervous tissues which functions to maintain homeostasis and to carry out those functions such as thinking, which distinguishes man from other beings. It is in this tissue that sensory perceptions are integrated and motor responses are initiated. **Sensory perceptions** (awareness) originate both internally within the organs and externally through complex receptors such as the eye and ear. Sensory perceptions keep the brain constantly aware of internal and external changes.

Cells, tissues and organs within the body respond instantly to the command of the nerve impulse. Nervous tissue is so specialized that it is found only within the brain and spinal cord and in the multitudinous branches of the peripheral nerves leading to and from these central structures.

The Neuron   You have learned that the basic cell of bone tissue is the osteocyte. The basic cell of nervous tissue is called the **neuron**. Supporting nerve cells form the **neuroglia**.

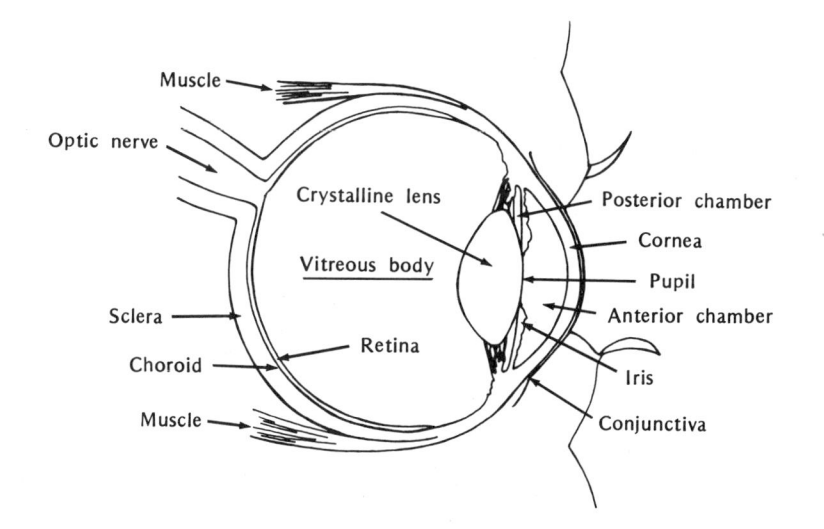

Figure 14-1:
Section of the eye showing the internal structures. It is a complex receptor for the sensory perception of light; *(courtesy of Ethicon, Inc.).*

The neuron, like all cells, has a nucleus, cell body (**perikaryon**), cytoplasm, and a selectively permeable cell membrane. Unlike other cells, the neuron has extensions. Some of these extensions branch out like tree limbs and are called **dendrites**. Some are like slender threads and are called **axons**. Neurons have a variable number of dendrites. The dendrites receive a stimulus that passes through the perikaryon and leaves the cell through its axon.

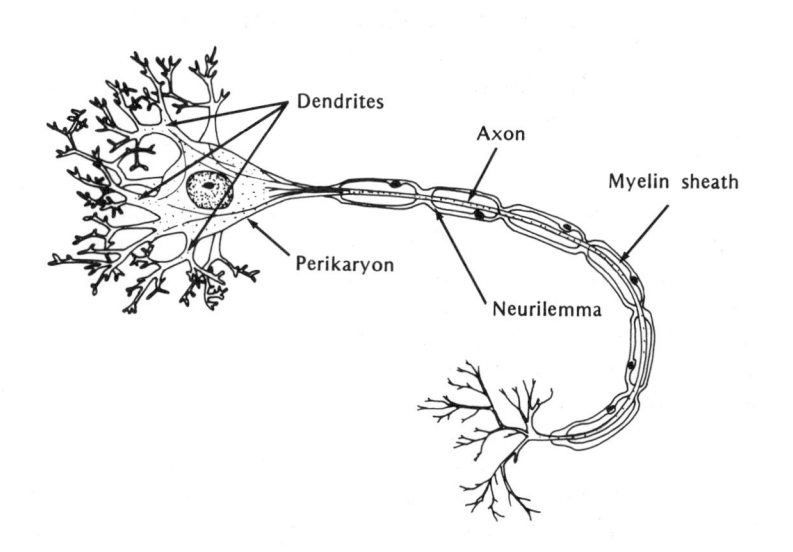

Figure 14-2:
The basic cell of the neuron's tissue is the neuron.

MEDICAL WORDS 225 *

Each neuron has only one axon. Since the axon of one neuron does not actually touch the dendrites of other neurons, a **neurotransmitter** (chemical) carries the stimulus across the space (**synapse**) between neurons. In this way, the stimulus can be carried by a series of neurons from a distant part such as the big toe, all the way to the brain in the cranium for interpretation.

Figure 14-3: Neurons do not actually touch but meet at the synapse. A neurotransmitter carries the message from one neuron to another.

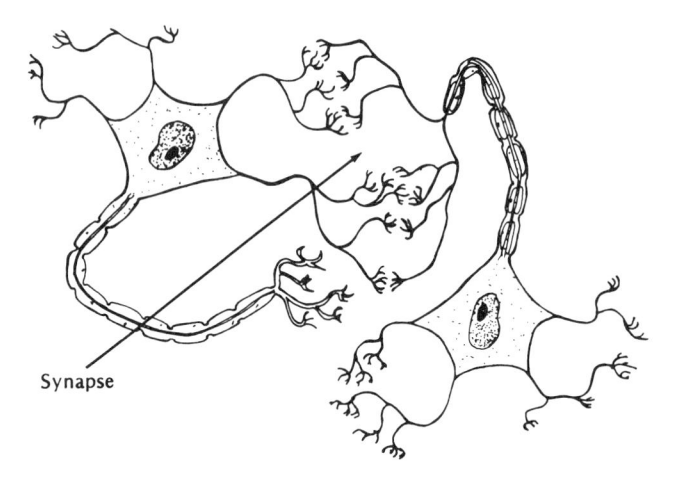

Another special characteristic of the neuron is its fatty insulation which is found around most axons and dendrites. This insulation is called the **myelin sheath**. An additional membrane, the **neurilemma**, is found around the myelin of peripheral nerves. The presence of myelin makes the nerve fiber white. When it is absent, the nervous tissue appears grey.

A **stimulus** is something which excites a nerve and causes it to transmit an impulse in the form of a wave of electricity along its length. Light, heat, cold, pressure and pain can each act as a stimulus.

The Stimulus

All neurons are not stimulated (**fired**) by the same type of stimuli. For example, sound waves stimulate the neurons of the ear but light waves stimulate the neurons of the eye. Receptors, nerve endings in certain areas of the skin, respond to heat. Others respond to cold. **Receptors** are peripheral nerve endings that are **sensitive** (responsive) to a specific stimuli. Other nerve endings that are found in the viscera are called **visceral receptors**. They give rise to sensations of pain or hunger or thirst.

Still others are found in the muscles and tendons. They carry information about the degree of stretch in these structures and are called **proprioceptors**. Each receptor is fired by a stimulus and carries its message to the spinal cord and brain where it

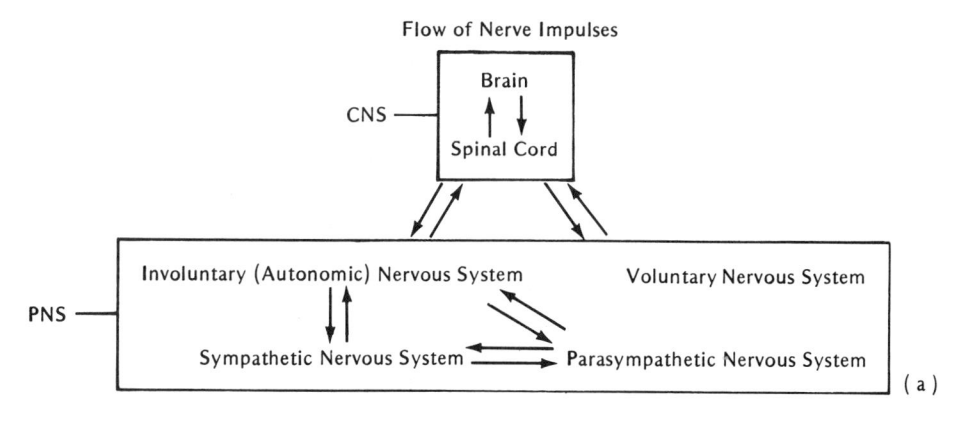

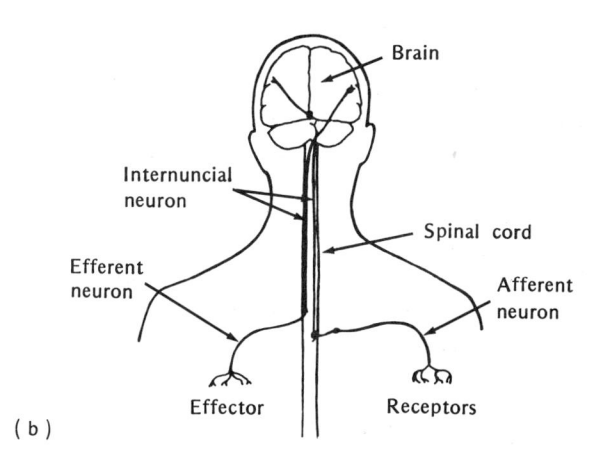

Figure 14-4:
(a) Flow of nerve impulses: afferent fibers carry messages toward the CNS. Efferent fibers carry messages away from the CNS; *(courtesy of Ethicon, Inc.);* (b) schematic flow of messages.

is interpreted as a specific sensation. Messages carried toward the spinal cord and brain are called **sensory** or **afferent**, and the nerves carrying them are called sensory or afferent neurons.

When the messages come from the body (**soma**) proper, the nerves are **somatic afferent fibers**. When the messages come from the organs, they are carried by **visceral afferent fibers**. The neurons within the brain and spinal cord (**central nervous system**) are called **central** neurons or **connecting** or **internuncial** neurons. These are the neurons that do the integration and interpretation of all sensory information.

Messages carried away from the central nervous system (CNS) cause activity in some part of the body. The part responding to the nervous stimuli is called an **effector** organ. The nerves (bundles of axons and dendrites) carrying the message to the effector organs are called **motor** or **efferent** neurons. Efferent neurons terminate in muscles which they cause to contract or

Effectors

MEDICAL WORDS 227 *

glands which they cause to secrete. They are called **somatic efferent fibers** if they go to skeletal muscles or **visceral efferent fibers** if they go to cardiac muscles or glands. The visceral efferent fibers make up the **autonomic** or involuntary nervous system (ANS).

Some autonomic fibers terminate in the myocardium where they alter the inherent rhythmicity established by the nodal tissue. There are two divisions of the autonomic nervous system: the **sympathetic** and the **parasympathetic**. Both divisions send fibers to the myocardium. Sympathetic fiber stimulation speeds the heart rate, parasympathetic slows the heart rate.

Reflex Arc

A **reflex** is the simplest nervous mechanism for making a rapid, involuntary response to an internal or external stimuli. The stimuli is carried to the spinal cord by an afferent neuron. The afferent neuron transmits the impulse across the synapse to the connecting neuron in the cord. The connecting neuron transmits the impulse immediately across the synapse to the efferent neuron. The efferent neuron stimulates the proper response. The entire sequence of events takes only a fraction of a second. It is known as the **reflex arc**.

Look at Figure 14-5 to see a cross section of the spinal cord. Learn the parts and see the relationship of the neurons which form the reflex arc. Remember that both sides of the cord have the same structures.

Figure 14-5: Cross section of spinal cord showing the pathway of the reflex arc; note that the cord has bilateral symmetry.

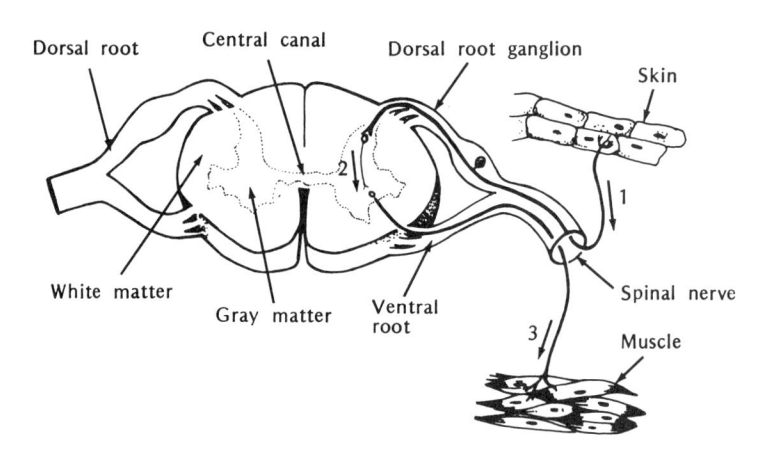

NERVOUS SYSTEM DIVISIONS

For easier study, the nervous system can be divided or described in several ways. The central nervous system is composed of the brain and spinal cord. The **peripheral nervous system** (PNS) is composed of the afferent and efferent fibers that make up the nerves leading to and from the brain and cord. The **cranial nerves** pass into and out of the brain. There are twelve pairs of these nerves.

Each of the cranial nerve pairs has both a name and number. They are just as frequently referred to by one as by the other. Table 14-1 lists the names and functions of some of the cranial nerves.

Table 14-1

Number	Nerve	Function
I	olfactory	sense of smell
II	optic	sense of sight
III	oculomotor	eye movements
V	trigeminal	chewing (**mastication**); sensations of face and head
VII	facial	facial expression; taste (**gustation**)
VIII	acoustic— branch of the Vestibulochochlear	hearing and sense of balance (**equilibrium**)
IX	glossopharyngeal	stimulation of the muscles of the tongue and throat for swallowing (**deglutition**)
X	vagus	supplies most of the viscera in the ventral cavity

As you can see, the names of the nerves give clues either to their function or to some special characteristic. The nerves from the eyes and the olfactory nerves from the nose describe their distribution. The name, trigeminal (triple), describes a special characteristic of this cranial nerve.

The trigeminal nerve, the largest of the cranial nerves, has three large branches leading to different areas of the face. The ophthalmic nerve is distributed over the eyes, the maxillary nerve passes over the cheek bone (**maxilla**), and the mandibular nerve follows the lower jaw bone, the mandible. When you experience a toothache, the sensation is being carried to the brain by one of the trigeminal branches. A severe neuralgia called **tic douloureux** can sometimes affect one or all of the trigeminal nerve branches. The etiology of this condition is not known.

The spinal nerves pass into and out of the spinal cord. There are 31 pairs of spinal nerves. The spinal nerves are **mixed nerves** because they contain somatic and visceral, afferent and efferent fibers. Most of the motor messages carried by the visceral efferent fibers are the result of complex reflex reactions and are not usually consciously directed. For this reason, the visceral efferent or autonomic system of fibers is also known as the **vegetative** or **involuntary** nervous system.

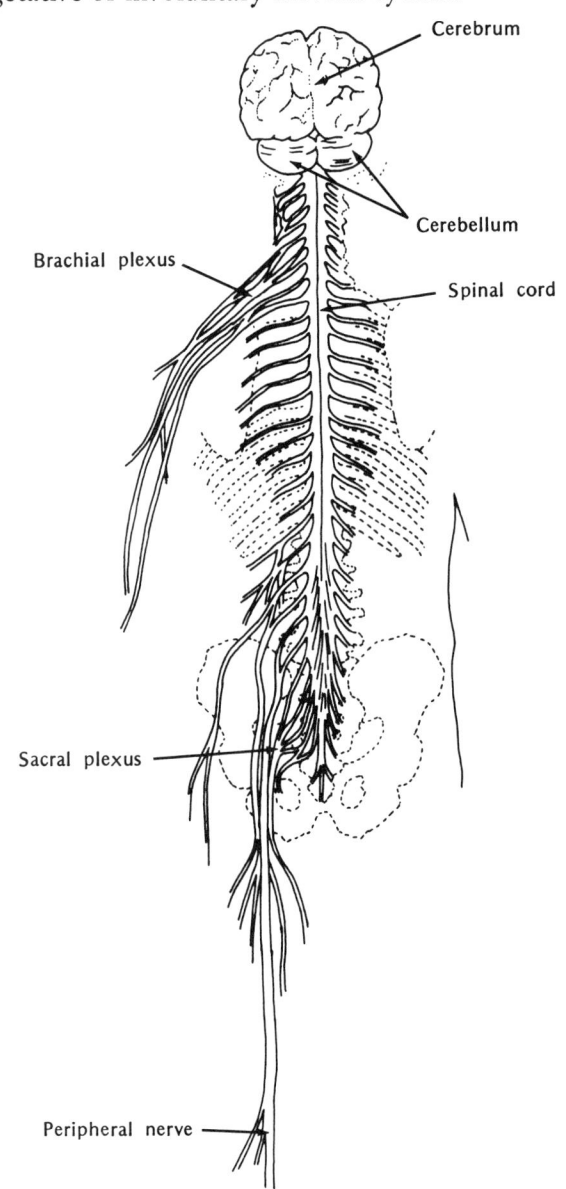

Figure 14-6: Central nervous system: messages to and from the brain travel along the spinal cord and nerves seen branching off the cord; *(courtesy of Ethicon, Inc.).*

*230 THE NERVOUS SYSTEM

The Central Nervous System

The central nervous system is located in the dorsal cavity. The brain is in the cranium and the spinal cord is in the vertebral canal which is formed by the bones of the spine. The dorsal cavity is lined by the three-layered membrane called the meninges. The outer layer is the dura mater, the middle layer is the arachnoid mater, and the innermost is the pia mater. There are also important spaces between the layers.

The biggest space is between the arachnoid mater and the pia mater. Remember, this subarachnoid space is filled with cerebrospinal fluid. Cerebrospinal fluid is very similar to tissue fluid in composition. A second potential space (**subdural**) is found between the dura mater and arachnoid mater. Subdural hematomas are associated with trauma to the cranium such as a fractured skull.

The cerebrospinal fluid is produced within cavities (the **ventricles**) of the brain as a blood filtrate. Between 400-500 ml are produced in a 24-hour period. Only about 100 ml is flowing through the ventricular system and subarachnoid space at any one time. As more cerebrospinal fluid is secreted, an equal amount is reabsorbed into the blood stream. A blockage in the system results in an accumulation of cerebrospinal fluid. The condition is called **hydrocephalus** (water of the head). The excess fluid increases the intracranial pressure putting stress on the soft brain tissue. The pressure traumatizes the delicate nervous tissue severely. Unless steps are taken to correct the situation, the damage will be permanent.

The Spinal Cord

The spinal cord (**myelon**) is a cone-shaped cylinder, a foot and a half long (42 cm). It extends in the vertebral canal, from the occiput to the level of the 1st or 2nd lumbar vertebra. The meninges, however, extend down to the coccyx where they are anchored.

The spinal nerves enter and leave the cord by two short roots; the anterior and posterior roots. The anterior root carries the motor fibers (axons) from their cell bodies out through the spinal nerve. The posterior root carries sensory fibers (dendrites) to their cell bodies, which are found in a small grey swelling on the nerve root called the dorsal root ganglion. A **ganglion** is a collection of nerve cell bodies or neurons. The axon of each neuron then extends into the cord.

Each pair of nerves is numbered and named according to the vertebra between which it emerges. For example, the first pair of spinal nerves passes out between the occiput and first cervical vertebra and is named Cervical 1 or C-1. C-2 comes out between cervical vertebra 1 and cervical vertebra 2. The cervical

Figure 14-7: Section of vertebral column: upper vertebrae have been removed to show location of the spinal cord within the canal; *(courtesy of Ethicon, Inc.)*.

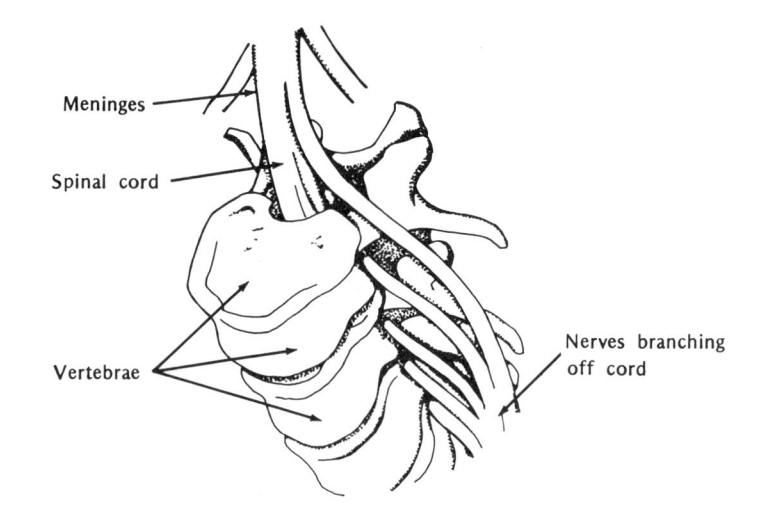

spinal nerve pairs are numbered 1 to 8, the thoracic spinal nerve pairs 1 to 12, the lumbar spinal nerve pairs 1 to 5, and the sacral spinal nerve 1 to 5. There is only one pair of coccygeal spinal nerves. Because the spinal cord is shorter than the vertebral canal, the lumbar, sacral, and coccygeal nerves all travel down the canal from the end of the cord to emerge between the proper vertebrae. This gives the mass of fibers a bushy appearance. The mass is called the horses tail (**cauda equina**).

Remember the spinal nerves are mixed nerves. That is, they carry both afferent and efferent fibers. Once the spinal nerves emerge, they interweave with one another to form a **plexus** (network). Large plexi are found in the cervical and lumbosacral parts of the cord. Look at the diagram of the cross section of the spinal cord to learn some additional information. Notice that the cord is **symmetrical** (two sides the same).

In the very center of the cord is a small hole, the **central canal**. Do not confuse this with the vertebral canal. Cerebrospinal fluid flows in the central canal. Surrounding the canal is a butterfly-shaped mass of **gray matter** consisting largely of cell bodies of internuncial neurons. The **white matter** surrounding the gray matter is composed of myelinated axons (**ascending sensory tracts**) which carry the messages up to higher centers and myelinated axons (**descending motor tracts**) which carry messages down from higher centers.

The Brain

The most complex and least understood mass of nervous tissue is the brain. The **brain** (encephalon) is composed of several parts that are continuous with each other and are extended upward from the spinal cord. Both gray matter and white matter make up the brain. Special areas of gray matter, called **nuclei** or **centers**, are responsible for controlling specific body functions.

The lowest part of the brain is called the **medulla oblongata**. The medulla oblongata is frequently referred to simply as the medulla. Very important centers are found in this part of the brain stem. They include the respiratory and cardiac centers which control the respiratory and cardiac rates. Above the medulla is the **pons varolii** and above the pons (bridge), the **midbrain**. Posterior to these structures is the cerebellum.

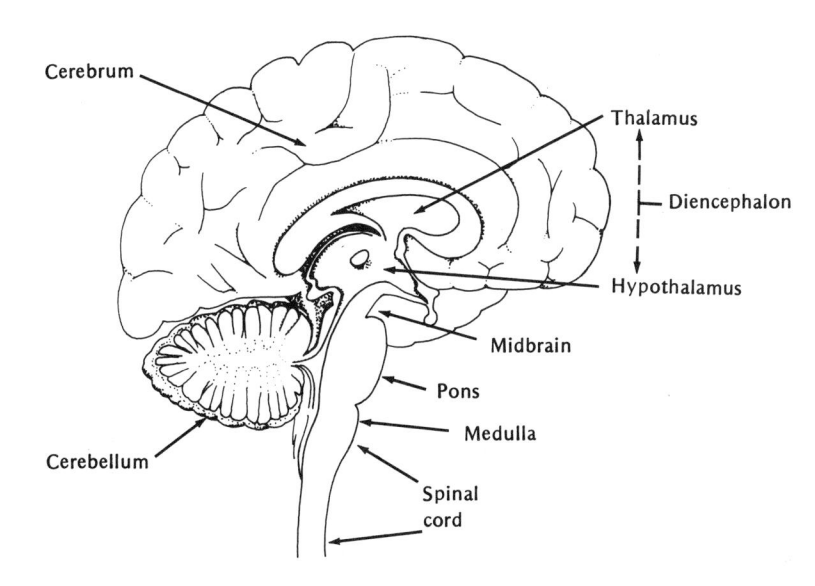

Figure 14-8: The brain.

The **cerebellum** is the second largest part of the brain. Among other activities, the cerebellum coordinates all voluntary movements. The top of the brain stem is the diencephalon. The **diencephalon** is made up of two important areas; the lower area or hypothalamus, to which the pituitary gland is attached, and the upper rounded portion or thalamus which caps the brain stem.

The **hypothalamus** functions is a reflex center for all visceral activities such as digestion and water balance. It manages these functions directly by nervous stimulation and indirectly by its relationship to the pituitary gland. The **thalamus** acts as a great relay center for all sensory input, redirecting the information to the proper centers for interpretation. The most superior, largest, most complex of all the brain structures is the cerebrum (**telencephalon**).

The **cerebrum** is a very elaborate structure. Its surface, the cortex, is composed of gray matter thrown into folds (**convolutions**). The rounded portion of each convolution is called a **gyrus**. The indentation between two gyri is called a sulcus. Deep grooves or fissures, divide the surface of the cerebrum into lobes and into a right and left **hemisphere**. The **longitudinal fissure** is found between the right and left hemispheres. The central fissure separates the frontal and parietal lobes. The lateral fissure separates the parietal and the temporal lobes.

Figure 14-9: Surface of cerebrum.

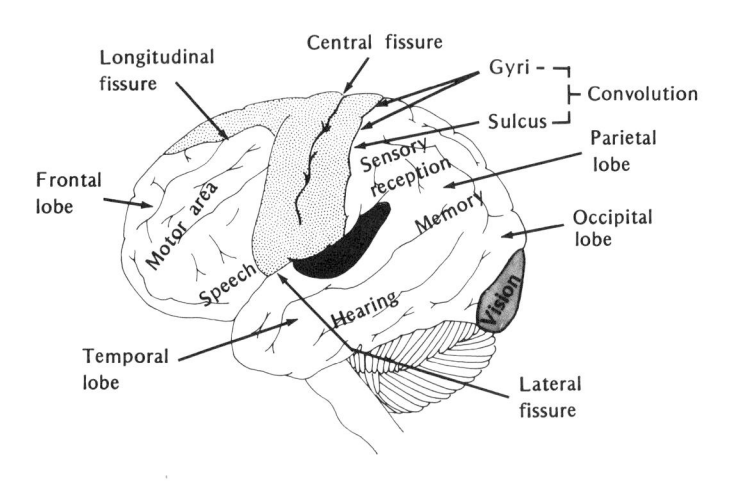

The names of the lobes correspond to the bones of the cranium, under which they lie. On each side there is a frontal, parietal, temporal and occipital lobe. Special centers for interpretation or control are located in the cortex. Study the diagram in Figure 14-9 in order to learn the location of some of the special centers on the surface of the cerebrum.

Loss of motor function is called **paralysis**. Loss of feeling or sensations is called **anesthesia**. Paralysis and anesthesia are not always total. **Paraplegia** means paralysis of the lower part of the body or of the legs. **Hemiplegia** means paralysis on one side of the body. Paraparesis means partial paralysis of the legs. The degree of paralysis or anesthesia depends upon the specific area of cerebral cortex involved.

Special Terminology

Special prefixes are associated with the nervous system. Neuro- or nervous, and encephal- or brain, have been introduced before. Study Table 14-2 which shows combined forms. See how many meanings you can recognize or analyze.

Table 14-2

Neuro-	Meaning
neurologist	a nervous system specialist
neuroma	nervous tissue tumor
neuromuscular	pertaining to nerves and muscles
neurotomy	surgical dissection of a nerve
neurosclerosis	abnormal hardening of nerve tissue
neurotropic	having a special affinity for nerves
neuritis	inflammation of a nerve
neuroparalysis	loss of function due to nerve damage
neuropathy	any disease of the nerve
neurofibroma	tumor of nervous tissue caused by excessive growth of binding connective tissue

Encephal-	Meaning
encephalitis	inflammation of the brain
encephalogram	X-ray picture of the brain
encephaloma	a brain tumor
encephalorrhagia	brain hemorrhage
encephalosclerosis	hardening of the brain tissue
encephalopyosis	brain abscess
encephalocele	protrusion of brain through an opening in the skull
encephalalgia	pain in the head
encephalatrophy	atrophy of brain tissue
encephaloid	resembling brain tissue

The prefix, **myelo-** means spinal cord. In the next table, see how many meanings you can recognize. Probably only one word in the series will be totally new.

Table 14-3

Myelo-	
myelomalacia	abnormal softening of the spinal cord
myelon	spinal cord
myelosclerosis	hardening of the spinal cord
myelodiastasis	disintegration of the spinal cord
myeloplegia	paralysis caused by a lesion of the spinal cord

Neuropathology

The nervous system is subject to the same pathologies as other systems. Tumors such as neuromas or **gliomas** (tumors of the neuroglia) can occur. Inflammation and infections such as encephalitis, meningitis, or neuritis do as much damage to nervous tissue as to any tissue in the body, and the effect may be more prolonged or permanent. Some pathologies such as tic douloureaux are specific to the nervous system. Read Table 14-4 and review some other specific nervous system diseases.

Table 14-4

Pathology	*Description*
epilepsy	a non-infectious disorder associated with **convulsions** (involuntary muscle spasms); the convulsions are sometimes associated with loss of consciousness or altered behavior
cerebral palsy	a group of disorders caused by damage to the cerebral motor areas; the disease is not progressive but is characterized by varying degrees of paralysis
sciatica	an inflammation on the root of the sciatic nerve, frequently from pressure; the sciatic nerve is a branch of the lumbosacral plexus; it is a mixed nerve to the legs
herpes zoster	a viral infection which attacks the dorsal root ganglion; vesicles develop on the skin along the paths of peripheral nerves
poliomyelitis	also called infantile paralysis; it is a viral infection that affects the motor cells of the spinal cord, although it can damage the cortex and brain stem; the disease causes flaccid paralysis of the skeletal muscles

The diagnosis was **cerebrovascular accident** (interrupted blood flow to the brain) but the nurse used the term "stroke" as she talked with the patient's husband and neighbor. Mrs. Concepción Garcia was the patient. The nurse took Mr. Garcia and his neighbor to a private room where they could talk quietly. From Mr. Garcia, the nurse learned the following facts.

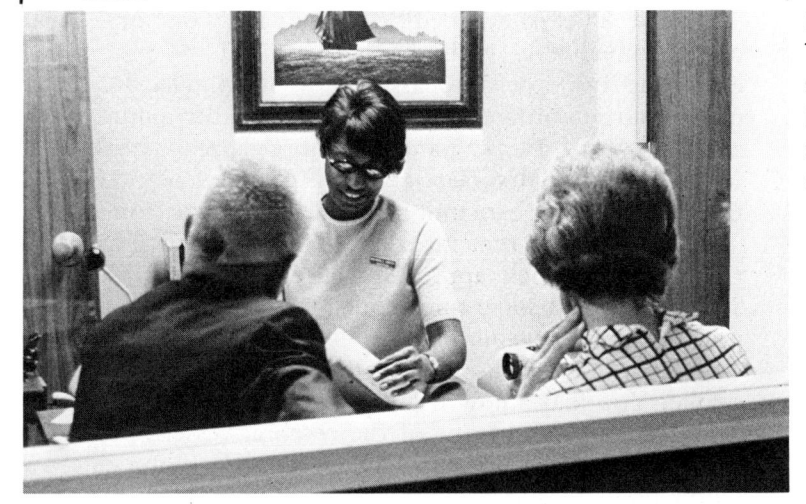

CASE STUDY

Figure 14-10: The nurse spent some time explaining the patients' situation in positive, supportive terms.

The patient, a sixty-year old secretary, has been treated in the past few years for hypertension. Recently, her husband said, she had been complaining of headaches, and double vision (**diplopia**). She sometimes forgot her blood pressure medication.

Just before her admission, the patient had prepared dinner for her husband and grandchild. Her husband, a retired mechanic, had a congestive heart condition so most of the household responsibilities were carried by the patient. In addition, because of their limited income and the responsibility for rearing their grandchild, Mrs. Garcia had had to continue working outside the home.

Mrs. Garcia had laid down to rest for a while before eating, complaining of a headache. A short while later, Mr. Garcia went to the bedroom to check on her. He found her apparently resting. But when he spoke to her she attempted to rise and said she felt weak. Her speech was slurred (**dysarthrea**), and she seemed confused and disoriented.

NERVOUS SYSTEM DIVISIONS 237

Swinging her legs over the edge of the bed, Mrs. Garcia attempted to stand, but instead slumped to the floor **unconscious** (not responsive to stimuli). Mr. Garcia thought she was in a faint (**syncope**), and when he couldn't rouse her, he called the paramedics. They found a hypertensive **comatose** (in coma) woman whose breathing was stertorous and who was slightly cyanotic.

One emergency medical technician communicated immediately with the hospital and the other established an airway to assist ventilation. The hospital physician ordered stat mask O_2 @ 3L per minute and an I.V. of 5% D/W and transport via ambulance to the hospital. Mrs. Garcia was admitted at once to the **neurovascular care unit** (NCU) for intensive care.

Mr. Garcia, remembering his own hospitalizations, was extremely **apprehensive** (fearfully anxious). The nurse spent some time explaining the situation in positive, supportive terms:

"The doctor suspects that your wife has had a stroke. You may know it as **apoplexy**. It may be due to a blocking off of one of the cerebral vessels, perhaps due to a clot. People who have a history of high blood pressure and atherosclerosis as your wife, are considered at risk for a **cerebrovascular accident** (C.V.A.). The effects of such a blockage can be very serious. Patients do recover but there may be some **residual** (lasting) effects such as problems with communication (**aphasis**) and some loss of movement or motor ability.

"Sometimes patients experience an inability to speak (**aphasia**) or to make sounds (**verbal apraxia**) but the speech therapist will work with her. An **occupational therapist** (O.T.) and a **physical therapist** (P.T.) and a social worker will all be available to assist your wife once she progresses beyond this first critical phase.

"The hospital has a very good rehabilitation department and Mrs. Garcia will be able to use their services on an out-patient basis after she returns home. The goal of everyone on the stroke team is to return your wife to her normal activities of daily living (ADL) so that she can do as much self-care as possible.

"Right now she is receiving the best possible care. The physician is performing a general physical and neurological examination. He has ordered a series of tests such as a urinalysis, complete blood count, electrocardiogram, chest films, a **lumbar puncture** (withdrawal of cerebrospinal fluid from the lumbar portion of the vertebral canal), a skull **plate** (X-ray), an **arteriogram** (arterial X-ray), and a **pneumoencephalogram** (an X-ray film of the brain after injection of gas into the subarachnoid space). After he has the results, he will be able to give you a more accurate picture of what to expect."

Mrs. Garcia recovered from the acute phase, regaining consciousness in about two days. She was **amnesic** (no memory of recent events) with right-sided hemiplegia. Her speech was slow and she had difficulty naming objects correctly. In three months, after intensive rehabilitation, she had made considerable progress and returned home. Mrs. Garcia is currently an out-patient in the stroke rehabilitation clinic three times a week and is making steady progress.

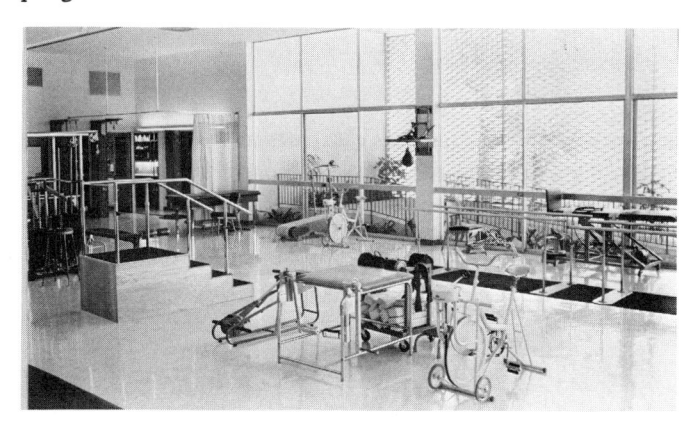

Figure 14-11: Mrs. Garcia visited the stroke rehabilitation clinic for post stroke therapy.

SUMMARY

The nervous system is composed of special tissue capable of conducting a nerve impulse. It conveys messages to and from the central nervous system by way of peripheral nerves. Through its complex network of nerves and its special relationship to the endocrine system, the nervous system maintains homeostasis. Nervous pathology results in loss of function or in loss of sensation in an area, and frequently in both.

PRACTICE & REVIEW Explain and define the new special terms you have been using. Remember, you learned how to pronounce them at the beginning of this chapter.

1. cerebrum _____
2. diplopia _____
3. encephalosclerosis _____
4. flaccid _____
5. gustation _____
6. mastication _____
7. myelodiastasis _____
8. neuroma _____
9. proprioceptors _____
10. sciatica _____

Now, double-check the meaning of the terms above by studying the brief definitions given in the Glossary-Index at the back of this text.

Test yourself quickly before going on to learn other medical and professional terms. Use these short review exercises to practice for your new work in health services. Your teacher will also help by recommending various other Study Activities.

A. The names of the cranial nerves give clues to their function or destination. Write the name for each of the following descriptions:

1. Carries sense of smell _____
2. Carries sense of vision _____
3. Supplies the face _____
4. Carries sound for sense of hearing _____
5. "Wanders" into the ventral cavity to supply the viscera _____

B. The prefix, neuro-, means nervous. Complete the five terms below by adding the proper ending to each:

1. nervous system specialist   neuro_____
2. surgical dissection of a nerve   neuro_____
3. loss of function due to nerve damage neuro_____
4. any disease of the nerves   neuro_____
5. having a special affinity for nerves neuro_____

C. Complete the ten statements below with the best word from this list:

equilibrium	opthalmic	dendrites
stimulus	amnesic	autonomic
myelon	efferent	ventricles
neuroglia	neuron	plexus
afferent		

1. Another name for the sense of balance is a _____ .
2. _____ is the supporting tissue of the nervous system.
3. An interweaving of spinal nerve fibers is called a _____ .
4. The fibers which carry the nerve impulse toward the Central Nervous System are called_____ .
5. The _____ nervous system is also known as the visceral efferent nervous system.
6. Light, pressure, and temperature variations can all act as a _____ to excite a nerve fiber.
7. The nerve cell is called a _____ .
8. Cavities within the brain that are filled with cerebrospinal fluid are called the_____ .
9. A person who has lost their memory is an _____ .
10. Another name for the spinal cord is the _____ .

D. The prefix, encephalo-, means brain. Complete the words at the right by adding the proper ending:

1. X-ray picture of the brain   encephalo_____
2. brain tumor   encephalo_____
3. brain hemorrhage   encephalo_____
4. brain abscess   encephalo_____
5. hardening of brain tissue   encephalo_____

After studying Chapter 15
The Gastrointestinal System
You should be able to:

* *Pronounce and define each of its new medical words and phrases and use the new technical jargon.*

* *Identify ten anatomical structures of the digestive system.*

* *Describe the function of the digestive system.*

MEDICAL WORDS

PRONOUNCE THESE TEN NEW WORDS WITH YOUR TEACHER:

alimentary tract (al″ĭ-men′tar-e) (trakt)
cholecystogram (ko″le-sĭs′to-gram)
choledocholithiasis (ko-led″o-ko-lĭ-thi′ah-sĭs)
colonopathy (ko″lon-op′ah-the)
enterocinesia (ĕn″tĕr-osi-ne″se-ah)

dyspepsia (dĭs-pep′se-ah)
gastric (gas′trĭk)
hepatalgia (hep″ah-tal′je-ah)
postprandial (post-pran′de-al)
proteases (pro′te-as-es)

The digestive system consists of the gastrointestinal tract (**alimentary tract**) and several accessory organs. It stretches from the mouth (**buccal** or **oral** cavity) to the anal canal. It is essentially a glandular tube system with smooth muscular walls and lined with mucous membrane.

Foods provide the **nutrients** (essential growth and repair elements) needed by the human body. Foods are complex, however, and the nutrients must be turned into simple forms before they can be **assimilated** (absorbed) from the digestive tract into the bloodstream. **Digestion**, the process of converting complex substances into simple, easily assimilated nutrients, is the vital role of the digestive system.

THE NUTRIENTS

Fats, proteins, and carbohydrates are three of the essential nutrients that must be broken down into simple forms before assimilation. Water, minerals and vitamins are also essential human nutrients, but they can be assimilated without further simplification by the alimentary tract.

Carbohydrates (**saccharides**) are the principal source of

energy. Complex forms are derived mainly from plant sources and are found in the form of starch (polysaccharide), a complex saccharide, double sugars such as **maltose**, a **disaccharide**, and simple sugars such as glucose, a **monosaccharide**. All carbohydrates must be broken down to monosaccharides by the digestive enzymes before they can be utilized by body cells. Glucose is the form in which sugar is found in the blood stream.

Fats come from plants and animal sources. They, too, provide energy but only when carbohydrates are unavailable. Fats also are necessary to the assimilation of fat soluble vitamins, such as vitamin D. The simplest form of fats are **fatty acids** and **glycerol**. It is in this form that they are assimilated.

Proteins also come from plants and animals. They are needed to build and repair tissues, but if necessary they can be utilized for energy.

The simplest form of proteins is **amino acid**. Changing nutrients from complex substances to simple ones is called **catabolism**. The use of the simple nutrients in forming new tissue is **anabolism**. The sum of all the chemical reactions of the body, including anabolism and catabolism of the nutrients, is called **metabolism**.

A well-balanced diet includes sufficient quantities of each of the six nutrients. Foods have been divided into four different food groups (**basic four**) to make the selection easier. The four groups include: the bread and cereal group, the milk group, the meat group, and the vegetable and fruit group.

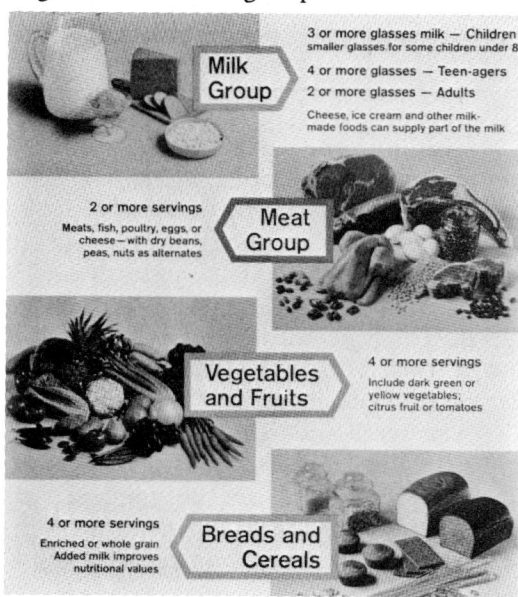

Figure 15-1: The basic four food groups; *(courtesy of The National Dairy Council).*

THE NUTRIENTS 243

Hospital Diets

Careful selection from each of the food groups is the basis for adequate meal planning in the hospital as well as in the home.

In the hospital, many different diets can be ordered for people with various illnesses. In general, the **regular** or **house** diets are **select** diets based on the basic four food groups and contain the same selections that you would make at home, but with fewer calories and fried foods. Look at Table 15-1 for some of the other special diets planned for hospital patients.

Table 15-1

Diet	Characteristics	When Ordered
clear liquid	chiefly water and carbohydrates	following surgery to provide fluids and energy
low sodium	eliminates salt from menu and curtails salty foods	congestive heart failure
high carbohydrates high protein	foods rich in carbohydrates and proteins	liver disease
low fat	foods not fried; fats limited	gall bladder disease
sippy	frequent feedings of milk and cream—gradually progresses to include eggs and custards	gastric ulcer

ALIMENTARY CANAL

The alimentary canal consists of several parts including the mouth, pharynx, esophagus, stomach, small intestines, large intestines (colon), and rectum.

The Mouth

Food enters the mouth where it is broken up mechanically by chewing. That is, it is masticated by the teeth and tongue and mixed with saliva. **Saliva** is a thin, watery liquid produced by the exocrine **salivary glands** whose ducts empty into the buccal cavity. Saliva contains an enzyme which begins the process of digesting carbohydrates.

The teeth (dentes) are embedded in the alveolar ridge of the mandible and maxilla. Each tooth sits in an **alveolus** (socket) surrounded by the **gingivae** (gums). The alveoli are lined with a **periodontal** (around a tooth) membrane which is an extension of the perioiosteum of the bones. **Gingivitis** is an

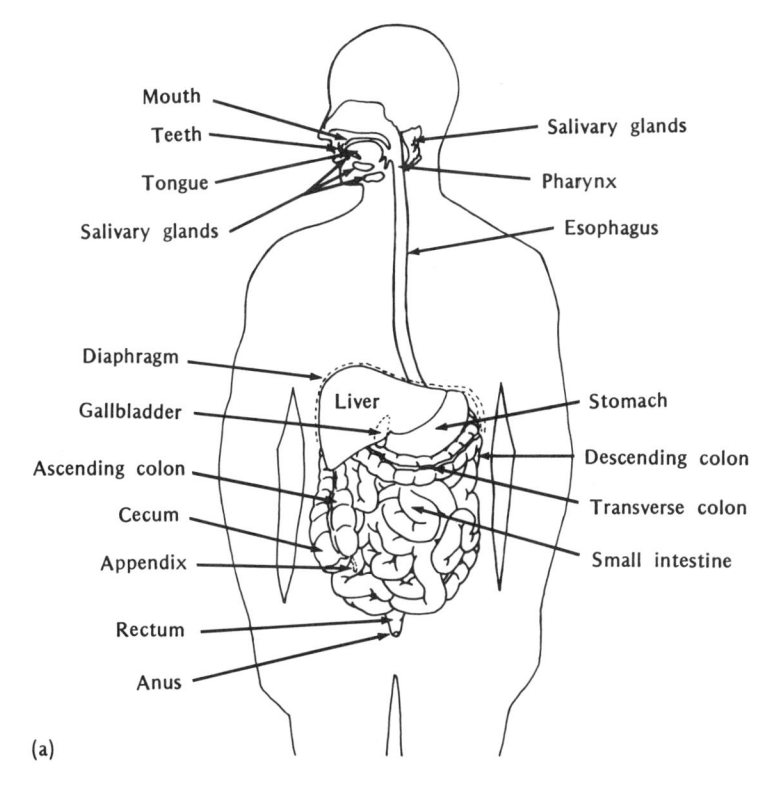

Figure 15-2: (a) The alimentary canal stretches from the mouth to anus; (b) the stomach and adjacent organs; *(courtesy of Ethicon, Inc.).*

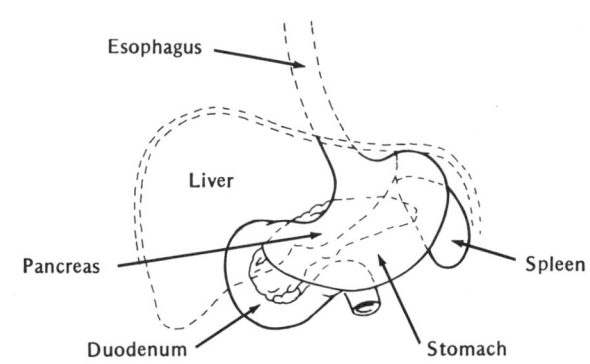

inflammation of the gums, which become swollen and tender. **Pyorrhea**, a discharge of pus from the alveolus, can result in a loosening of the teeth.

Each person has two natural sets of teeth (**dentitions**) in his/her lifetime. The first set, the **deciduous** teeth (baby teeth), are 20 in number. The second set of teeth, the **permanent set**, number 32 and can remain throughout an individual's life if

Figure 15-3:
The oral or buccal cavity; *(courtesy of Picker Corp.).*

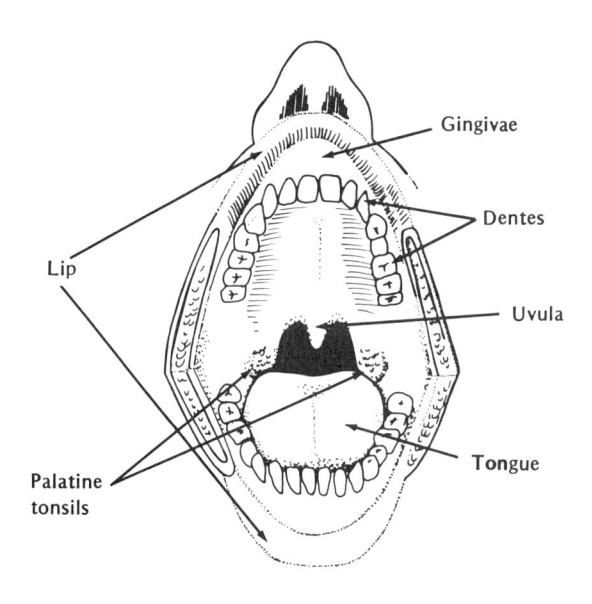

proper **dental** (referring to teeth) **hygiene** (healthy practices) is carried out. Dental **caries** (cavities) are a frequent problem when there is poor hygiene. Subsequent loss of teeth may necessitate the use of artificial teeth (**dentures**).

From the oral cavity, the **bolus** (soft mass) of food is propelled backward to be swallowed (**deglutition**). This bolus continues its passage downward through the approximately 30 foot long (9 meters) digestive tract; first into the pharynx and then into the esophagus. The pharynx is a common passageway for food and air.

The **esophagus** is a collapsible muscular cylinder extending from the pharynx to the stomach. It is located in the mediastinum and is posterior to the trachea. From mouth to stomach, the passage of food takes approximately 4 to 8 seconds. The esophagus is 10 inches (23-25 cm) long and is separated from the stomach by a round, circular muscle, the **cardiac sphincter**. Rhythmic waves contract the smooth muscular walls of the digestive tract and help move the bolus into the stomach. This **peristalsis (enterocinesis)** consists of waves that occur the entire length of the alimentary tract, propelling the digested material onward toward the **anus** (terminal opening).

The bolus of food is retained from 3 to 4 hours in the **stomach**, a J-shaped, dilated portion of the gastrointestinal tract (G.I.). There the bolus is churned back and forth by the peristaltic waves until it becomes a liquid called **chyme**.

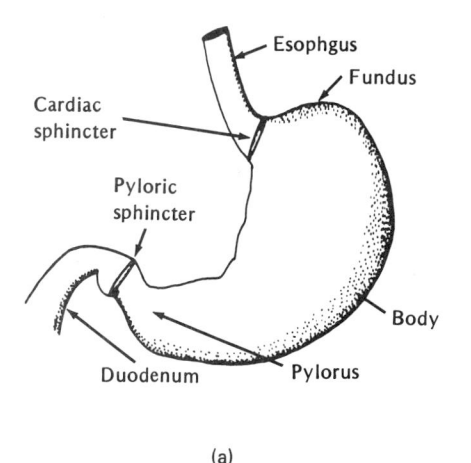

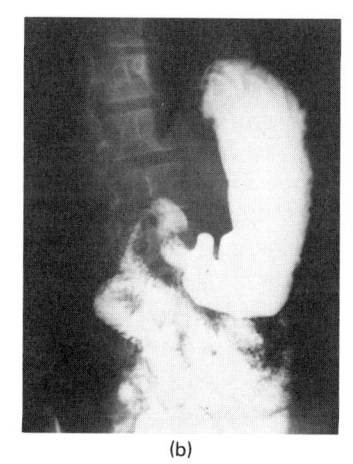

Figure 15-4:
(a) The stomach;
(b) the X-ray shows the J-shaped contour of the stomach after the structures were filled with contrast media.

The Stomach

The stomach divides into a fundus (rounded base) near the cardiac sphincter, a body (a large central portion) and a narrowed area, the **pylorus**, which connects to the small intestine.

Food is maintained in the stomach by contraction of the cardiac sphincter and the **pyloric** sphincter, another sphincter muscle is at the end of the pylorus. **Gastric** (pertaining to the stomach) glandular secretions include mucous, **hydrochloric acid** (HCl), and pepsin. **Pepsin** is an enzyme which begins the chemical breakdown of the proteins that nourish the body.

Remember the prefix "gastro-" means stomach. Look at the list of combined forms that use this prefix. Some should be familiar to you.

Gastro (Stomach)	Meaning
gastralgia	stomach pain
gastritis	inflamed stomach
gastrectomy	excision of the stomach
gastrology	study of the stomach
gastroparalysis	paralysis of the stomach

Excessive production of HCL (**hyperacidity**) in the stomach causes great discomfort and is described by most patients as a burning sensation. A feeling of fullness (**bloat**) or **distention** (stretching) that is experienced is related to excessive gas (**flatus**) in the tract.

The Small Intestine   The small intestine is about 1 inch (2.5cm) in diameter and approximately 10 to 12 inches (3m) long. It is divided into three parts, the **duodenum** or the first 10 inches (25cm), the **jejunum** which is the next 3/4 inch (1m), and the **ileum** which is 6 to 7 feet or 2 meters long. The ileum terminates with the ileocecal valve. The **ileocecal valve** is a one-way valve that prevents material from moving from the colon back into the small intestine.

Figure 15-5: The small intestines.

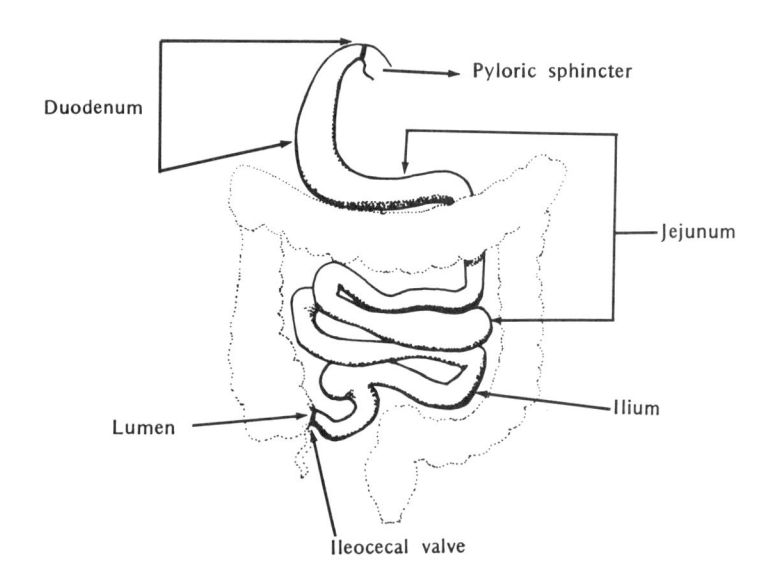

The major digestion of food takes place in the small intestine, and it is through the wall of the small intestine that assimilation of the nutrients occurs. Millions of microscopic **villi** (finger-like projections) line the **lumen** (tube, cavity) of the small intestine. There nutrients reduced to the simplest forms diffuse through the villi into the blood stream.

The exocrine glandular cells of the intestinal **mucosa** (mucous membrane lining) secrete several digestive enzymes which act on different nutrients. Nutrients called disaccharides are broken down into monosaccharides by three specific enzymes. For instance, the enzyme, **maltase**, converts the disaccharide, maltose, to a monosaccharide. The enzymes, **sucrase** and **lactase**, act in a like manner on the disaccharide sugars, **sucrose** and **lactose**. Other enzymes called **peptidases** convert proteins to amino acids.

Accessory organs, such as the liver, gall bladder, and pancreas, also empty exocrine secretions into the lumen of the duodenum. The **cystic** duct, **hepatic** duct, and **common bile** duct bring the secretion, **bile**, from the gall bladder and liver to emulsify fats. The **pancreatic duct** brings digestive enzymes such as **amylase** to break down carbohydrates, **protease** to break down proteins, and **lipase** to break down fats in the small intestines.

The prefix, **entero-** means intestine. It is used in a wide variety of combinations. Five are listed here for your consideration:

Entero	*Meaning*
enterectomy	excision of a portion of intestine
enteritis	inflammation of intestine
enterodynia	pain in the intestine
enterogenous	arising within the intestine
enterocentesis	puncture of intestine to withdraw gas or a fluid

The Large Intestine

The large intestine is also made up of continuous segments: the cecum, the ascending colon, the transverse colon, and the descending and sigmoid colon. The final 6 to 8 inches (20cm) of the alimentary tract is the **rectum**, which terminates in the anus or opening to the outside. A circular muscle, the **anal sphincter**, guards this exit.

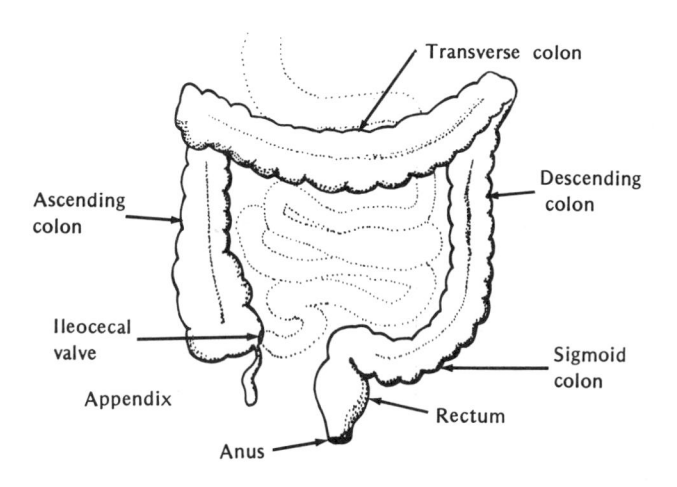

Figure 15-6: The colon.

ALIMENTARY CANAL 249 *

The large intestine, extending from the cecum to the rectum, is called the colon. It averages 5 inches (1.5m) in length and has a 2½ inch (6.5cm) diameter. Several important functions are carried on in the lumen or channel of the colon.

Bacteria that live in the large intestine synthesize some of the vitamins that then pass through the intestinal wall into the blood stream. Water is also reabsorbed into the body through the wall of the colon so that the chyme is dehydrated and turned into a semi-solid waste called **feces**. These feces continue along the canal and are finally eliminated (**defecated**) from the body through the anus.

The **appendix** is a small finger-like pouch which extends out of the **cecum** (beginning section of the colon). The appendix is somewhat vulnerable to infection and can become inflamed. Then it must be removed surgically or the consequences are serious. One serious complication is called **peritonitis** (inflammation of the peritoneum).

Much of the gastrointestinal portion of the alimentary tract is contained within the peritoneal membrane. Recall that this is an important double-walled membrane whose parietal layer lines the cavity and whose visceral layer is deflected over the organs.

Extensions of the visceral peritoneum are attached in such a way as to stabilize the digestive organs. One partition, the **lesser omentum** helps join the stomach and duodenum to the liver. The **greater omentum** hangs down like an apron over the intestines. It contains large quantities of adipose tissue. Still another extension of the peritoneum is called the **mesentery**. It is attached to the posterior abdominal wall and binds most of the intestines to that wall. The large blood vessels, the lymph vessels, and the lymph nodes that serve the area are located in the mesentery.

Several prefixes indicate colon. They include **coli**, **colo**, **colon**, and **colono**. Study the list for examples of their use:

colic	pertaining to the colon
colonitis (*colitis*)	inflammation of the colon
colocentesis	surgical puncture of the colon
colonopathy	disease of the colon
coloclysis	irritation of the colon

ACCESSORY STRUCTURES

The teeth, tongue, and salivary glands are accessory structures of the mouth. The liver, gall bladder, and pancreas are accessory structures of the intestinal tract.

The Liver

The **liver (hepar)** is the largest glandular organ in the body. It has 4 lobes and weighs approximately 3 to 4 pounds (1.8 kg). It is a vital organ and carries out many critical functions.

Figure 15-7: The biliary apparatus.

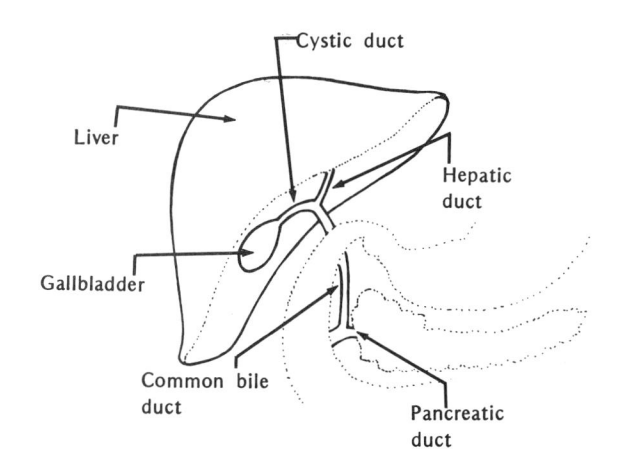

Some of the liver functions include: converting glucose to the storage form of glycogen, producing blood proteins such as prothrombin and fibrinogen, removing harmful or toxic substances from the blood stream and producing bile.

Bile (gall) is a yellowish-brown or greenish-yellow liquid produced by the liver. Approximately 1½ pints to 1 quart (800-1000 ml) of bile are produced daily. This bile is drained from the liver by the hepatic duct and into the gall bladder by the cystic duct where it is stored and converted.

The **gall bladder** is a small sac which lies on the posterior inferior hepatic surface. It can hold approximately 2 ounces (60 ml) of bile at a time and releases it into the common bile duct to the duodenum upon endocrine command. The endocrine command comes in response to the presence in the duodenum of unemulsified fats. The hepatic duct, cystic duct, and common bile duct are referred to as the **biliary apparatus** since they serve in the transport of bile.

Concretions (stones) of bile may occlude the biliary apparatus anywhere along the tract causing obstruction to the biliary flow. Since bile is formed from substances extracted from the blood stream, these substances accumulate and can cause a person to become jaundiced.

Three very important prefixes are associated with these structures. **Hepat**, for liver, **chol** or **chole**, for gall or bile, and **choledocho** for common bile duct. Look at the combining terms with which each prefix has been used.

Hepat- (Liver)	Meaning
hepatitis	inflammation of the liver
hepatectomy	surgical removal of part of the liver
hepatalgia	pain in the liver
hepatodynia	pain in the liver
hepatolith	a gall stone in the liver
hepatologist	a liver specialist

Chol- (Gall Bladder)	Meaning
cholecystectomy	excision of the gall bladder
cholecystitis	inflammation of the gall bladder
cholepathia	disease of the gall bladder
cholemesis	vomiting of bile
cholerrhagia	excessive bile flow
cholecystogram	X-ray record of gall bladder function

Choledocho- (Common bile duct)	Meaning
choledochitis	inflammation of the common bile ducts
choledocholithotomy	incision of the common bile duct to remove stones
choledochal	pertaining to the common bile duct
choledochotomy	incision of the common bile duct.
choledochoduodenostomy	anatomosis of the common bile duct and the duodenum

The pancreas, a flat, glandular organ, is found within the peritoneum. The head portion is in the curve of the duodenum while its body and tail extend posterior to the stomach. A long duct, the pancreatic duct, carries the exocrine secretions which are digestive enzymes into the duodenum. There the enzymes act on its contents, the chyme. Remember that this gland is also an endocrine gland, secreting insulin and glucogen directly into the blood stream.

Tumors and inflammations can occur anywhere along the alimentary tract and in its accessory organs. A major problem is that of obstruction to the normal passage of materials or secretions. Read the following case study to learn about one of the commonly seen problems.

Pathology of the Alimentary Tract

CASE STUDY

Roberta Gutiérrez, a fair-skinned blonde, 48 yrs. old, and moderately obese, was admitted to the Brachmoor Community Hospital for diagnosis and treatment. Her symptoms included indigestion (**dyspepsia**), **flatulence** (excessive gas), severe, intermittent pain in the upper right quadrant and right shoulder, slight jaundice, an intolerance to fatty foods, and a history of **postprandial** (after meal) nausea, and vomiting.

Her admission diagnosis was cholecystitis. To confirm the diagnosis, a cholecystogram was ordered. **Cholecystography** is a technique in which the patient eats a fat-free meal and then, postprandial, swallows some tablets of a special dye. The tablets dissolve and eventually fill the gall bladder with a dye that can be seen with X-rays.

The cholecystography confirmed the presence of stones in the gall bladder (**cholelithiasis**) and a rather large stone in the common bile duct (**choledocholithiasis**). The patient was scheduled for a cholecystectomy and a choledochal exploration (E.C.D., exploration of the common duct).

Pre-operatively, the patient had a gastrointestinal tube **passed** (inserted) through the nose and down into the intestines to relieve the abdominal distention and flatulence. She was given **enemas** (introduction of fluid into the rectum) to clear the lower **bowel** (intestine). It was noted that external **hemorrhoids** (varicose veins of the rectum) were present and this fact was reported. She expressed some relief following

Figure 15-8: The gastrointestinal tube was passed into the nose and down into the jejunum; *(courtesy of American Hospital Supply).*

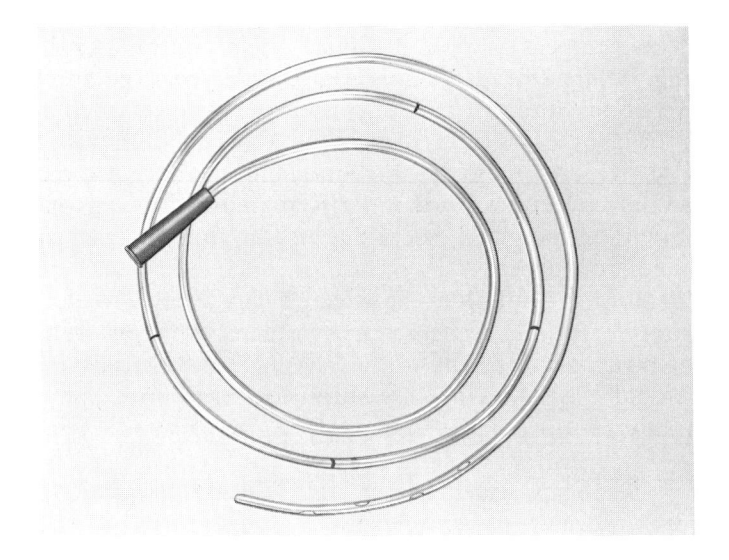

the enemas, explaining that **constipation** (difficult defecating) had been a problem for her for some time. The surgery, a cholecystectomy with choledochotomy and **choledocholithotripsy** (crushing of gall stone in the common duct) was successful.

Post-operatively, the patient responded well to all therapy. Within two weeks, she was able to be discharged, to return home.

SUMMARY

The alimentary tract and its associated organs change foods from complex substances into basic nutrients that can be assimilated by the body. The body cells utilize the nutrients for energy, growth, and repair. Solid waste products are eliminated from the tract in the form of feces.

The digestive system is primarily a tube system and some of its most common pathologies involve lumen obstruction.

PRACTICE & REVIEW

Explain and define the new special terms you have been using. Remember, you learned how to pronounce them at the beginning of this chapter.

1. alimentary tract _____
2. cholecystogram _____
3. choledocholithiasis _____
4. colonopathy _____

5. enterocinesia _____

6. dyspepsia _____

7. gastric _____

8. hepatalgia _____

9. postprandial _____

10. proteases _____

Now, double-check the meaning of the terms above by studying the brief definitions given in the Glossary-Index at the back of this text.

Test yourself quickly before going on to learn other medical and professional terms. Use these short review exercises to practice for your new work in health services. Your teacher will also help by recommending various other Study Activities.

A. Complete the statements below with the best word from this list:

saliva	peristalsis	maltose	cholemesis
caries	enterocentesis	sippy	anus
mucus	villi	omentum	glucose

1. One example of a monosaccharide is _____ .
2. A diet consisting primarily of milk and cream is called a _____ diet.
3. The fluid produced by the salivary glands is called _____ .
4. Dental cavities are also known as dental _____ .
5. The terminal opening to the gastrointestinal tract is the _____ .
6. Rhythmic waves of contraction which propel the food along the digestive tract are called _____ .
7. Microscopic finger-like projections lining the intestinal tract are called the _____ .
8. Puncturing the intestines to withdraw gas or fluid is called _____ .
9. Segment of peritoneum that hangs like an apron over the intestines is called the _____ .
10. The term used to mean vomiting bile is _____ .

B. Gastr- or gastro- are common prefixes meaning stomach. Complete the words below by adding the proper ending according to meaning:

1. Stomach pain   Gastr _____
2. Inflamed stomach   Gastr _____
3. Removal of the stomach   Gastr _____
4. Study of the stomach   Gastr _____
5. Paralysis of the stomach Gastro _____

ALIMENTARY CANAL 255 *

C. In the following list, there are various terms which pertain to the digestive system. Define the underlined prefix, combining words, or suffix.

1. <u>enter</u>itis _____
2. <u>hepat</u>itis _____
3. col<u>itis</u> _____
4. <u>cholecyst</u>itis _____
5. <u>choledoch</u>itis _____

D. Match the words on the right with the best statement on the left:

____ 1. Another name for the oral cavity   a. deglutition
____ 2. The process of swallowing   b. nutrients
____ 3. A feeling of fullness   c. lumen
____ 4. Pain in the intestines   d. enterogenous
____ 5. Semi-solid waste   e. amylase
____ 6. Enzyme which acts on carbohydrates   f. dentes
____ 7. Cavity of a tube organ   g. lipase
____ 8. Arising within the intestines   h. enterodynia
____ 9. Essential substances for growth   i. bloat
____ 10. Another word for teeth   j. feces
   k. buccal
   l. urine

E. The following words are introduced in this chapter's case study. Define them in the space provided:

1. cholecystography _____
2. cholelithiasis _____
3. bowel _____
4. hemorrhoids _____
5. enema _____

After studying Chapter 16
The Urinary System
You should be able to:

* *Pronounce and define each of its new medical words and phrases and use the new technical jargon.*

* *Identify ten structures of the urinary system.*

* *Describe the production of urine.*

PRONOUNCE THESE TEN NEW WORDS WITH YOUR TEACHER: MEDICAL WORDS

albuminuria (al-bu″mĭ-nu′re-ah)
glomerulonephritis (glo-mer′u-lo-nĕ fri′tis)
hemodialysis (he″mo-di-al′ĭ-sis)
hyponatremia (hi″po-na-tre′me-ah)
nephroptosis (nef″rop-to′sĭs)

renopathy (re-nop′ah-the)
uromancy (u′ro-man′se)
hyperkalemia (hi″per-kah-le′me-ah)
emaciated (e-ma″se-a-ted)
hematuria (hem′ah-tu′re-ah)

Excessive accumulation of the waste products of metabolism is not compatible with life. In fact, regular continuous **excretion** (elimination) of these substances must be assured for health.

Several organs and systems in the body are concerned with this function. For example, you have already learned that the skin eliminates water and salts through perspiration. Perspiration tastes salty because it contains **sodium chloride**. Sodium chloride is but one of the many different salts found in the body.

Salts, minerals, or crystalloids in the body dissolve in the body fluids and break apart (**dissociate**). Substances that so dissociate are called electrolytes because they **ionize** or develop electrical charges when they are dissolved in water. The individual components or particles of these substances have an electrical charge and are called **ions**. Some ions are positively charged (+) and some are negatively charged (−) electrically. For example, the salt, sodium chloride, dissolves in solution into sodium ions and chlorine ions. **Electrolytes**, then, are salts

Figure 16-1: Salts that dissociate are called electrolytes. When sodium chloride is placed in water, it dissociates to form electrically charged sodium and chlorine ions.

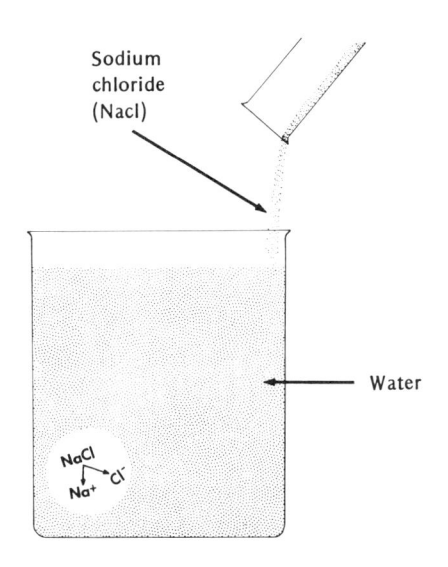

or other compounds, or combinations of elements, such as acids or bases which ionize in solution. Very simply, acids contain **hydrogen ions** and bases contain **hydroxyl ions**.

The next list illustrates some of the ions in the body that are vital to normal physiology:

Name of Ions	Symbol & Electrical Charge
Sodium	Na^+
Potassium	K^+
Calcium	Ca^{++}
Hydrogen	H^+
Hydroxyl	OH^-
Chlorine	Cl^-
Bicarbonate	HCO_3^-

ENZYME SYSTEMS

The enzyme systems of the body can only operate within narrow parameters or limiting measures of ionic concentrations and acid base balance. **Base** is another word for alkaline. The pH or acid base level of body fluids is dependent upon the presence of hydrogen ions. An excess of hydrogen ions lowers the pH

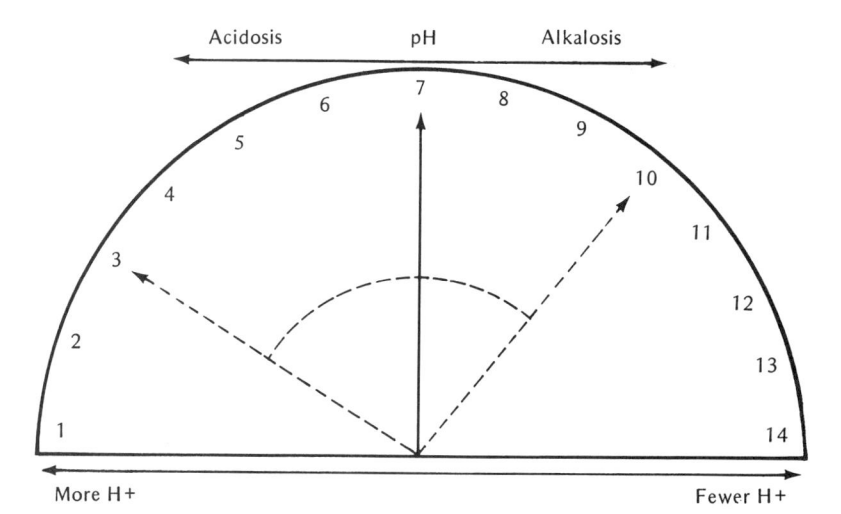

Figure 16-2: Enzyme systems of the body will only operate if the ionic concentrations of body fluid are balanced.

and leads to acidosis or **acid intoxication**. Too few hydrogen ions raises the pH and leads to **alkalosis** (excess alkalinity). Too many sodium ions lead to **hypernatremia**; too few to **hyponatremia**. Too many potassium ions lead to **hyperkalemia**; too few potassium ions to **hypokalemia**. Each of these disturbed ionic concentrations can prove life threatening.

Other organs that eliminate waste products include the lungs which excrete carbon dioxide and water, the intestines which eliminate solid wastes in the form of feces, and the liver which excretes substances in the bile. The major organs responsible for fluid and electrolyte balance are the two kidneys. They filter the blood and produce the liquid waste product called urine.

Urine normally is a clear yellow acid liquid slightly heavier than water. It contains various concentrations of electrolytes as well as metabolic wastes such as **uric acid**, urea, **creatinine**, and **ammonia**. **Urinalysis** (urine examination) frequently discloses abnormal constituents such as blood (**hematuria**), sugar, the protein, albumin (**albuminuria**), ketones (**ketonuria**), pus (**pyuria**), and casts. **Casts** (sediments) are made up of salts which have precipitated out of solution and formed in the shape of little tubes. These concretions can accumulate and form stone in the kidneys.

Although small (4 to 6 ounces), the kidneys are marvelously complex organs. Managing much of the blood chemistry, they excrete approximately 1,000 to 1,800 ml or from 2 to 3½ pints of urine in a 24-hour period. The character and composition of the urine reflect the composition of the blood. For example, as calcium ions in the blood rise to excessive levels (**calcemia**), the amount of calcium excreted in the urine also rises (**calciuria**). In a like manner, if the body becomes **dehydrated** (excessive water loss), the urine becomes more **concentrated** (contains less water), as part of the attempt to conserve water to meet body needs.

THE KIDNEYS

The **kidneys** are two reddish-brown organs approximately 4 inches long (11.25 cm), 2 to 3 inches wide (5–7.5 cm), and one inch thick (2.5 cm). Each is shaped like the dark red "kidney bean" and has a hilum or notch on its medial border. Blood vessels, nerves, and the ureter enter and leave each kidney through that hilum.

Figure 16-3: The urinary system organs; *(courtesy of Ethicon, Inc.).*

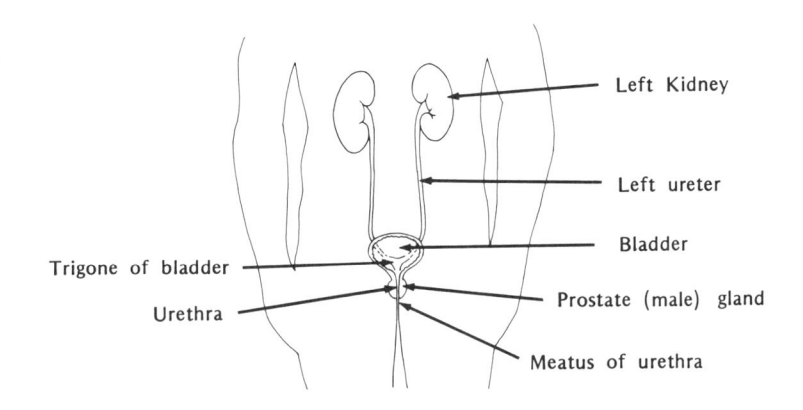

- Left Kidney
- Left ureter
- Bladder
- Trigone of bladder
- Urethra
- Prostate (male) gland
- Meatus of urethra

The kidneys have a fibrous capsule (**renal fascia**) and are embedded in **perirenal** (around kidney) fat. The fat pad and the pressure of the adjacent organs hold the kidneys in place between the 12th thoracic vertebra and the 3rd lumbar vetebra in the retroperitoneal space.

The urine produced in the kidneys passes into the **ureters**. There are two ureters, each approximately 10 to 12 inches long (25–30 cm). They are lined with mucous membrane and have smooth muscular walls. Peristaltic waves assist gravity in moving the urine into the urinary bladder (**urocyst**) for storage and elimination from the body.

The urocyst has a maximum capacity under normal circumstance of 750 ml of urine. The urge to empty the bladder (**void**) is felt when there is approximately 250 ml of urine present. Emptying the bladder is called **urinating**, **voiding**, or **micturating**.

The urinary bladder is found in the pelvic cavity, just posterior to the pubic bone. In the male, it lies just anterior to the rectum but in the female, it lies anterior to the uterus or womb. A sack-like organ, it is lined with mucous membrane and has smooth muscular walls. The urine passes from the bladder through a round muscle (**urinary sphincter**) which guards the entrance to the bladder. It then passes to the outside and is excreted through the urethra. Through a **cystoscope** (instrument to view the bladder) the ureters and urethra are seen as three tiny openings in the base of the bladder. They form a rough triangular area (**trigone**) in which **calculi** (stones) tend to collect.

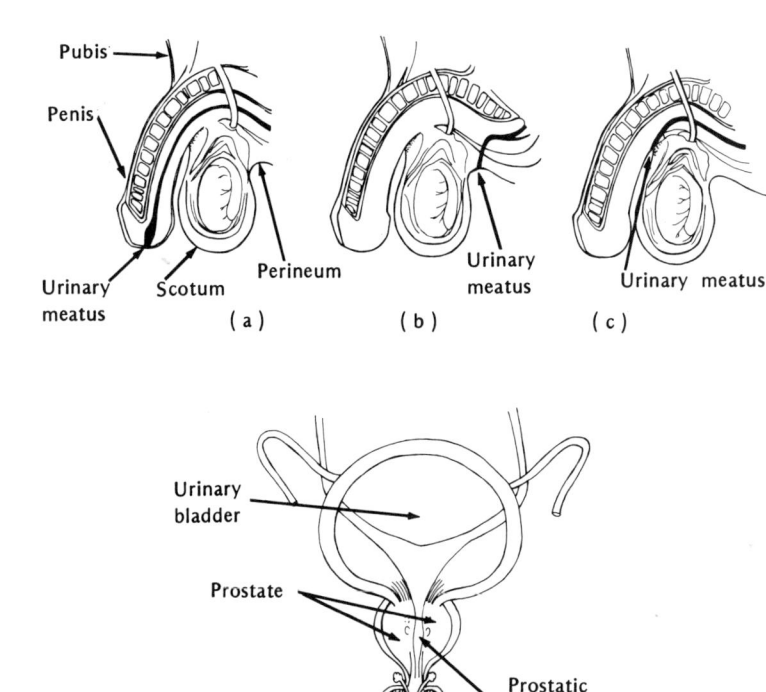

Figure 16-4:
(a) Normal urinary meatus;
(b) hypospadias—urinary meatus opening on perineum;
(c) hypospadias—urinary meatus opening on under surface of penis;
(d) the male urethra passes directly through the prostate gland. Hypertrophy of the pros prostate can obstruct the flow of urine; *(courtesy of Picker Corp.).*

THE KIDNEYS 261 *

Figure 16-5: Each condition prevents continuous flow of urine: (a) nephroptosis; (b) stricture due to inflammation; (c) atresia due to congenital lack of development.

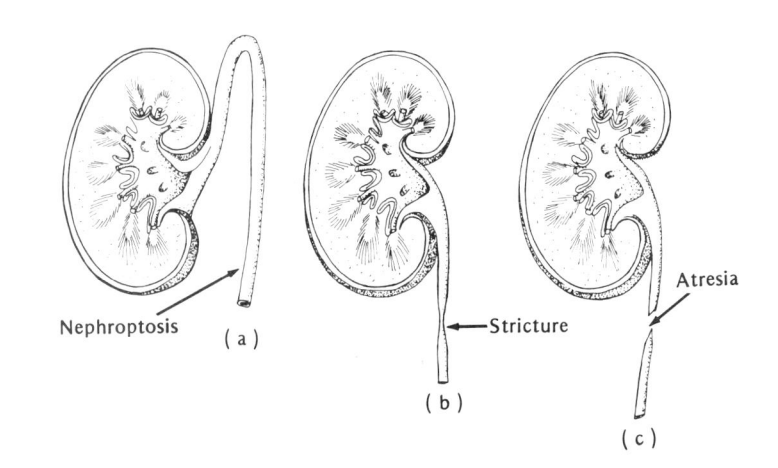

The **urethra** is a narrow mucous-lined canal or tube which leads from the bladder to the outside. In the female, the urethra is approximately one and a half inches long (3.8 cm) and the urinary meatus opens just anterior to the vagina. The male urethra is nearly 8 inches long (20 cm). It passes from the urinary bladder through the floor of the pelvis and travels the length of the male penis. Near the base of the male bladder, the urethra is surrounded by the prostate gland.

The male external urinary meatus normally is found at the distal tip of the penis. Sometimes the male external urinary meatus congenitally fails to extend to the penile tip. If the urethra opens on the underside of the penis or on the **perineum** (area between the anus and scrotum), the condition is known as **hypospadias**.

The tube system for draining, storing, and eliminating urine must be maintained in a **patent** (open) state. Obstruction to the flow of urine in the ureters can result from either congenital **atresia** (lack of development), or from **strictures** (narrowing) due to inflammations, from the presence of renal calculi, from kinking due to downward displacement of the kidneys (**nephroptosis**), or from occlusion due to some pressure or pathology in adjacent organs. For example, a tumor of the small bowel wall could extend posteriorly and compress the ureter in the area. Hypertrophy of the prostate can also occlude the urethra which passes through it, and so obstruct the flow of urine.

Urine Production

The production of urine occurs in the microscopic tubule units of the kidney called the **nephrons**. To locate them, one must first section the kidney longitudinally and inspect the gross internal renal structures. Look at the diagram in Figure 16-6 to identify the **cortex** or outer portion, the **medulla** or middle portion, and the pelvis or inner portion of the kidney.

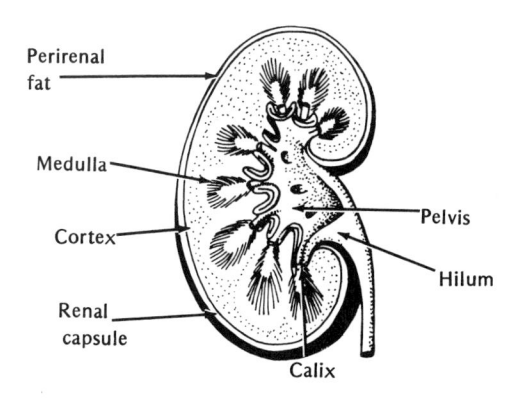

Figure 16-6: Gross structures of internal kidney.

The pelvis of the kidney is an expanded extension of the ureters. These subdivisions or recesses reach into the substance of the kidney toward the medulla as cup-like **calices**. The medulla is formed of multiple tubules (**collecting tubules**) which are piled together in such a way as to form microscopic mounds called the **pyramids**. The collecting tubules drain the urine formed in the cortex into the calices and then into the pelvis to the ureters.

The cortex of each kidney contains approximately one million nephrons. Each **nephron** is made up of blood vessels and tubules—the **glomerulus** (tuft of capillaries), a surrounding tubule (**Bowman's capsule**), and a series of twisted tubules, the proximal **convoluted** and the distal **convoluted** tubules, and **Henle's loop**. The distal convoluted tubules are continuous with the collecting tubule of the medulla.

Urine production (**uropoiesis**) actually begins when blood is brought to the cells of the nephron in the cortex by branches of the renal artery. The terminal branches of the renal artery are called the **afferent vessels**. These carry blood into each glomerular capillary bed where water and waste products pass through the vascular walls and into Bowman's capsule. At this point, the solution is known as the **filtrate**. The fluid is not urine until it enters the collecting tubules of the medulla.

Many changes occur in the composition of fluid as it passes through the tubular system. Blood from each glomerulus, minus the fluid and solutes that pass into the tube system, flows into the **efferent blood** vessels. These efferent vessels form a second capillary bed (**efferent** or **tubular capillary bed**) whose vessels

Figure 16-7: The nephron, a microscopic renal structure in which urine is produced.

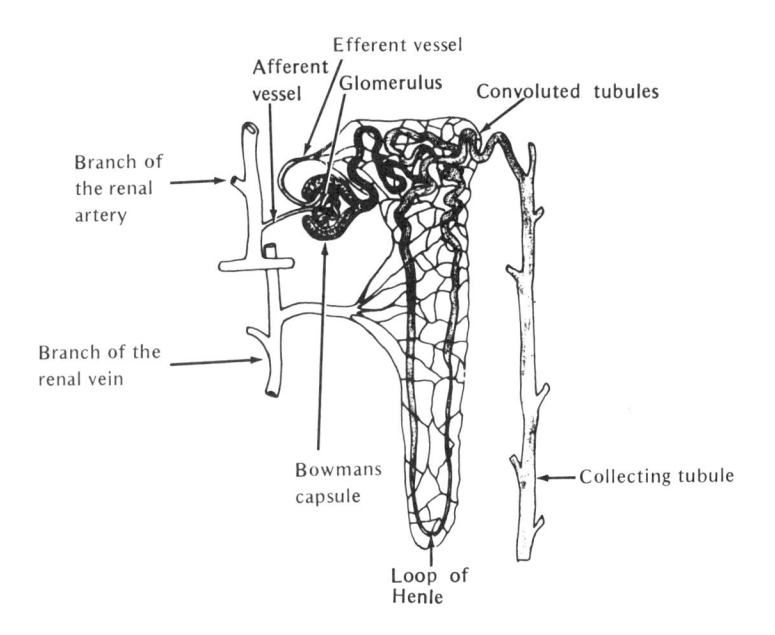

wind themselves around the convoluted tubules and the loop of Henle. At this point, substances such as ions and water pass into the filtrate from the blood or return from the filtrate into the blood stream.

The direction of ion movement is directly related to the physiologic need of the body to maintain the proper pH. For example, if the blood becomes too acid, hydrogen ions move into the filtrate and are eliminated from the body in the urine. If the blood becomes too alkaline, hydrogen ions move in the opposite direction back into the blood from the filtrate.

Remember, **dialysis** means the separation of substances in solution due to passage of some of the substances through a semipermeable membrane. Urine production depends in part on filtration osmosis, and in part, on dialysis.

Two hormones greatly influence urine production. One is ADH and the other is aldosterone. Aldosterone is produced in the cortex of the adrenal gland. Hormones also influence the work of the kidney. The kidney cells themselves, in addition to regulating blood chemistry and water balance, influence the activity of other organs. The kidneys are vital organs but since there are two, the loss of one is not fatal.

Renin, an enzyme secreted by the renal cells, affects the size of blood vessels, causing them to constrict as needed. Constriction of blood vessels raises the blood pressure. But an excessive level of renin results in the high blood pressure that contributes to hypertension. A second substance, the hormone **erythropoietin**, is also believed to be produced by the kidney cells. Erythropoietin stimulates the release of erythrocytes from the bone marrow when the number of circulating erythrocytes falls below normal.

Two important prefixes that mean kidney are **nephro-** and **reni-**. Review the two lists of words which follow in order to understand some of the terms used about kidney-related health problems:

Prefix Reni	Medical Term
renopathy	any disease of the kidneys
renography	X-ray study of the kidney
renal	pertaining to the kidney
renipelvic	pertaining to the kidney pelvis
renitis	inflammation of the kidney

Prefix Nephro	Medical Meaning
nephrogram	X-ray film of the kidney
nephrolith	kidney stone
nephrectomy	removal of a kidney
nephritis	inflammation of a kidney
nephropexy	surgical fixation of nephroptosis

The combining form **uro-**, **ur-**, or **uria**, denoting relationships to urine, can be used as a prefix or suffix or in other combined forms. Review some combined forms in the list that follows:

Combining Form Ur, Uria, Uro	Medical Meaning
urologist	urinary specialist
urodynia	painful urination
oliguria	scant urine in relation to fluid intake
anuria	no urine excretion
uromancy	prognosis based on urine examination

In addition to obstructions, various inflammations and tumor formations can cause **nephropathy** (kidney pathology).   Pathology

Chronic nephropathy can eventually lead to kidney failure (renal **suppression**) so that dangerous waste products accumulate (**uremia**) in the body. Five other major pathologies of the urinary tract have been summarized for you in the following list:

Pathology	Medical Meaning
glomerulonephritis	inflammation of the glomeruli, frequently following a hemolytic streptococcal infection
pyelitis	inflammation of the renal pelvis associated with pyuria
hydronephrosis	distention of the renal pelvis and tubules with urine
cystitis	inflammation of the urinary bladder; associated with dysuria (painful voiding)

CASE HISTORY

Randolph Hunt, age 67, is dying of uremia. His **emaciated** (appearing wasted) body is almost motionless in the hospital bed except for the fingers of his right hand which seem to pick at the bedding. Tubes of various kinds can be seen entering and leaving his body orifices. A nasogastric tube has been passed and now contains brownish fluid drainage. An intravenous bottle hangs over the bed, with 200 ml of solution still to be **infused** (introduced) into a vein by gravity. A urinary retention **catheter** (tube) is inserted in his bladder and drains into the bedside bag. Its contents show oliguria.

For over two years, Mr. Hunt has been treated with **hemodialysis** (blood dialysis) but in the last three months, his condition has deteriorated. He is disoriented, experiencing cheyne-stokes respirations, feeble tachycardia, and a white, powdery substance (**uremic frost**) is present on his skin. The latest blood chemistries indicate acidosis. He has been visited by his priest and by his family.

* * *

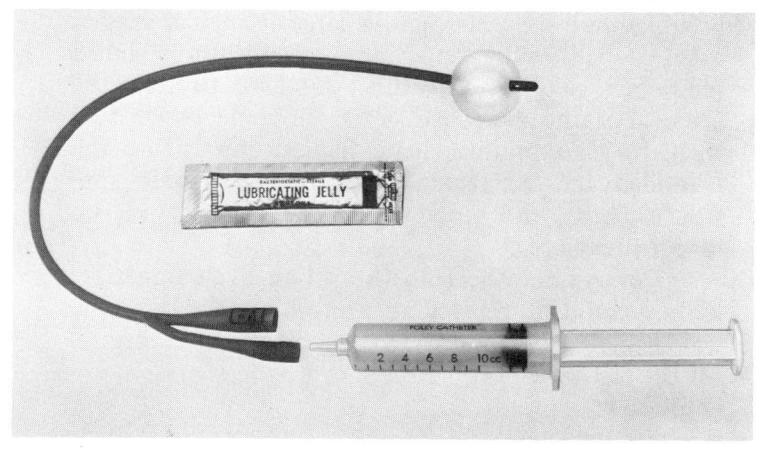

Figure 16-8: A lubricated catheter is passed into the bladder through the urethra. The catheter balloon is then inflated with water with a syringe. The baloon retains the catheter in the bladder for continuous drainage; *(courtesy of American Hospital Supply).*

What circumstances brought this once vital man to his present **moribund** (dying) state? They consist of a long history of nephropathy that gradually produced a chronic uremic state and finally total renal failure. When Mr. Hunt was twelve years old, he was injured in a motorcycle accident with a resulting left nephroptosis. Kinking of the ureter had already caused a left hydronephrosis with kidney damage by the time a nephropexy was performed.

At 54 years of age, complaining of a severe pain in his right flank, Mr. Hunt made an appointment with the hospital's staff urologist. The pain was diagnosed as **renal colic** (acute paroxysmal intermittent pain). Urinalysis revealed **hematuria**, pyuria, albuminuria, and casts. The physician, suspecting renal calculi, admitted Mr. Hunt to the hospital. There he was prepared for a **cystoscopy** (bladder inspection) and **retrograde pyelogram** (nephrogram with dye introduced from below). The cystoscopy was performed by introducing a cystoscope into the urinary bladder. During the cystoscopy, a small ureteral catheter was threaded up into each ureter and a contrast media was injected. It filled the pelvis of the kidney, then drained down into the bladder as X rays were taken. This procedure confirmed the suspected diagnosis—renal colic due to renal calculi. The calculi then present were crushed and finally excreted (**passed**) in the urine.

Despite dietary adjustments, the following ten years saw repeated episodes of renal colic. At one point, about six years ago, a large triangular-shaped calculus had to be removed by nephrotomy and a temporary nephrostomy tube was used to drain the urine. For the next two years, he came twice each week to a community hemodialysis unit to use the **hemodialyzer,** a machine that removes toxic substances from the blood when the kidneys can no longer function.

For a time Mr. Hunt hoped that a compatible kidney could be transplanted into his body, but none was available. A month ago, he entered the hospital for the last time.

SUMMARY

The urinary system carries out the important function of secreting urine, a liquid waste. In the process of urine formation, fluids and electrolytes are balanced and the homeostasis of blood chemistry is maintained.

PRACTICE & REVIEW

Explain and define the new special terms you have been using. Remember, you learned how to pronounce them at the beginning of this chapter.

1. albuminuria _____
2. glomerulonephritis _____
3. hemodialysis _____
4. hyponatremia _____
5. nephroptosis _____
6. renopathy _____
7. uromancy _____
8. hyperkalemia _____
9. emaciated _____
10. hematuria _____

Now, double-check the meaning of the terms above by studying the brief definitions given in the Glossary-Index at the back of this text.

Test yourself quickly before going on to learn other medical and professional terms. Use these short review exercises to practice for your new work in health services. Your teacher will also help by recommending various other Study Activities.

*268 THE URINARY SYSTEM

A. In each of these ten statements, a word has been underlined. Encircle the number of those that are false after you read them carefully:

1. <u>Excretion</u> is another word for elimination.
2. <u>Dissociate</u> means to cling together.
3. Ions which have a negative charge are indicated by the symbol "<u>±</u>".
4. Acids contain <u>H^+</u>.
5. Excessive hydrogen ions leads to <u>alkalosis</u>.
6. <u>Hyponatremia</u> means too many sodium ions are present.
7. <u>Urine</u> is a semi-solid waste product.
8. <u>Perirenal</u> fat found around the kidney helps hold the kidney in place.
9. Another name for the kidney is <u>urocyst</u>.
10. Congenital lack of development is called <u>atresia</u>.

B. Nephro- and ren- are two prefixes that mean the same thing, kidney. Complete the terms at the right correctly:

1. kidney stone — nephro _____
2. X-ray film of the kidney — nephro _____
3. surgical fixation of nephroptosis — nephro _____
4. pertaining to the kidney — ren _____
5. pertaining to the kidney pelvis — reni _____
6. removal of a kidney — nephr _____
7. inflammation of the kidney — nephr _____
8. inflammation of the kidney — ren _____
9. X-ray study of the kidney — ren _____
10. any disease of the kidney — ren _____

C. Three terms meaning "eliminating urine from the bladder" have been introduced in this chapter.
They are: 1. _____ ; 2. _____ ; 3. _____ .

D. The list below has the names of some of the important ions in the body. In the space provided, write the symbols for each ion:

1. potassium _____
2. calcium _____
3. sodium _____
4. hydrogen _____
5. chlorine _____

E. Each of the following words indicates the presence of some substance in the urine. Define each in the space provided:

1. hematuria _____
2. glycosuria _____
3. pyuria _____
4. ketonuria _____
5. albuminuria _____

F. Match the words on the right with the best statement in the left column:

____ 1. Presence of too many potassium ions
____ 2. Excessive water loss
____ 3. Term which means "narrowing"
____ 4. Urethra opening on under surface of penis
____ 5. Area between anus and scrotum
____ 6. Area in base of bladder between openings of ureters and urethra
____ 7. Another term for urine production
____ 8. Microscopic unit which secretes urine
____ 9. Deficiency of potassium ions in the blood
____ 10. Scant urine

a. oliguria
b. hypokalemia
c. hyperkalemia
d. hyponatremia
e. perineum
f. nephron
g. hypospadias
h. dehydrated
i. ammonia
j. stricture
k. trigone
l. uropoiesis

After studying Chapter 17
The Reproductive System
You should be able to:

* *Pronounce and define each of its new medical words and phrases and use the new technical jargon.*

* *Identify eight female reproductive organs.*

* *Identify four male reproductive organs.*

PRONOUNCE THESE TEN NEW WORDS WITH YOUR TEACHER: MEDICAL WORDS

aneurysm (an'u-rĭzm) hysteropathy (his″te-rop'ah-the)
chancre (shang'ker) menarche (mē-nar'ke)
colporrhaphy (kol-por'ah-fe) phimosis (fe-mo'sĭs)
amenorrhea (a-men″o-re'ah) prostatectomy (pros″tah-tek'to-me)
epididymitis (ep″ĭ-did″ĭ-mi'tĭs) spermatogenesis (sper'mah-to-jen'e-sis)

The reproductive organs in both male and female serve a dual role. They function as part of the reproductive system by producing the gametes which unite to form new human beings, and as part of the endocrine system by supplying the body with specific hormones.

Although the reproductive organs of both sexes originate from the same embryonal tissue, the mature reproductive structures (**genitals**) are unalike. The dissimilarity differentiates male from female. Both systems consist of a series of tubes and glands—the external and internal genitalia. The female organs house the fetus until birth and then deliver the baby to the outside. The male organs have a single passageway for both the reproductive cells and urine, although they cannot function at the same time.

The internal female reproductive organs include the ovaries, fallopian tubes, uterus (**womb**), and vagina. The external female genitalia are called the vulva. The **vulva** includes the mons pubis, THE INTERNAL FEMALE ORGANS

Figure 17-1:
(a) Female reproductive tract—lateral view;
(b) internal female reproductive structures showing ovulation.

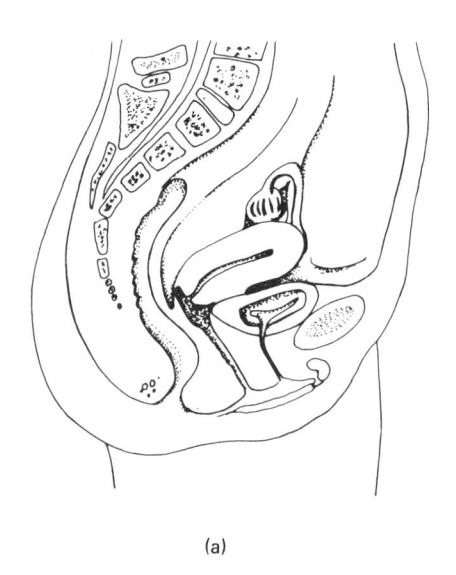

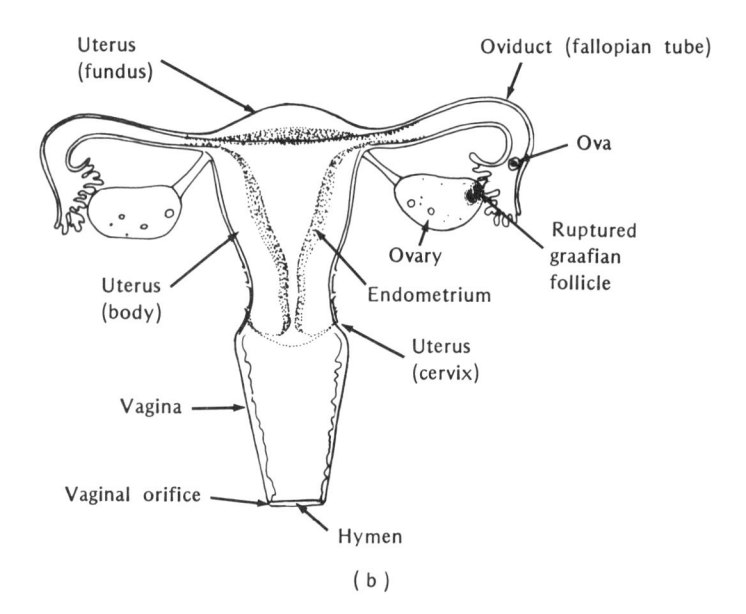

(a)

(b)

the clitoris, labia majora, labia minora, external vaginal orifice, and the perineum.

The **ovaries** (female gonads) are two oval-shaped glandular organs found deep in the pelvis. After puberty, most women extrude (**ovulate**) an **ovum** (egg) on a fairly regular basis that is determined by the length of their menstrual cycle. That **menstrual cycle** (length of time between menses) is under the control of two pituitary hormones—FSH (follicle stimulating hormone) and LH (luteinizing hormones). Both of these hormones influence the ovaries. The ovaries in turn secrete two hormones, estrogen and progesterone, which act upon the uterus.

The **oviducts** or **fallopian tubes** (**salpinges**) serve as passageways for both ovum and sperm. Conception or fertilization of the ovum takes place either before the ovum enters an oviduct or soon after it enters one of them. The two oviducts are approximately 4 inches (10 cm) long. Conception must take place normally within the lateral one-third of the tube to be viable. Their free-moving ends or cilia near the ovary are thought to help move the ovum.

The **uterus** is a hollow, pear-shaped organ approximately 3 inches (7.5 cm) long and 2 inches (5 cm) wide. It is found between the urinary bladder and rectum. It is normally slightly flexed in an anterior position. Sometimes the anterior flexion is quite pronounced (**anteflexion**). Sometimes the body and the fundus of the uterus are bent backward (**retroflexion**) and sometimes the entire uterus is tipped backward (**retroversion**). The uterus is held in place by ligaments. Sometimes these ligaments weaken so that the uterus drops out of place and descends (**prolapses**) into the vagina (**procidentia**). Surgery to resuspend the uterus in its proper position is called **hysteropexy** (uterine suspension).

The uterus has three parts; the area above the attachments of the oviducts called the **fundus**, a middle section called the body, and a slender neck-like portion called the **cervix** which hangs into the vagina. The external cervical **os** (mouth or opening) leads into the uterine cavity. The walls of the uterus consist of a smooth muscle (**myometrium**) that is capable of the great distention needed to accommodate pregnancy. Its lining is called the **endometrium**. This endometrium is the vascular tissue lining of the uterus which is periodically shed during and in the menstrual flow. As you can see, three organs are involved in the menstrual cycle—the pituitary gland, the ovaries, and the uterus.

The **menstrual flow** (**menses**) begins about every four weeks in the absence of pregnancy. It is a recurring discharge of blood and tissue fluid and of the mucous membrane that makes up the endometrium. The average menstrual cycle spans approximately 28 days. But many factors can cause wide variances in the regularity and length of each woman's normal cycle. Emotional and physical stress as well as frank pathology may also alter the usual periodic rhythm.

Look at the diagram in Figure 17-2 to review the course of

The Menstrual Cycle

Figure 17-2: (a) The menstrual cycle: days 1-11 FSH stimulates development of ova in Graafian follicle. Ovary produces estrogen which stimulates the endometrium; (b) the menstrual cycle: days 11-14 LH produced by pituitary. Day 14, ovulation; (c) days 14-28—after ovulation, corpus luteum forms and produces progesterone which makes the endometrium ready for implantation of the ova. Day 28 is followed by menstruation;

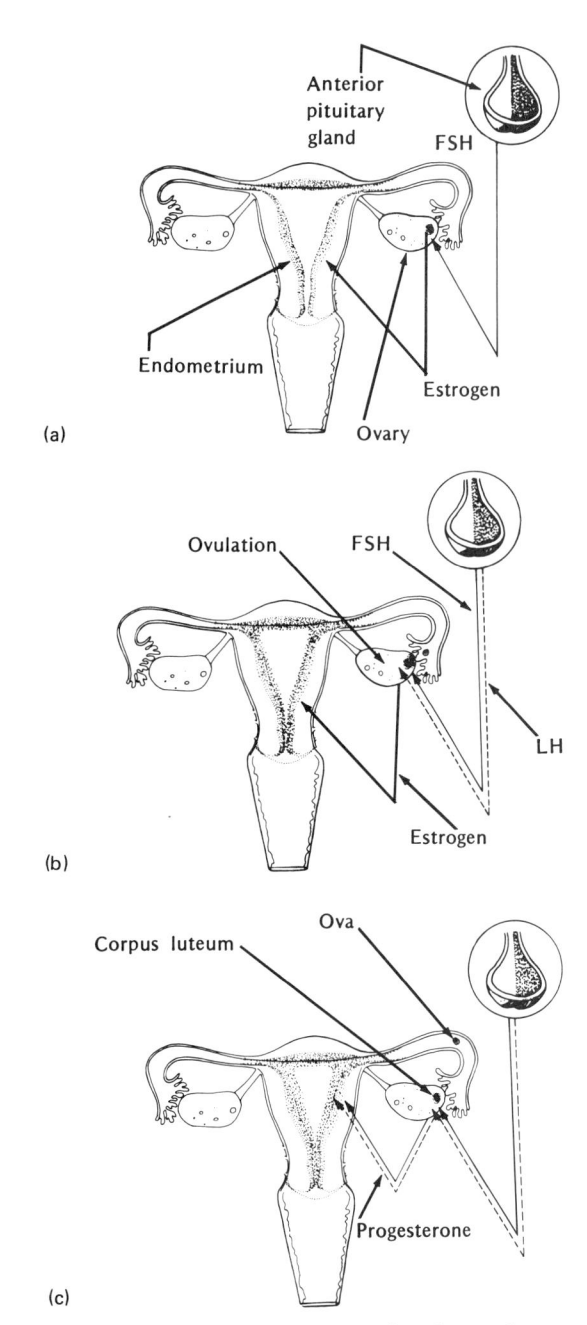

the menstrual cycle. On the first day in the cycle, the endometrium begins to be shed and the pituitary gland begins to secrete increasing amounts of FSH. The FSH hormone reaches the ovary by way of the blood stream. It stimulates the special ovarian cells, called collectively the **graafian follicle**, so that it matures an ovum. In their turn, the cells of the graafian follicle secrete estrogen, a hormone that prepares the genitalia for fertilization. By the 3rd to the 5th day of the cycle, if there is no fertilization, the endometrium is lost and the **menses** (menstruation) again takes place.

Then, as the estrogen level gradually rises again, the lining of the uterus begins to develop once more. The tissue becomes thicker and new blood vessels grow in the area.

About the 11th day of the cycle, pituitary LH levels begin to rise and exert a synergistic effect on the graafian follicle development. About the 14th day, the ova break free of the follicle (**ovulation**) leaving a yellow mass of cells behind called the **corpus luteum** or yellow body.

The cells of the corpus luteum secrete progesterone as the levels of LH remain high. This progesterone is carried to the uterus where it enables the endometrium to become soft and sticky, ready for the implantation of a fertilized ovum. The high levels of progesterone have a depressing effect on the levels of luteinizing hormone which begins to diminish. As the luteinizing hormone levels lower, the corpus luteum disintegrates and the levels of progesterone drop. Lowered progesterone levels result in the termination of the cycle and menstruation begins. If pregnancy takes place, the placenta secretes progesterone in sufficient levels to prevent ovulation and to maintain the endometrium.

The menstrual cycle continues from puberty at about the twelfth year (**hebetic age**) to the menopause (**climacteric**) at about age 55. The age for the climacteric varies with the individual woman. Many terms are associated with the menstrual cycle, since changes in the menses are often a sign of **gynecological** (pertaining to female reproductive) pathology. Study the list below to learn some of them:

Term	Description
menarche	first menstrual cycle (**period**)
menorrhagia	excessive menstrual flow
metrorrhagia	irregular menstrual flow
dysmenorrhea	painful menstruation
amenorrhea	absence of menses

Many words relating to the uterus are formed by combining the prefixes **metra-** or **hyster-** with other forms. Analyze and learn some terms formed in this way:

Term	Description
hysterectomy	surgical removal of the uterus
hysterodynia	pain in the uterus
hysterology	study of the uterus
hysterometer	instrument for measuring the uterus
hysteropathy	disease of the uterus
metrectomy	surgical removal of the uterus
metrodynia	pain in the uterus
metritis	inflammation of the uterus
metropathy	uterine disease
metrorrhea	an abnormal uterine discharge

Do not be fooled; some words in medicine and science can be deceptively similar. "Metro-" and "metra-" do mean uterus and "ology" does mean study of. But it might be somewhat disconcerting if you don't realize that **metrology** is the study of weights and measurements. That is because "metron-" (also from the Greek and meaning "measure") loses its "n" in modern English. Be sure to consider the context and check for sense when you encounter unfamiliar terms that you must use.

The vagina is a hollow muscular tube approximately 4 inches (10 cm) long which leads to the outside of the body. It is located between the urethra and rectum. Its entrance is guarded by a thin membrane, the **hymen**. Two small glands, **Bartholins glands**, pour their secretions into the anterior vagina. Words relating to the vagina begin with the prefix **colp-** or **colpo-**. For example, removal of the vagina is a **colpectomy** and repair of the vaginal wall, a **colporrhapy**.

The vagina is the female organ for **copulation** (sexual intercourse) and also serves as the birth canal. Painful copulation is called **dyspareunia**. The shared wall between the vagina and rectum may become weakened, although ordinarily there is no actual communication between them. If part of the rectum protrudes into the vagina, the condition is called a **rectocele**.

A weakening of the anterior vaginal wall, between the vagina and urethra and bladder, results in a **cystocele**, a herniation or protrusion of the bladder backward. The surgery to correct the rectocele is called a posterior colporrhaphy. The surgery to correct the cystocele is called an anterior colporrhaphy. In medical jargon, the procedure is called an **A&P repair**.

THE EXTERNAL FEMALE GENITALIA

The external female genitalia are collectively known as the **vulva** or **pudendum**. The upper part of the vulva is a rounded pad of hair-covered fat, resting over the pubic bone. This area is called the **mons pubis** or **mons veneris**.

Two folds or lip-like structures, also covered with hair, run backward from the mons pubis toward the rectum on either side of the pudendal cleft. These bordering folds extend posteriorly and rejoin at the perineum. Beneath these **labia majora**, also starting just below the mons pubis, are two hairless lips or folds called the **labia minora**. The clitoris is at this anterior junction.

The **clitoris**, a small cylindrical mass of tissue resembling the penis, is very sensitive and highly **erotic** (responsive to sexual stimulation). It is partially covered by a sheath of tissue, the **prepuce**. The area protected by the labia minora is called the **vestibule**.

This vestibule encloses the external urinary meatus and the external vaginal orifice. The perineum is the area between the external genitalia and the anus in both male and female. It helps to form the floor of the pelvis.

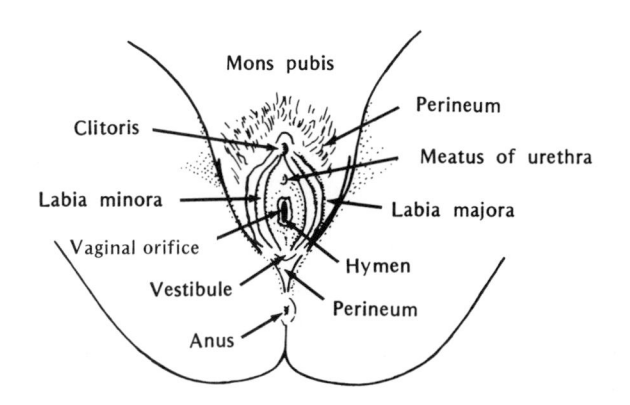

Figure 17-3: External female genitalia; *(courtesy of Ethicon, Inc.).*

THE MALE GENITALIA

The male genitals are also both internal and external. The most visible structures are the penis and scrotum.

Figure 17-4: Lateral view of male reproductive organs; *(courtesy of Ethicon, Inc.)*.

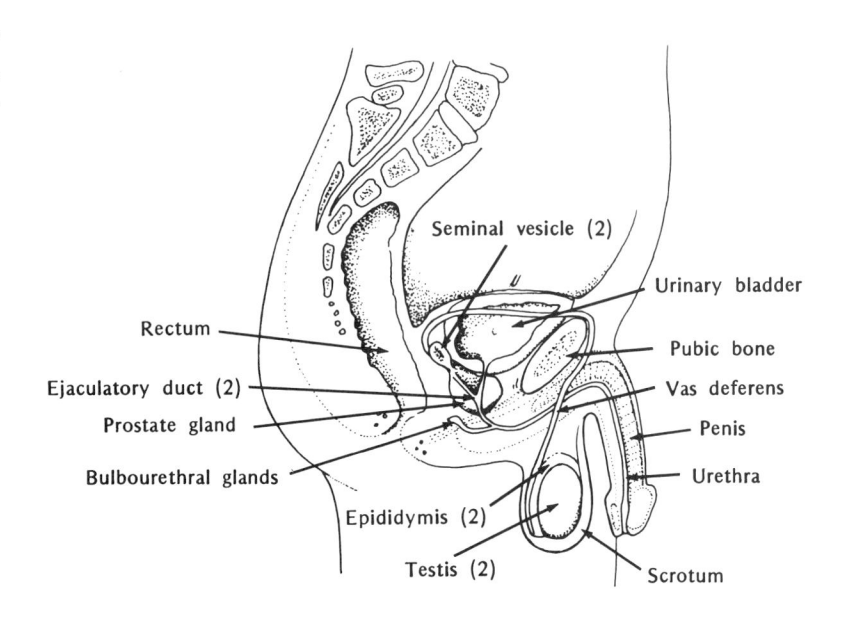

The **scrotum** is a sack-like pouch that holds the male gonads, the testes, and the tubes leading from them which are called the epididymides and vas deferans. The internal structures include the ejaculatory duct, the seminal vessicles, the bulbouretheral glands, and the prostate gland.

The **penis** is the male organ of copulation. It is approximately 6 inches (15 cm) long and composed of a special spongy tissue called cavernous erectile tissue. During sexual stimulation, this tissue fills with blood and becomes enlarged, very firm (**turgid**) and erect. The slightly enlarged tip of the penis is called the **glans**. A prepuce (**foreskin**) extends over the length of the penis and glans. Sometimes the foreskin is difficult to retract or pull back. This condition is known as **phimosis**. Phimosis prevents proper cleaning around the glans. **Circumcision** is a surgical procedure which removes the excess foreskin and corrects the phimosis.

The urethra travels the length of the penis and carries both urine and seminal fluid, but not at the same time. A sphincter at the base of the bladder prevents urine from passing during copulation.

The **seminal fluid** or **semen** is a composite of sperm, mucus and other alkaline secretions. The discharge of semen through the tube system during intercourse is known as **ejaculation**.

There are two testes, or male gonads. Small, oval glands approximately 2 inches (5 cm) long, they function in sperm production (**spermatogenesis**) and in hormone production. Spermatogenesis begins at puberty. Like the ovaries, the testes are stimulated by a pituitary hormone into activity. But unlike the ovaries, there is no dramatic cyclical rise and fall.

The male hormone, testosterone, is responsible for the secondary male characteristics. Both activities may continue until death since there is no climacteric as in the female. But normally there is a gradual decrease of sexual activity after middle age.

Occasionally, the testes, which develop in the fetal pelvis, fail to descend into the scrotum (**cryptorchidism**). If this condition is not corrected before puberty, that person will be **sterile** (unable to reproduce). But that same person may not be **impotent** (unable to perform sexually) since testosterone is still produced.

The **seminiferous tubules**, which form the testes and in which the sperm are produced, culminate in two 20 foot (6 m) long tubules, the **epididymides**. One epididymis is coiled tightly atop each testis. There the sperm are stored and mature until they are propelled through the reproductive tract for ejaculation. Each epididymis leads into the **vas deferens** or **ductus deferens** on its own side.

The ductus deferans, along with nerves and blood vessels, compose the **spermatic cord**. This cord passes through the abdominal wall and into the pelvis and down along the base of the urinary bladder, joining the **ejaculatory** duct on its own side. The pouch-like **seminal vessicles** lie at the base of the bladder and secrete part of the seminal fluid into the ejaculatory duct.

Three other glands, the small paired pea-shaped **Bulbourethral (Cowpers) glands**, and the large, single **prostate gland**, also contribute to the semen just before it enters the urethra. Removal of a diseased part of the prostate gland (**prostatectomy**) is a fairly common surgical procedure, especially in older men.

VENEREAL DISEASE

Venereal disease (V.D.) is a name given to a group of infectious, communicable diseases that are easily transmitted through direct sexual intercourse. Although there are many of these diseases, the two most commonly seen are gonorrhea and syphilis. These two venereal diseases can have most serious consequences.

Gonorrhea is caused by the gonococcus organisms. They are parasites and do not live long away from the moisture of body tissues. The gonococcus is pyogenic, causing an acute inflammatory process in the mucous membrane of the reproductive tract. In the male, the infection is accompanied by a urethral discharge and burning on micturition. The female may show no infection until an acute inflammatory pelvic disease (P.I.D.) develops.

In either male or female, the infection can result in the scarring of the tube systems to such an extent that the gametes cannot meet. That person is therefore made sterile. **Urethritis** (inflammation of the urethra), **vaginitis** (inflammation of the vagina), **salpingitis** (inflammation of the oviducts), and **epididymitis** (inflammation of the epididymides) and **orchitis** (inflammation of the testes) are common infections of the reproductive tract.

If the female becomes pregnant and then contracts gonorrhea, the baby may contract the disease as it passes through the cervical os and vagina during delivery. If unsuspected and/or untreated, gonorrhea will destroy the sight of a newborn. For that reason, medication is placed in the eyes of most newborn babies as a preventative technique.

Syphilis is caused by a corkscrew-shaped bacterium (a spirochete), the *Treponema pallidum*. Like the gonococcus, this microorganism is a parasite that requires living tissue for its own life. The initial site of invasion by the microbes results in a primary lesion called a **chancre**. Chancres are painless ulcers that are frequently found on the glans penis, cervix, and vagina. Such a chancre is a sign of primary syphilis. The lesion heals spontaneously. The spirochetes then enter the body systematically and reproduce (**secondary syphilis**).

Signs of this second stage of syphilis are sometimes exhibited in a body rash, sore throat, and general malaise. Sometimes, however, many years may pass before identifiable evidence of systemic involvement is seen. By that time, the disease process is in the third stage (**tertiary syphilis**). Then there may be cardiovascular and neurological involvement: **aneurysms** (weakened wall of blood vessels) which may rupture, **tabes dorsalis** (progressive wasting of the spinal cord) leading to paralysis, and **general paresis** (degeneration of the brain) leading to loss of mental powers. These are among the life-threatening consequences of syphilis. Both gonorrhea and syphilis are world-wide in their distribution.

CASE STUDY

Ricky Malone, seventeen years old and a high-school senior was a popular boy, well-liked by classmates and teachers. Nevertheless, he was obviously uncomfortable one morning as he stopped by the school nurse's office. Although her office was a favorite place with students who liked to stop and chat, Mrs. Cadwall, an R.N., sensed immediately that this visit was different.

She and Ricky went into the inner office and sat down. After much hesitation, Ricky confided to her that he thought he had caught the "**clapps**" (jargon for gonorrhea). He said he had met a new girl and "lost his head." He had been intimate with her last weekend and now, four days later, he had a yellowish discharge from his penis and it "burned" when he urinated. He wanted the nurse to give him "something" and begged her not to let anyone "know." He said he "knew" it wasn't serious.

Mrs. Cadwall was an experienced nurse who had worked with teenagers for many years. She quietly explained that it was important for Ricky to go to the V.D. clinic at the city health department right away for an urethral smear. She told him that the doctor would take a sample of the discharge, smear it on a glass slide, and stain it. He would look for the small microbes that cause gonorrhea. If he found them, as she suspected he would, he would order penicillin as treatment for the infection. She further explained that gonorrhea is an infectious venereal disease that is usually transmitted through copulation and that it can have serious consequences.

Right now, Mrs. Cadwall said, it seemed to be what was causing his urethritis. But without prompt treatment, such an infection could lead to cystitis, epididymitis, orchitis, and sterility. She explained that it was equally important for him to identify all his sexual contacts so that they could also be examined. Girls often are unaware that they are infected since their symptoms are not as pronounced. They, too, can develop venereal infections, particularly salpingitis. When that happens pus forms (**pyosalpinx**) in the fallopian tubes and that in turn may lead to sterility.

Figure 17-5: Cases of gonorrhea are on the increase throughout the nation.

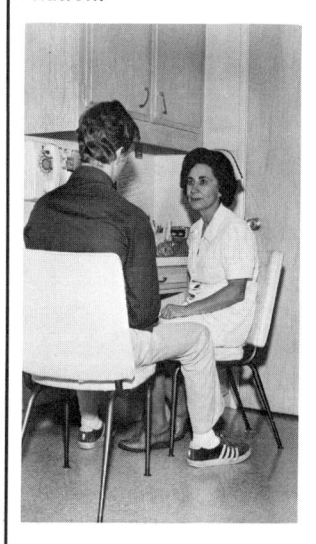

VENERAL DISEASE

It took some convincing but Ricky finally agreed to go to the V.D. clinic for diagnosis and treatment, and to name all his contacts. He only agreed to the latter after he was assured that his name as the informant would be kept confidential.

SUMMARY

The reproductive system has a dual role in the body; first, to reproduce the human species and secondly, to secrete the hormones that serve as part of the endocrine system. Venereal diseases are highly communicable, infectious diseases of the reproductive system that are transmitted primarily through direct sexual contact. Today, the morbidity rate for gonorrhea, one of the most serious venereal diseases, is remarkably high. Prompt treatment and case-finding offers the best hope for reduction in the number of cases and the severity of its consequences for human health.

PRACTICE & REVIEW

Explain and define the new special terms you have been using. Remember, you learned how to pronounce them at the beginning of this chapter.

1. aneurysm _____
2. chancre _____
3. colporrhaphy _____
4. amenorrhea _____
5. epididymitis _____
6. hysteropathy _____
7. menarche _____
8. phimosis _____
9. prostatectomy _____
10. spermatogenesis _____

Now, double-check the meaning of the terms above by studying the brief definitions given in the Glossary-Index at the back of this text.

Test yourself quickly before going on to learn other medical and professional terms. Use these short review exercises to practice for your new work in health services. Your teacher will also help by recommending various other Study Activities.

A. Match the words on the right with the best statement on the left:

___ 1. Excessive menstrual flow
___ 2. Sexual intercourse
___ 3. Painful menstruation
___ 4. Vulva
___ 5. Sack which holds the testes
___ 6. Study of weights and measures
___ 7. Protrusion
___ 8. Disease of the uterus
___ 9. Removal of the vagina
___ 10. Pain in the uterus

a. hysteropathy
b. dysmenorrhea
c. menorrhagia
d. metrodynia
e. copulation
f. herniation
g. pudendum
h. scrotum
i. metrology
j. prepuce
k. ejaculation
l. colpectomy

B. Complete the ten sentences below with terms from this list:

ovulation   climacteric   hymen   urological
ejaculation myometrium   hebetic   procedentia
dyspareunia gynecological endometrium   oviducts

1. Another name for the fallopian tubes is the _____ .
2. Extrusion of an ova from the ovary is called _____ .
3. The _____ is the muscular layer of the uterus.
4. Prolapse of the uterus into the vagina is called _____ .
5. The menopause is also called the _____ .
6. The menstrual cycle continues from the age of puberty or the _____ age until menopause.
7. The term _____ applies to female reproductive problems.
8. The vaginal orifice is guarded by a thin membrane called the _____ .
9. The term meaning painful copulation is _____ .
10. The passage of semen through the male reproductive tubes during intercourse is called _____ .

C. The prefixes, hyster- and metra-, both mean <u>uterus</u>. Complete the terms below by adding the proper ending:

1. Pain in the uterus   hystero _____
2. Study of the uterus   hyster _____
3. An abnormal uterine discharge   metr _____
4. Instrument for measuring uterus   hystero _____
5. Surgical removal of the uterus   metr _____

VENERAL DISEASE 283 *

After studying Chapter 18

Respiratory Care

You should be able to:

* Pronounce and define each of its new medical words and phrases and use the new technical jargon.

* Identify five medical gases.

* Name four methods by which oxygen may be administered.

* Describe five techniques used in chest physical therapy.

MEDICAL WORDS   PRONOUNCE THESE TEN NEW WORDS WITH YOUR TEACHER:

adjuvants (ad′joo-vants)
asphyxia (as-fik′se-ah)
hemoptysis (he-mop′tĭ″-sis)
laryngectomy (lar″in-jek′to-me)
nebulizer (neb′u-liz″er)
dysphagia (dĭs-fa′je-ah)
ventilators (ven″tĭ-la-tors)
hypercarbia (hi″per-kar′be-ah)
compliance (kom-pli′ans)
perfusion (per-fu′zhun)

There are always some irritants in the **ambient** (surrounding natural atmosphere) air we breathe. Substances such as pollens float in the atmosphere seasonably. They often irritate sensitive mucous membranes and can cause even more serious consequences in the allergic individual.

In our modern technological society, urban man lives in a sea of gaseous pollutants. Industry spews its contaminants into the air and the automobile contributes noxious toxic materials through fuel combustion. Cigarette smoke is also a recognized source of air pollution. Even in less well-populated places, such as rural and suburban areas, pollens and grasses may also contribute heavily to the accumulation of irritating materials in the air. As population densities increase, the amounts of microbial contaminants and pollutants also increase.

Air is essential to life. It is a solution of gases (vapor-like state of matter that is neither solid nor liquid). Air consists mainly of oxygen and nitrogen. It also includes carbon dioxide, argon, neon, and other gases.

Oxygen is essential for life and is the essential agent in air. It enters the body through the respiratory tract. Therefore, **anoxia** (absence of oxygen) is incompatible with life. This condition can result in either hypoxia or hypoxemia. Hypoxemia (deficiency of oxygen in the blood) or hypoxia (too little oxygen available to the tissues) are both life-threatening.

Nitrogen is equally important but it enters the body primarily through food—as protein nutrients. Nitrogen forms about four-fifths of common air but it is not taken into the body in great quantities through the respiratory tract as oxygen. Mainly, nitrogen is washed into the soil from the air and is combined into protein nutrients through a very complex process known as the nitrogen fixation cycle.

AIR POLLUTANTS

Open as the respiratory tract is to the environment, pollutants in the air can gain entrance even to the deeper regions of the lungs. So the natural mechanisms of mucous secretion and cilia may not always be sufficient to protect the body from damage. Many persons today suffer from the effects of having breathed air pollutants over long periods of time. Chronic pulmonary pathologies are exacerbated by air pollutants and recurrent infections.

One of the most rapidly rising types of pulmonary pathology is emphysema. In emphysema, chronic obstructions and infections cause a breakdown in the walls between the pulmonary alveoli with a subsequent loss of distensibility (**compliance**). Expiration becomes the major difficulty. The condition is progressive, ultimately leading to congestive heart failure.

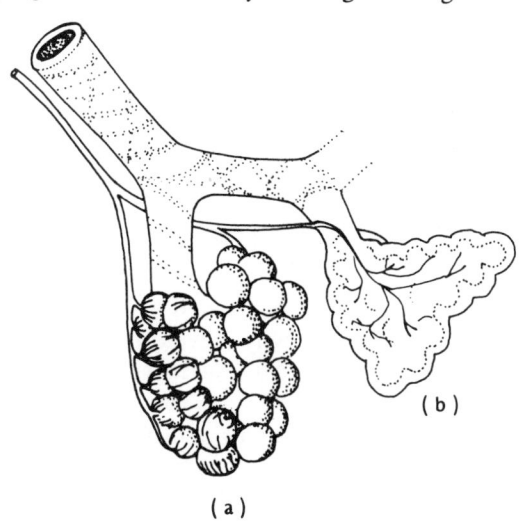

Figure 18-1:
(a) Healthy alveoli with definite walls between;
(b) lung with emphysema; Elasticity of alveoli is lost as the interalveolus wall is broken down;
(courtesy of The American Lung Association).

Because the cardiovascular network is so interrelated with the pulmonary mechanism, pathology in either system is mirrored in stress on the other system and substantial loss of function in both. Long standing cardiovascular problems such as atherosclerosis increases the work load of the lungs just as chronic asthma and an obstruction in the airways increase the resistance to pulmonary blood perfusion. Heart disease developed secondarily to lung pathology is known as **cor pulmonale**.

In the last few years, a new worker has joined the health team to specially meet the respiratory needs of the cardiopulmonary patient. Like many of the new interdisciplinary health workers, the respiratory care therapist begins his education with a general medical and scientific preparation. He has, in addition, a highly developed expertise in the care of patients with ventilation problems. Ventilation, which means moving air into and out of the lungs, is probably one of the most important words in the vocabulary of the respiratory technician.

Figure 18-2: The Respiratory Care therapist monitors the patient on the "Gill I Volume Ventilator" *(courtesy of Chemetron Healthcare Systems Medical Products Division).*

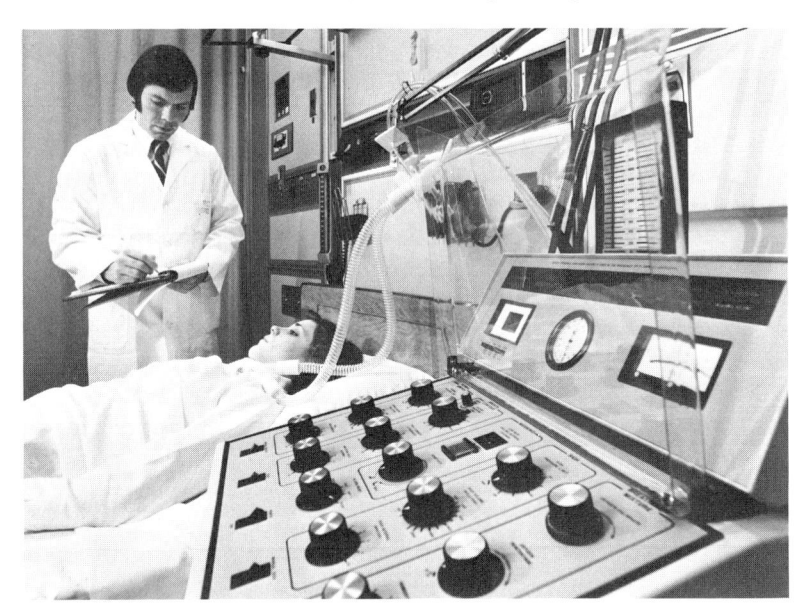

Both by using techniques borrowed from other medical disciplines and by introducing newly developed techniques, the skilled respiratory therapist helps in evaluating the respiratory **status** (condition) of patients and in preventing respiratory disease. These technical workers help establish a diagnosis by using sophisticated techniques and instruments to perform pulmonary function tests.

Known pulmonary disease conditions are treated with **medical gases** (gases used in medicine), **aerosols** (fine mists of medicine), **humidification** (moisturization), and various forms of **chest physical therapy**. Chest physical therapy includes techniques designed to loosen pulmonary secretions that would otherwise remain to obstruct the airways. Chest pulmonary therapy and pulmonary rehabilitation techniques help patients utilize their muscles for maximum ventilatory support.

Since respiratory care involves a great deal of complex evaluation and therapy, two kinds of skilled workers have evolved as medical technology has developed: the respiratory care therapist and the cardio-pulmonary technician. Their technical skills and functions overlap, but the respiratory care therapist (**inhalation therapist**) focuses more on direct supportive patient care while the cardio-pulmonary technician spends more time evaluating patients through pulmonary function assessments. He works closely with the physician, using those diagnostic techniques that clearly define the parameters of the patient's pathology and respiratory limitations.

Neither of these technicians works in a totally independent manner. Both work as an integral part of a coordinated team effort. Such respiratory personnel work in both routine and critical care areas and are found in hospitals and clinics, working both with in-patients and out-patients.

Figure 18-3: Fine aerosols of medication are delivered into the patient's airways loosening thick secretions *(courtesy of Mead Johnson Laboratories).*

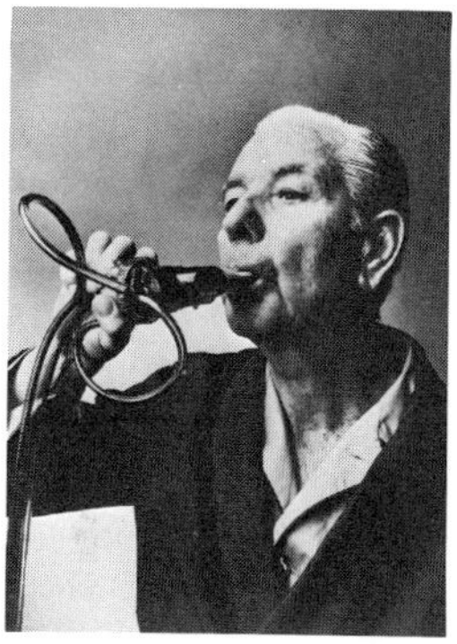

PULMONARY FUNCTION TESTS

Recall that the purpose of the respiratory system is threefold: 1) to deliver a sufficient quantity or volume of air into the alveoli, the diffusing membranes of the lungs; 2) to provide an avenue of gaseous exchange; and, 3) to provide a pathway for the elimination of carbon dioxide from the body.

(Re-read Chapter 10 quickly before you go on with this chapter. It is important that you review your information on the respiratory system so that you can easily see the reason for many therapeutic procedures.)

Two results of this tri-part respiratory function that can be readily studied are the overall effectiveness of ventilation and the volumes of gases that are moved in and out during it. The overall effectiveness of ventilatory effort is demonstrated in the patient's blood chemistry. Adequate ventilation, diffusion, and perfusion are all essential to the maintenance of **homeostasis** (stability). The level of homeostasis in turn is reflected in the pH of the blood and in the levels of gases in the arterial blood. One way to determine both is by studying a sample of the arterial blood. The sample is drawn from an artery. Usually

Arterial Blood Gas Studies

either the brachial artery, or the radial artery, or the femoral artery is used as the puncture site.

Blood samples are processed in an **arterial blood gas analyzer**. Arterial blood gas (ABG) studies are critical in determining the effectiveness of either natural or assisted ventilation. Ventilation may be assisted by various machines called **ventilators**. A series of before-and-after blood gas studies give good indications of the effectiveness of whatever therapy is being employed.

Figure 18-4: The arterial blood gas analyzer determines the levels of blood gases and pH in a sample of arterial blood *(courtesy of Instrumentation Laboratory, Inc.).*

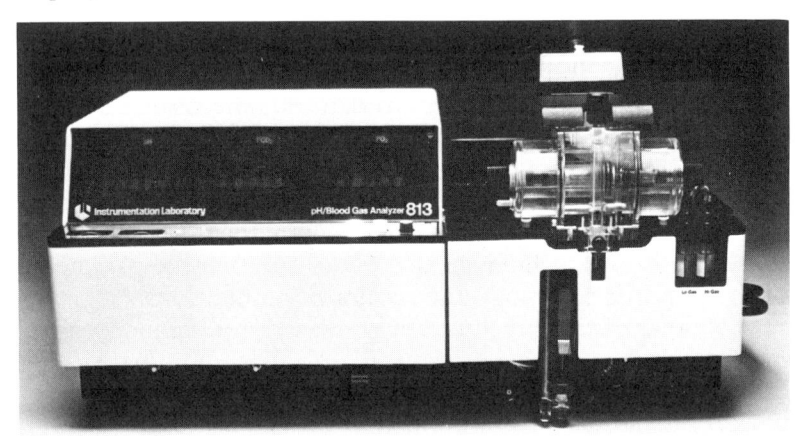

Ventilation is measured in terms of the volume of **gas** that is moved with varying degrees of respiratory effort. A spirometer is the instrument used to measure and record respiratory volumes. Cases of **hypoventilation** (under ventilation) or **hyperventilation** (excessive ventilation) can be detected with this machine by comparing the readings with established norms. Total volume, complemental volumes, and supplemental volumes are frequently determined in this way.

Hypoventilation can result in **hypercapnia** or **hypercarbia** (accumulation of CO_2 in the blood). Unchecked hypercapnia leads to acidosis. Hyperventilation can deplete the blood of carbon dioxide (**hypocapnia** or **hypocarbia**). Unless hypocarbia is relieved, it leads to alkalosis.

Spirometry readings taken of the ill patient are compared with normal findings and then used to evaluate the patient's functional capabilities. Special techniques have been developed to evaluate both pulmonary diffusion and perfusion **capacities** (capabilities). These pulmonary function tests are an important part of pulmonary diagnosis. They provide an initial baseline of pulmonary function and a method for evaluating the progress of therapy.

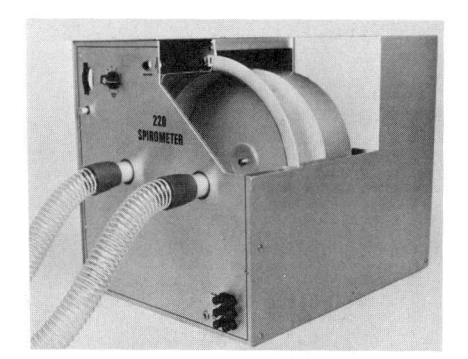

Figure 18-5:
A "spirometer" is used to measure respiratory volumes *(courtesy of Cardio-Pulmonary Instruments Corporation).*

MEDICAL GASES

Several gases are utilized in medicine. Some of the medical gases commonly used include **compressed air** (air under pressure), oxygen, nitrogen, **nitrous oxide**, carbon dioxide, **cyclopropane**, and **helium**. Medical gases are stored and dispensed in cylinders or "tanks" of various sizes. Some tanks are small enough to be carried about. Such portable tanks may be strapped to an oxygen-dependent patient so that he/she can remain ambulatory.

Tanks are color coded for easier identification. For example, oxygen is found in green-colored tanks and air in yellow tanks. In health care facilities, gases are often dispensed from a central area through pipes to individual patient rooms or therapy areas. Administration of gases to either location requires the use of an accurate mechanism (**flow meter**) which controls the rate at which the gas flows. These gases are commonly measured by liter, the basic unit of capacity in the metric system.

Medical gases such as compressed air and oxygen are used to improve lung inflation and aeration. Oxygen inhalation therapy was introduced almost two hundred years ago. Today, nitrogen, helium, and oxygen combinations are also frequently employed in pulmonary function testing. Such gases as cyclopropane, nitrous oxide, and helium are used in combinations either as anesthetic agents or as **adjuvants** (assistants) to other primary forms of anesthesia. Medical gases are administered in a variety of ways. For example, oxygen or compressed air can be delivered by means of masks, nasal cannulas, tents, and nasal catheters, as well as through tubes introduced into the trachea. Tracheal **intubation** (passing a tube) may either be inserted through the mouth and larynx into the trachea (endotracheal) or directly into the trachea through a **tracheostomy** (opening into the trachea).

Regardless of how a medical gas is administered, it must be moisturized (**humidified**) to prevent dehydration damage to the

Figure 18-6:
This patient has had an airway established through oral intubation *(courtesy of Olympic Medical Corporation).*

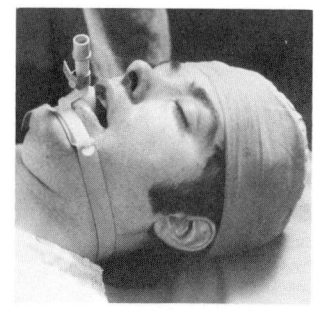

Figure 18-7: "Gases must be humidified" *(courtesy of Ohio Medical Products, Division of Airco, Inc.)*.

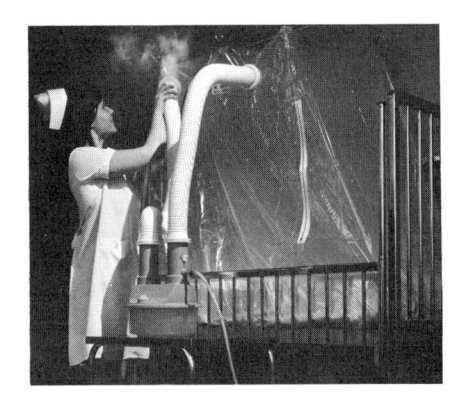

mucous membrane of the **airway** (air passageway from atmosphere to alveolus). Humidifiers are attached to gas lines in such a way that the gas is moisturized before it reaches the patient. Oxygen supports combustion as well as life; therefore, very strict safety regulations are always employed wherever it is used to prevent fires and explosions. Safety signs must be conspicuously posted to this effect whenever oxygen is administered.

AEROSOLS

Aerosols are suspensions of solids or liquids in a gas. Aerosols are delivered to the patient as a fine mist. The drug or solution to be administered is placed in a **nebulizer** or **atomizer** that converts it into a fine spray. Either oxygen or compressed air is usually given by cannula, mask or tent when a patient needs a higher level of either but is able to breathe independently of a machine.

The same gases may be administered by means of various mechanical ventilators to patients needing ventilatory assistance.

Figure 18-8: (a) Oxygen delivered by nasal cannula *(courtesy of American Hospital Supply Corporation)*. (b) The mask as a means of administering oxygen.

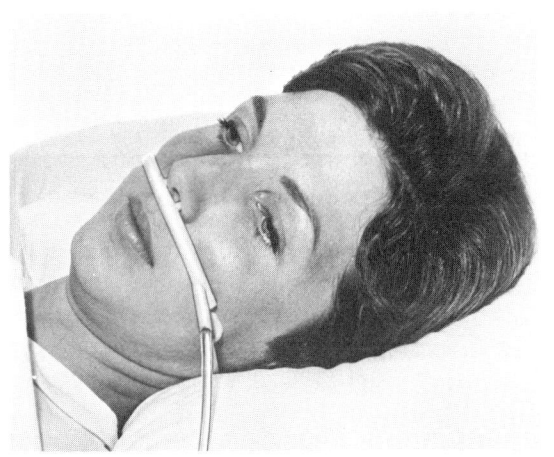

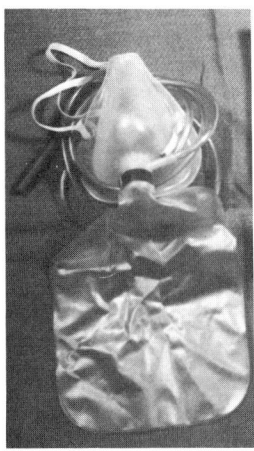

*290 RESPIRATORY CARE

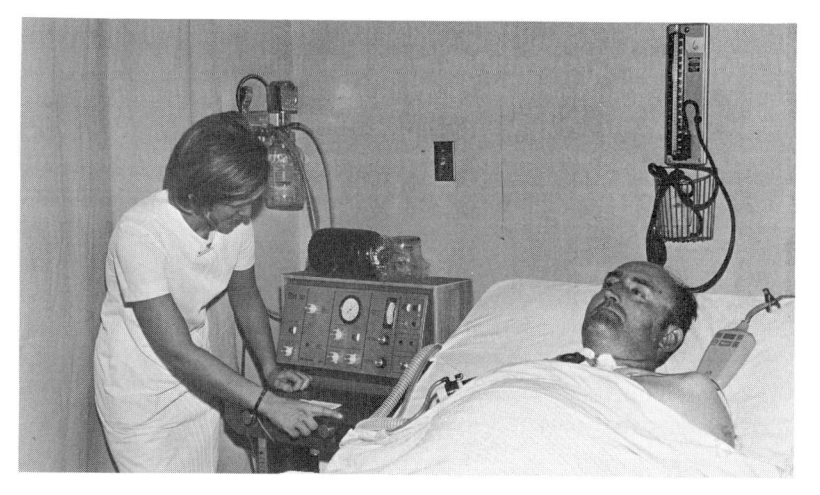

Figure 18-9: The volume ventilator delivers a specific volume of air or oxygen through the endotracheal tube through the tracheostomy *(courtesy of Ohio Medical Products, Division of Airco, Inc.).*

For example, a **volume ventilator** can deliver a specified amount of gas to the patient so that it assists his inspiratory efforts. One of these, the Intermittent Positive Pressure Breathing (IPPB) machine delivers the gas under pressure during the inspiratory phase in order to help increase lung expansion. Expiration is not assisted by the machine. But, during IPPB treatments, aerosol **mucolytic** (mucous thinning) drugs are frequently administered. They loosen thick, tenacious mucous secretions so they can be coughed up and **expectorated** (expelled from the airway by spitting).

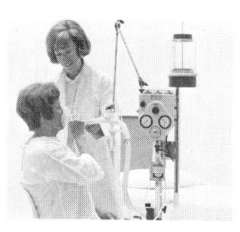

Figure 18-10: The IPPB Machine delivers gas to the patient under pressure during the ensperatory phase.

CHEST PHYSICAL THERAPY

In many chronic pulmonary disease states, the patient's ventilation is hampered by weakened musculature as well as by excessively thick mucus secretions that adhere to airway walls and obstruct air flow. So chest physical therapy is directed toward improving muscular action and to clearing the air passages.

Several techniques for this include chest tapping, breathing exercises, coughing techniques, and postural drainage. These all increase the patient's ventilation in proportion to his exertion.

The diaphragm is the major muscle of respiration, assisted by the intercostal muscles and the abdominal muscles. When respirations are difficult, several auxiliary muscles can be trained to help fill and empty the lungs.

The major emphasis in muscle retraining is on the abdominal muscles. In therapy sessions these muscles are exercised against a mild resistance to gradually increase their strength. As tolerance to these basic muscle-strengthening exercises is gained, general muscular exercises, such as walking are added. Some-

Figure 18-11: Pursed lip breathing is a technique which patients use to improve expiration.

times low levels of oxygen are also administered during the exercise periods.

Pursed lip breathing is another breathing technique that is taught to many patients. Retraining with this type of respiratory pattern allows the patient to more completely empty his lungs. Pursed lip breathing is especially helpful for the patient with emphysema whose major difficulty involves inadequate expiration.

Other respiratory control techniques such as counting "one" on respiration and "two," "three" on expiration, puts the emphasis on the expiratory phase. Adequate coughing is also important for clearing the air passages. Coughing techniques are taught to patients who have had **IPPB** treatments with mucolytic aerosols or after chest tapping (**cupping**).

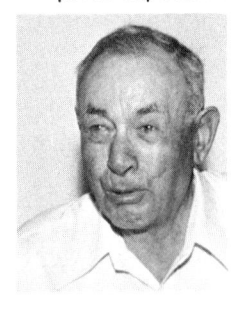

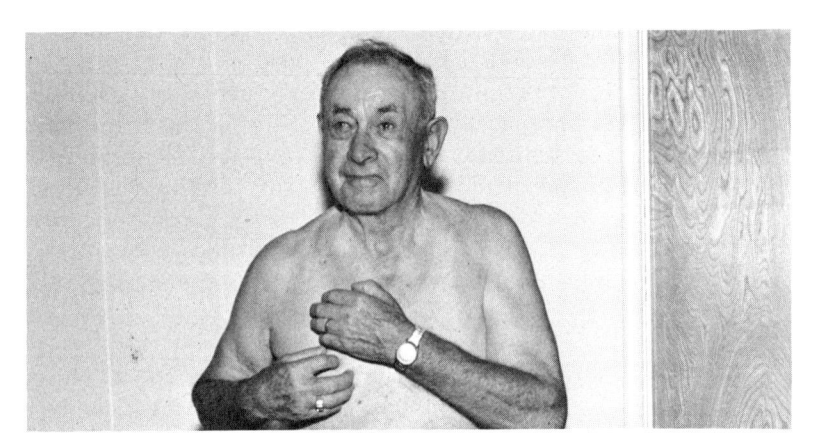

Figure 18-12: Chest physical therapy loosens the secretions in the respiratory tree.

The cupping treatment is done to patients, but it can also be taught to them so they can do it for themselves. The hand is flexed like a cup and the thumb and fingertips are used to strike the chest in the affected area, loosening the secretions. Such chest cupping is followed by some form of postural drainage.

Postural drainage puts the patient's head and thorax downward in a dependent position—below his lungs. This means that gravity is used to promote drainage of the chest. When these techniques are employed successfully, more complete **aeration** (exchange of carbon dioxide for oxygen) of the lungs is possible. These activities are very fatiguing, however, so care must be taken not to overtax the patient.

Typical Respiratory Care Therapists

Roberta Rooker and Cesar Marhakian were high school classmates. Both seniors hoped to enter some sort of health care work. Neither had any specific plans, although Roberta was leaning toward a career in nursing. On "Career Day," representatives of several colleges visited the campus, including a respiratory therapist from the local community college. He described the field, its possibilities, and opportunities for a career. Both students were really "turned on" by what they heard and decided respiratory therapy was the field of medicine for them.

After two years of rigorous training, education, and clinical experience they were prepared to enter the field as beginning workers. Roberta found work at a large metropolitan hospital in the Respiratory Rehabilitation Department which cared for patients with chronic cardio-pulmonary problems. Cesar was also hired by the same hospital. He was assigned to the Respiratory Intensive Care Unit (RICU). They both immediately became very occupied with the patients who comprised their case loads.

Meeting in the staff dining room about six weeks later, they shared some of their experiences. Before hearing about their patients, it is important that you understand some of the basic pathology. The conditions they discussed are summarized in the following list:

Pathology	Description
anaphylactic shock	severe, allergic reaction leading to shock, unconsciousness; untreated, may be fatal
carbon monoxide poisoning	carbon monoxide is a gas which combines permanently with the hemoglobin, preventing union with oxygen; leads to hypoxemia
laryngeal adenocarcinoma	a malignant tumor of the larynx, frequently necessitating **laryngectomy** (removal of the larynx)
histoplamosis	lung infection caused by mold; can result in a pneumonectomy and may spread to other organs of the body
bronchiectasis	abnormal permanent dilation of the bronchi and bronchioles; usually develops following prolonged chronic obstruction due to infections; excessive mucous is secreted leading to obstruction and further infection and obstructions
atelectasis	collapse of the alveoli associated with pneumothorax and accumulation of fluid in the chest (**hydrothorax**)

Three of the patients Roberta and Cesar discussed were currently in the RICU unit. Cesar had assisted with their care. The other two were patients Roberta had encountered in the Respiratory Rehabilitation Clinic.

CASE STUDY 1

Vera Szczpaniak is a 45 year-old woman, who had been stung by a bee while on a camping trip with her family. Within a very short period of time, she began to have wheezing respirations as if she were having an asthmatic attack. Her body became cold and clammy. Her family transported her to the nearest hospital immediately for emergency care.

It was apparent that she was severely sensitive to the insect bite and had gone into anaphylactic shock. By the time Mrs. Szczpaniak reached the Emergency Room she was suffering from acute ventilatory **insufficiency** (inadequate air supply). Tracheostomy and intubation were required to sustain ventilation. Oxygen, antihistamines, and other drugs were administered and she was placed on a volume respirator with orders for continuous positive pressure breathing (CPPB). The nurses and respiratory care therapist monitored her condition carefully and **suctioned** (withdrawing or **aspirating** of fluid) the tracheostomy tube regularly.

Unless supportive and therapeutic measures had been taken at once, the most likely outcome would have been death. The emergency over, the physician on duty wrote an order to have the chief therapist evaluate the patient's pulmonary status. The therapist examined the patient, drew blood for arterial blood

Figure 18-13: Placed on the volume respirator, under the careful supervision of professional personnel, the patient responded to therapy. *(courtesy of Ohio Medical Products, Division of Airco, Inc.).*

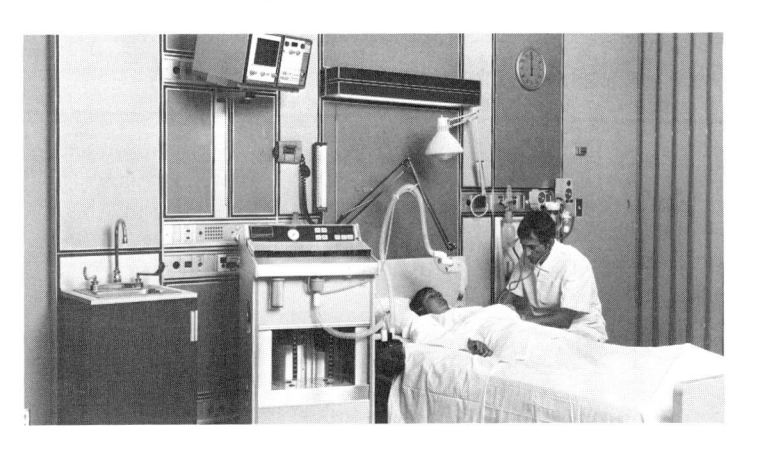

* 294 *RESPIRATORY CARE*

gas studies, and reviewed her history. Together the chief respiratory therapist and the physician are now planning the therapy for Mrs. Szczpaniak.

CASE STUDY 2

Carlos Ramirez, 57 years old, had complained of difficulty swallowing (**dysphagia**) and a **hoarseness** (roughness) in his voice. **Laryngoscopy** (visualization of the larynx) revealed a nodular mass on his vocal cords. Subsequently, a **bronchoscopy** (visual examination of the bronchus) and a **bronchogram** (a bronchographic X-ray) both indicated the pathology was probably localized and did not involve the **tracheobronchial tree** (conduction passageways).

Several days later, a **laryngectomy** and tracheostomy were performed. The final diagnosis was laryngeal adenocarcinoma. He, too, was intubated and is receiving ventilatory assistance with a volume respirator.

Ventilator care is a supportive measure only. Gradually, Mr. Ramirez will have to be **weaned** (taken off) from the ventilator and assume independent ventilation. Weaning is a gradual process, of course, so Mr. Ramirez will be able to adjust to his changed circumstances.

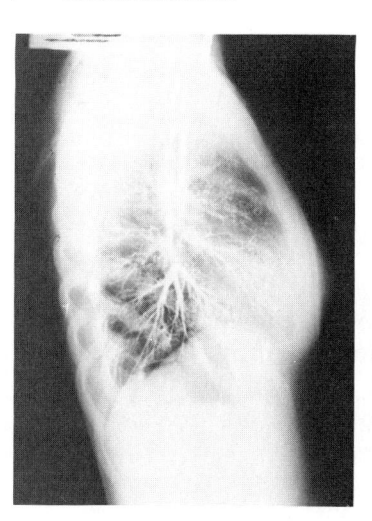

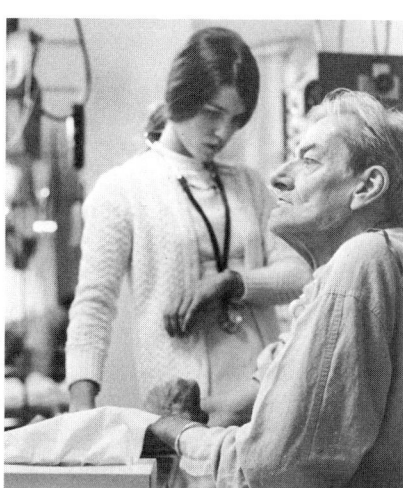

Figure 18-14: (left) Lateral view of chest showing filled bronchi during bronchogram.

Figure 18-15: (right) The nurse checks the patient for tachycardia, an indication of hypoxemia as he is gradually weaned from the ventilator. *(courtesy of American Lung Association).*

CASE STUDY 3

Peter Podlesky, 17 years old, is also a patient in the respiratory intensive care unit. Paramedics brought him to the hospital after his mother found him lying under his car in the garage with the motor running and the garage door closed.

As soon as they saw his cherry-red face, the paramedics suspected carbon monoxide poisoning. They administered oxygen by mask immediately. On admission to the hospital, Peter was placed in the **hyperbaric** (under greater than atmospheric pressure) oxygen chamber where oxygen could be delivered to his hypoxic tissues under high pressure, both through his respiratory tract and directly into the tissues.

Peter's condition was critical but now he seems to be improving and has been transferred to the RIC unit. He is still receiving oxygen therapy by mask.

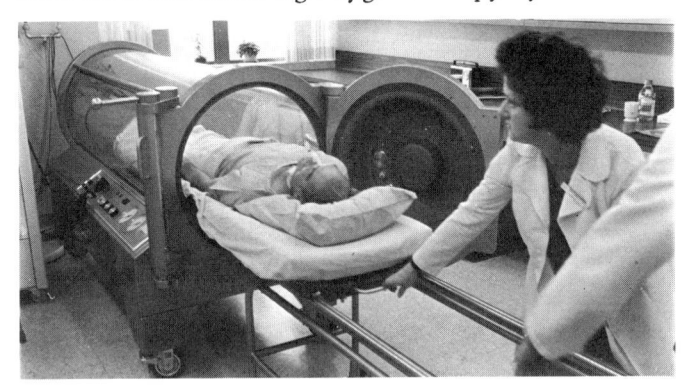

Figure 18-16: The hyperbaric oxygen chamber delivers greater than atmospheric pressure oxygen to the patient's lungs and tissues.

CASE STUDY

Henry Murphy and Isaac Rubin are no strangers to the respiratory rehabilitation clinic. Mr. Murphy, 76 years old, is a regular out-patient. Many years ago when he lived in an Ohio River Valley town, he was infected with histoplasmosis. (Histoplasmosis is endemic in parts of the Midwest.) The infection had **infiltrated** (invaded) his lungs and left behind pulmonary scars which decreased his pulmonary **compliance** (elasticity). Mr. Murphy gradually developed bronchiectasis since repeated infections plagued him through the years. He also suffers from chronic ventilatory failure. Until now he has been able to remain at home, using a portable IPPB machine and taking **expectorants** (medication to aid spitting). He has also been taught at the clinic how to do chest cupping and postural drainage, and he used mucolytic agents in a nebulizer to **insufflate** (blow up or into) his lungs and thus thin and loosen excessive secretions.

Still, coughing and expectorating the thick phlegm is weakening. Recently he has also noted some **hemoptysis** (spitting up blood) and his sputum is more copious than ever. Mr. Murphy says that his normal activities seem to take more and more effort and to leave him more fatigued than ever before. So he has come into the clinic with a friend, Isaac Rubin, this week for progress evaluation. Arterial blood was drawn for analysis, a spirometry reading was made and he was started on some muscle strengthening exercises. Mr. Murphy has also expressed his constant fear of **asphyxia** (death due to cessation of ventilation) and dreads being along.

Isaac Rubin who regularly drives his friend, Henry Murphy, over to the clinic also has an interesting history. He owned and operated an all-night liquor store until his forced retirement a year ago. Late one evening last winter, two armed men came in and held him up. One of the gunmen panicked when a customer came in during the holdup and shot both the customer and Mr. Rubin. The customer died instantly, but the gravely wounded proprietor was rushed by police ambulance to a city hospital.

X rays revealed that the bullet lodging in Mr. Rubin's chest had fractured a rib. A lung had also been punctured, either by the bullet fragments or by the fractured rib. So a right pneumothorax and atelectasis were diagnosed. Following surgery to remove the bullet fragments, a chest tube was inserted to help reinflate his right lung and remove the accumulated fluid (**hydrothorax**). After a few days in the hospital's respiratory intensive care unit he spent some time in the general pulmonary unit. He is now well recovered and is in good health presently. Both he and Mr. Murphy live in a rooming house across town and since Henry Murphy can no longer drive, Isaac Rubin not only supplies transportation but also much of the emotional support needed by his friend.

CASE STUDY 5

The fields of respiratory testing and care are rapidly growing branches of medicine. The expansion of these specialties is due mainly to the rising numbers of cases of both acute and

SUMMARY

chronic pulmonary diseases affecting the population. Microbial invasion and the pervasiveness of air pollutants are among the causes contributing to the alarming increase of pulmonary pathologies.

PRACTICE & REVIEW   Explain and define the new special terms you have been using. Remember, you learned how to pronounce them at the beginning of this chapter.

1. adjuvants _____
2. asphyxia _____
3. hemoptysis _____
4. laryngectomy _____
5. nebulizer _____
6. dysphagia _____
7. ventilators _____
8. hypercarbia _____
9. compliance _____
10. perfusion _____

Now, double-check the meaning of the terms above by studying the brief definitions given in the Glossary-Index at the back of this text.

Test yourself quickly before going on to learn other medical and professional terms. Use these short review exercises to practice for your new work in health services. Your teacher will also help by recommending various other Study Activities.

A. Complete the ten statements with the best word from the list provided below:

tracheostomy	carbon monoxide	postural drainage
anaphylactic shock	aeration	cupping
atelectasis	histoplasmosis	bronchiectasis
airway	volume ventilator	mucolytic

1. Passageway from atmosphere to alveolus is called the _____ .
2. Machine delivering a specific amount of gas to a patient is called a _____ .
3. Mucous thinning drugs are called _____ .

* 298 *RESPIRATORY CARE*

4. The technique of placing the patient's head and thorax in a dependent position to drain mucous secretions is called _____.

5. The exchange of carbon dioxide for oxygen in the lungs is called _____.

6. Gas which forms a permanent bond with hemoglobin is _____.

7. _____ is a lung infection caused by a mold.

8. _____ is an abnormal permanent dilation of the bronchi and the bronchioles.

9. An opening into the trachea is called a _____.

10. The term used when discussing the technique of chest tapping is _____.

B. Match the words on the right with the best statement in the left column:

____ 1. Moisturized air
____ 2. Letters standing for arterial blood gas
____ 3. Excessive ventilation
____ 4. Within the trachea
____ 5. Mechanism for controlling gas flow rate
____ 6. Moving air into and out of the lungs
____ 7. Depletion of carbon dioxide
____ 8. A word meaning condition
____ 9. Accumulation of CO_2 in the blood
____ 10. Heart disease following lung disease
____ 11. Another word for inadequacy
____ 12. Visualization of the bronchus
____ 13. Means "invaded"
____ 14. Means "to blow up"
____ 15. Lung collapse
____ 16. Air conduction passageways
____ 17. Withdrawing fluid
____ 18. Rough voice quality
____ 19. Means greater than atmospheric pressure
____ 20. Refers to blood flow

a. cor pulmonale
b. ventilation
c. status
d. ABG
e. hyperventilation
f. hypocarbia
g. hypercapnia
h. nitrogen
i. flow meter
j. endotracheal
k. humidification
l. BGA
m. suctioning
n. hemotysis
o. asphyxia
p. atelectasis
q. perfusion
r. hoarseness
s. tracheobronchial tree
t. hyperbaric
u. insufficiency
v. infiltrated
w. insufflate
x. bronchoscopy

After studying Chapter 19
Radiology and Radiotherapy
You should be able to:

* *Pronounce and define each of its new medical words and phrases and use the new technical jargon.*

* *Describe the safety precautions necessary in the use of roentgen rays.*

* *Describe the four basic radiographic positions.*

MEDICAL WORDS   PRONOUNCE THESE TEN NEW WORDS WITH YOUR TEACHER:

radioactive (ra'de-o-ak'tive)
roentgenography (rent"gĕ-nog'rah-fe)
radiolucent (ra"de-o-lu'sent)
radiopaque (ra"de-o-pah'k)
irradiation (ĭ-ra"de-a'shun)
craniocaudad (kra'ne-o-kaw'dad)
fluoroscopy (floo"or-os'ko-pe)
pneumoencephalography (nu"mo-en-sel"ah-log'rah-fe)
tomography (to-mog'rah-fe)
scintiscanner (sin'tĭ-skan-r)

Recent technological events have made us all increasingly aware of the importance of solar energy to life on our planet. The sun's rays also furnish heat and light that is being captured and intensified for use in space and on the ground in numerous ways. Other forms of pure energy given off by matter are also important. Certain chemical elements, for instance, transmute into other elements and give off or spread (**radiate**) electromagnetic energy in the form of invisible waves or particles. Radium is one of these naturally radioactive elements that releases rays of pure energy.

During the past eighty years particularly, scientists and technologists have developed many ways to control and use such energy in sophisticated industry and in clinical medicine. Several forms of radiant energy are widely used in diagnostic radiology, in **radiotherapy**, and in **nuclear medicine**.

Gamma rays, **X rays**, ultraviolet rays and the **alpha** and **beta particles** are all forms of electromagnetic radiations. Radiology (study of radiation) for the diagnosis of pathologies, and radiotherapy for the treatment of certain tissue and blood malignancies, are increasingly used. Radiations can be captured or generated mechanically on various wave lengths. In general, the shorter their wave length, the more the waves are able to penetrate into and be absorbed by substances. X rays have very short wave lengths and are able to penetrate relatively **dense** (thick) substances such as soft body tissues. Some gamma rays have even shorter wave lengths, with even greater penetrating power. Both are very useful in radiotherapy.

CHEMICAL ELEMENTS

Chemical elements are primary substances that cannot be decomposed by chemical means and are made up of atoms which are alike in their electronic configurations and in their chemical properties. A large number of elements have been identified, each with its own characteristics and weak or strong radioactive properties. Iron, for example, is an element that most of us know. Its symbol is Fe and it is present in the body in minute quantities. Some important elements also present in the body are calcium, sodium, and chlorine.

Elements are composed of submicroscopic particles called **atoms**. Each atom in turn has been found to be made up of electrically charged particles called protons, electrons and neutrons. The **protons** are positively charged, the **neutrons** are neutral and unchanged; the **electrons** have a negative charge. Protons and neutrons are found together in the center (**nucleus**) of each atom where the electrons form a cloud of rapidly moving negative charges in orbit around the nucleus.

Atoms

Each atom has a specific number of protons, neutrons and electrons. The combination of protons and neutrons gives each atom its atomic weight. Some **stable** elements have atoms with a specific relationship between the protons and neutrons that keeps them together in the nucleus. Some **radioactive** elements do not have the special proton to neutron ratio and give off nuclear particles until that special relationship is reached.

The release of radioactive particles changes the atom and the element and is accompanied by the release (**emission**) of radiations in the form of alpha and beta particles and gamma rays. Radioactive elements have an atomic weight that is greater or less than that of the original element and are called **isotopes**. Some are used in medicine.

In the atom of an element, the number of electrons equals the number of protons. This means that the number of negative electrical charges equals the number of positive electrical charges. The electrical charges of an atom are thus balanced.

Figure 19-1:
The atom.

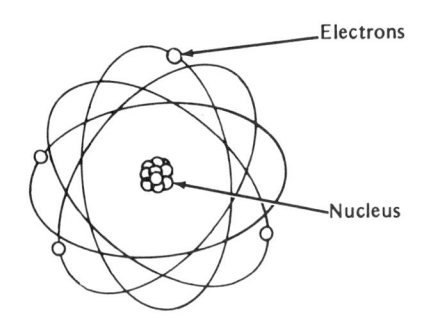

During chemical reactions, the atoms interact with other atoms, exchanging or sharing electrons to form new substances called compounds. A salt, such as sodium chloride, is a compound. Remember, sodium chloride is called an electrolyte because in the body it ionizes to form ions. Ions are negatively and positively charged particles that are very important to human physiology. The ions become electrically charged when the balance between protons and electrons is upset. That is, the ionic particle is positively charged when there are fewer electrons than protons in it. It is negatively charged when there are more electrons than protons.

DIAGNOSTIC RADIOLOGY

The primary form of radiation for diagnostic purposes is the X ray. X rays were accidentally discovered in 1895 by Wilhelm Roentgen, a German physicist. Because of their unknown nature, he called them X rays. These **roentgen rays** (R) or X rays are the controlled streams of short-wave radiant energy used most in radiography.

Roentgen rays have penetrating power. The more intense they are or the closer the radiation source is to the substance to be penetrated, the more effect the radiation has. Penetrating power is only one of the properties of X rays. X rays act like light rays on photographic plates, producing an **image** (picture) that can be viewed after the film is developed.

Roentgenography or photography by X-ray, is also called **radiography**. It is a widely used diagnostic technique. The body part to be radiographed is positioned between the film-containing cassette and the X-ray source. Special photographic film is placed in a lightproof holder (**cassette**). Cassettes are made of a **radiolucent** (permits passage of X rays) material with a lead backing to absorb and stop the rays. Also, in the cassette, are **intensifying screens**, which supplement production of the image by the X-ray energy. High voltage X rays are directed toward the area, passing through it to the film to produce a **radiogram**

Figure 19-2:
The cassette is a lightproof holder for the radiographic film *(courtesy of Picker Corp.)*.

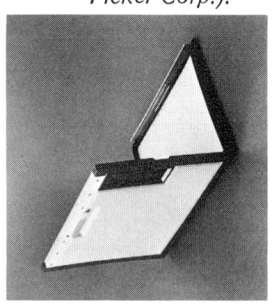

(X-ray picture) or image. The process is sometimes referred to as an "imaging technique." The extent of penetration depends on the voltage used to produce the radiation and on the varying densities of the structures. As the X rays strike the film, its surface is changed and patterns appear showing what the rays travel through. Then the latent (hidden) image or picture is developed photographically.

Originally coated glass plates were used by radiologists, hence the still-used jargon which refers to the procedure as taking a "**plate**." For example, you may hear the radiologic technician say he is taking a "chest plate" when he radiographs the thorax. Actually, thin, coated sheets of light-sensitive plastic (film) are now used. This exposed film, still in its cassette, is put into a two-sided **pass box** (transfer cupboard) built into the wall of the room where the X-ray camera is used. The cassette is placed in the side of the pass box marked "exposed" and the door on the "X-ray side" is tightly closed. The cassette is then removed from the opposite side of the box (the "dark room side") for developing. Cassettes with fresh film are also placed in the "unexposed side" of the pass box ready for the technician to remove and use.

Figure 19-3: The "passbox" is used to transfer an exposed film into the darkroom for developing without allowing light into the darkroom.

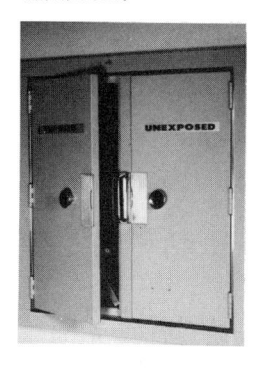

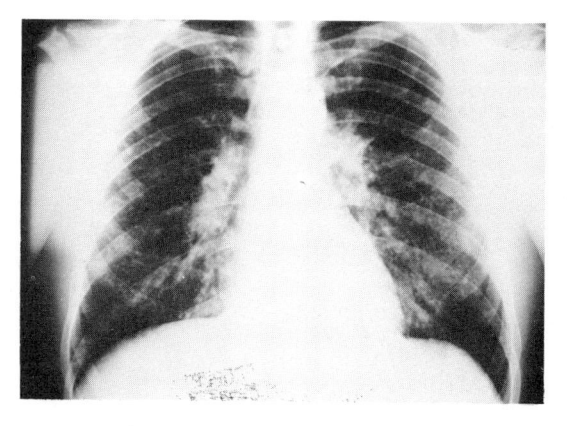

Figure 19-4: Chest X-ray. Note dense areas appear light and less dense areas appear darker.

The X-ray Image

The X-ray picture or image is unlike the usual continuous tone black and white photograph. It consists of shadows in varying degrees of gray. The less dense the tissue penetrated, the darker the color represented in an X-ray image. The more dense or **radiopaque** (impervious to radiation) the object is, the lighter and whiter it appears. For example, air in the thorax is not dense. Hence it appears dark gray on the film. But bones, such as the ribs, which are very dense appear almost white. You can see then that the completed **roentgenogram** (radiogram) is really a shadowy representation of the varying densities of the tissues being examined.

It takes great skill to do radiography properly and to correctly interpret the images that are formed on the radiogram. Skilled radiologic technicians prepare and position the patient for optimum results and then actually "take" the roentgenogram by accurately directing high voltage rays to the area.

The radiologist is a physician specially trained in radiologic techniques. He "reads" the radiogram by placing the film on a **view box** (film illuminator) which lights it from behind. Then he looks for differences in density, for **discrete** (very distinct) areas, and for **rarefied** (lessened density) areas. Many pathologic states such as tumors or fractures are **radiable** (capable of X-ray examination).

Figure 19-5: (left) The Radiologic Technologist and Radiologist are both part of the Radiology Team *(courtesy of Picker Corp.)*.

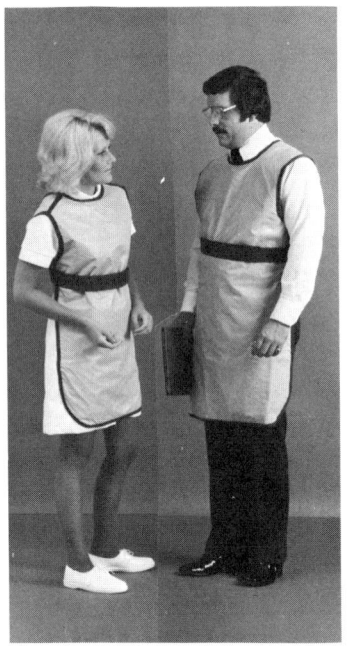

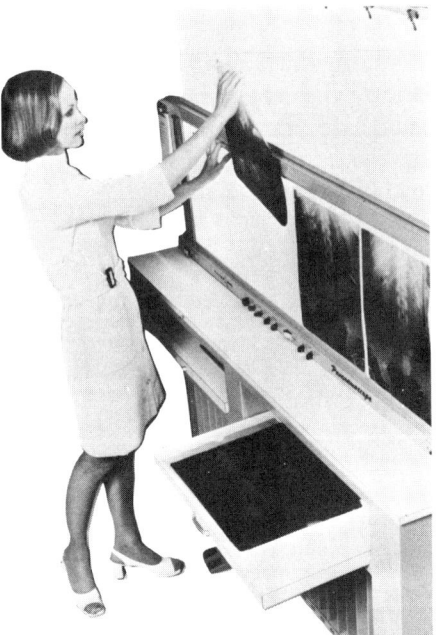

Figure 19-6: (right) The Radiologic Technologist places the radiographs on the illuminator for easier viewing *(courtesy of Radx Corp.)*.

Radioscopy, or examination of the deep body structures by X-ray is usually enhanced by the addition of a **contrast media** of radiopaque material. Radiologic examinations of structures such as the stomach are more effective when the organ is first filled with such a radiopaque substance. The radiopaque contrast media outlines the organ so that defects are more easily discernible. Frequently, a **scout** (preliminary) **film** is taken prior to the introduction of the contrast media. This scout is used as comparison "control." Air can sometimes be used as a contrast media rather than a radiopaque substance like barium preparations. Barium is a metallic element which, in a compound such as barium sulfate, is swallowed as a "meal" that makes certain hollow organs easier to "read." Any air filling an organ also shows on the film as rarefied or less dense than the surrounding tissues.

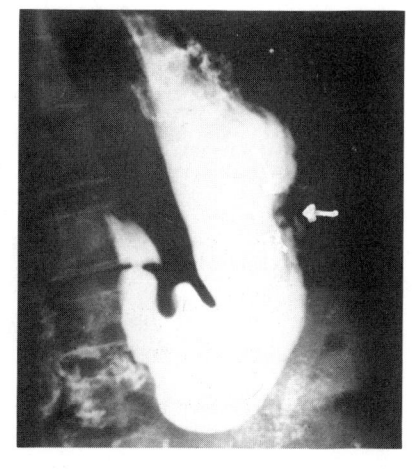

Figure 19-7: Contrast media outlines the organ for greater visibility. Arrows indicate presence of lesion.

The injudicious or excessive use of roentgen rays can result in tissue damage to both patients and health personnel. But if the voltage is properly handled, the X rays used for diagnostic studies should prove no threat to the patient. Proper **shielding** (protection from radiation) must also be done at all times.

Repeated, unnecessary radiographic exposures must always be avoided. This is best accomplished by correctly positioning the patient the first time, by using sandbags or other immobilization equipment adequate for maintaining the best position, and by being absolutely accurate as to patient identification, equipment operation, and part exposure.

Rapidly growing and reproducing cells such as those found in the gonads, the bone marrow, and the lymph nodes are most sensitive to the effects of **irradiation** (radiant energy emissions) so shields are used to protect these tissues. The shields are made of materials impervious to medical X rays. Lead is most commonly used, but concrete and barium plaster can also be used.

The greatest danger from the effects of radiation are to the radiologic technician and to the radiologist. These dangers can be minimized if the general radiation precautions are carefully and conscientiously carried out. These precautions include the use of dosimeters.

SAFETY PRECAUTIONS

Figure 19-8: Radiopaque contrast media of barium sulfate which the patient drinks *(courtesy of Picker Corp.).*

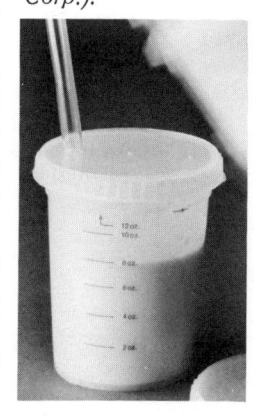

Figure 19-9: Shields protect the radiologic personnel from accidental exposure to radiations *(courtesy of Picker Corp.)*

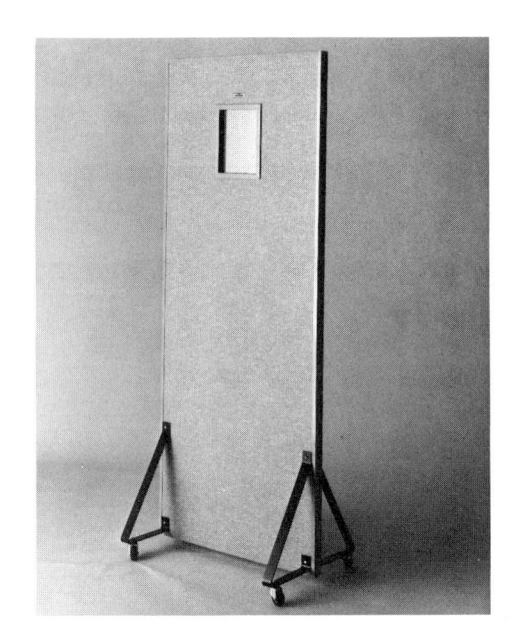

Dosimeters or **electroscopes** are instruments which record the intensity and level of radiation exposure and thus give warning when dangerous limits are near. One type of dosimeter is the **film badge**, which is worn on the outer clothing by all the personnel involved with radiation in any way. Another type is the pocket dosimeter carried in either a shirt or trouser pocket. It also detects degrees of exposure.

Laboratory monitors keep track of overall radiation build-up in the area. Lead screens are used to separate personnel from any radiations that may escape during radiography. Lead aprons (Figure 19-5) and gloves can also be worn to protect the health worker. Periodic blood counts are performed on all radiologic workers since excessive radiation exposure can result in blood dyscrasias. The blood counts do not measure radiation levels but they do indicate whether or not there is any apparent radiation damage.

X-ray Positioning Techniques

Diagnostic roentgenograms are made by directing a stream of X rays toward a specific area by means of an X-ray tube. X rays travel in a straight line from the X-ray tube, diverging only as they move forward. The radiologic technician directs the central beam at the part to be radiographed.

For proper **exposure** (filming) of the body part, the patient must be positioned with that body part closest to the cassette, and the central beam must be correctly directed. Several terms are used which describe the manner or direction of the filming.

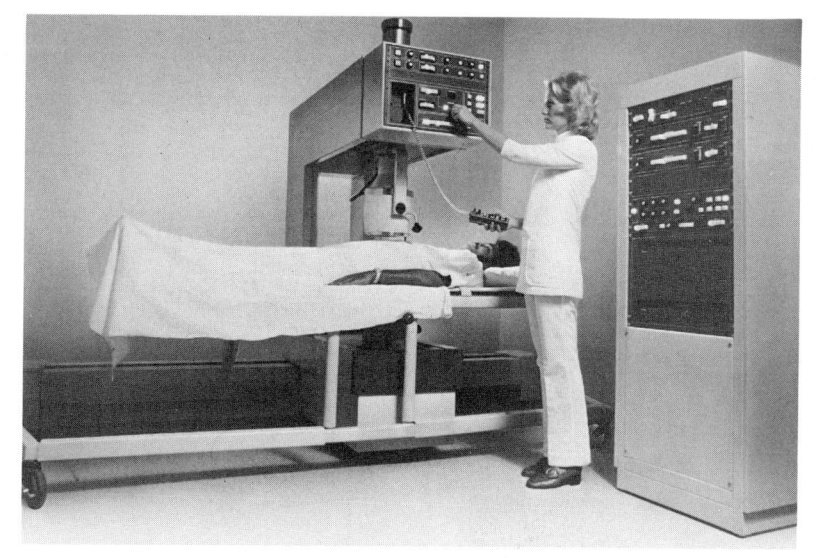

Figure 19-10: Whole Body Scanner; a special radiologic machine *(courtesy of General Electric Company).*

The X-ray **view** (**projection** or **position**) takes into consideration the position of the patient and the direction of the central beam. Many of the terms are familiar, but now you will be using them in a somewhat different context.

Four basic radiographic positions are used to line up the large body surfaces with the X-ray tube: **A-P** (anterior-posterior) when the beam is directed from front to back, **P-A** (posterior-anterior) when the beam is directed from back to front; the **lateral** when the beam is directed from one side, and the **oblique** when the beam is directed at an angle.

Table 19-1

Body Section	Direction of Central Beam
axillary	toward the axilla
mediolateral	from the midline toward the side
supine mediolateral	from the midline toward the side and with the patient lying face upward
craniocaudal	from superior to inferior levels (from head to tail, the craniocaudad)

Before the film is shot, markers are affixed to the cassette to indicate the projection view and patient identification. That marker becomes part of the permanent image so that there can be no mix-up.

SAFETY PRECAUTIONS

Figure 19-11:
(a) Mammography—sitting axillary view;
(b) mammography—recumbent mediolateral position;
(c) mammography—sitting craniocaudal view *(courtesy of G.H. Fischer, Inc.)*.

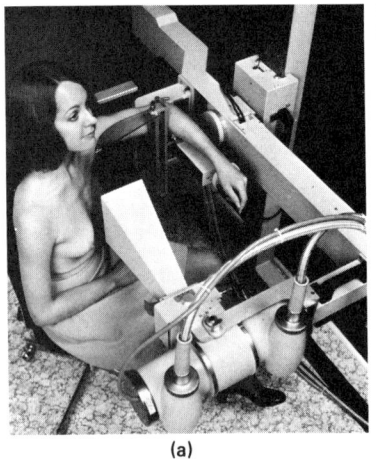

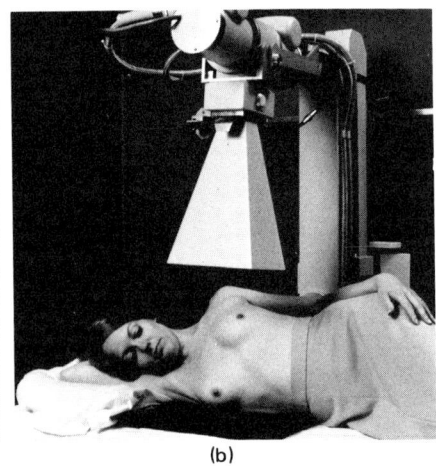

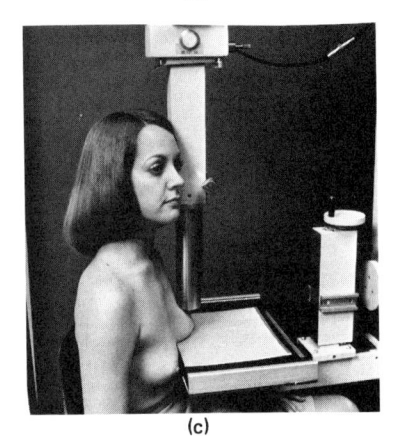

Figure 19-12: Markers used to indicate radiographic projection, view or position *(courtesy of Picker Corp.)*.

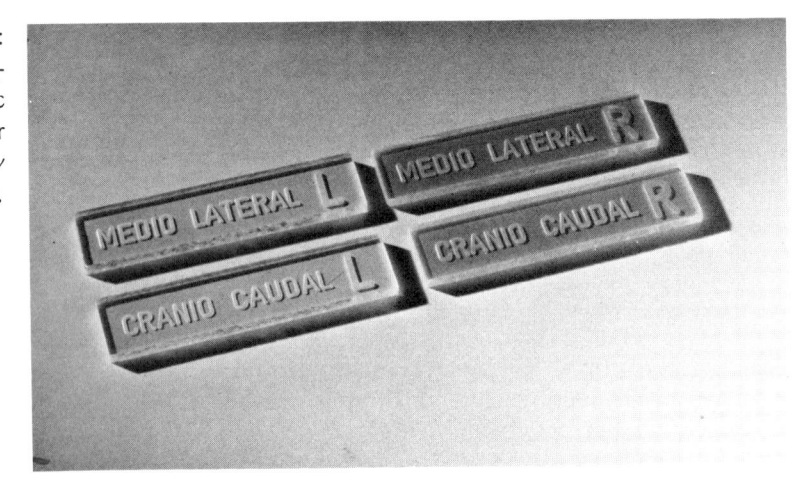

FLUOROSCOPY

Radiologic technicians also assist in fluoroscopic techniques. **Fluoroscopy** (radioscopy) is a visual examination of the deep body parts with a fluoroscope. Fluoroscopy is a special X-ray technique that produces a temporary image of the body when it is placed between the X-ray source and a special screen in a darkened room. The screen is coated with crystals that emit light (**fluorescence**) which they have absorbed from another source.

The original fluoroscopic technique required absolute darkness and the radiologist had to wear special red goggles for at least 20 minutes prior to the examination. That dilated (**enlarged**) the pupils of his eyes so that he could better see density variations necessary in the total darkness. That is, his vision accommodated to the special light.

Modern fluoroscopy employs an electronic image intensifier which takes the weak image and increases it so that total dark is not required and dark adaptation with goggles is no longer needed. This newer technique is also accomplished with reduced radiation. The patient is placed in front of the fluoroscopic device, usually after a contrast media has been introduced. The radiologist is then able to observe functioning viscera or certain other organs as the X rays cause the crystals on the screen to fluoresce.

Look at Table 19-2 to review the five roentgenographic procedures in which contrast media are used:

Table 19-2

Special Technique	Picture Obtained	Kind of Roentgenogram
bronchography	*bronchogram*	of lungs after instillation of contrast media
arthrography	*arthrogram*	of joint after injection of contrast media
myelography	*myelogram*	of the spinal cord after injection of contrast media
pneumo-encephalography	*pneumo-encephalogram*	of brain after injection of air
cholecystography	*cholecystogram*	of the gall bladder after ingestion of radiopaque media

A special roentgenographic technique, called **tomography**, produces a **tomogram** of thin body sections as the X-ray tube is moved. This radiogram is a picture of internal structures produced on a specially sensitized film. It allows for more detailed study of body planes. Many of the new, fast machines are also computer assisted so that clear multiple images are combined as aids to diagnosis.

RADIOTHERAPY Radiotherapy or **roentgenism** is the use of ionizing radiation in the treatment of tissue diseases. At certain strengths, radiation in the form of X rays, gamma rays, or alpha and beta particles converts the atoms of cellular elements wholly or partly into ions. This ionization of cellular atoms disrupts normal cellular function and eventually causes cellular death. So X rays directed toward malignant cells cause them to ionize; therefore, they become disorganized and cannot reproduce. In this way, the cellular elements that make up malignant tumors can be treated and destroyed.

Ionizing radiations can have the same ionizing effect on healthy tissue, of course. But healthy tissues are less **radiosensitive** (affected by radiations). The **recuperative** (recovery) powers of healthy cells are also greater than those of malignant cells. So the key to radiotherapy is to irradiate or bombard the tissues with radiation doses strong enough to permanently damage abnormal tissues while simultaneously causing no irreparable damage to surrounding healthy tissues.

Unfortunately the high levels of radiation needed in tumor therapy often have various side effects on body tissue, including hair loss (**depilation**), skin shedding (**desquamation**), hemopoietic dysfunction, and chromosomal changes. Both the intended and the side effects of ionization radiation are cumulative. Therefore, the safety precautions already discussed must be conscientiously followed.

Comparatively low-voltage X ray is used to irradiate surface lesions while ultra-high voltage radiation is used on deeper lesions. This form of radiotherapy is used in combination with other tumor therapies such as surgery and chemotherapy.

NUCLEAR MEDICINE Nuclear medicine is an extension of radiotherapy. It uses various radioactive elements that give off or emit the radiations of electromagnetic waves such as gamma waves and alpha and beta particles. Some elements such as **radium** are naturally radioactive. Radium spontaneously emits radiations. Because of this, small amounts of radium in the form of seeds or needles (**implants**) can be inserted (**implanted**) into a tumor mass. There, for a prescribed period of time, the elctromagnetic radiations are able to act on and destroy the abnormal cells.

Radioactive or unstable elements can also be produced artificially. Called radioactive isotopes, they are made by bombarding certain elements with streams of neutrons which upset the proton-neutron ratio of that atomic nucleus. As the isotope strives to reestablish the nuclear ratio, large amounts of gamma rays are emitted.

Produced and controlled in sophisticated machines, these radioactive isotopes (**radionuclides**) are the foundation of nuclear therapy and diagnosis. **Radioactive iodine**, **radioactive cobalt**, and **radioactive phosphorus** are three radioactive isotopes widely used in nuclear medicine.

Many techniques have been developed to use these substances in studying the body. For example, **teletherapy** (radiation ionization from a distance) is the technique of directing the gamma rays of a radioactive isotope such as cobalt 60, from a shielded unit placed some distance from the patient.

Radioisotope **scanning** (detailed successive examining of small or isolated areas) produces a two-dimensional picture representing the gamma rays emitted by a radioactive isotope concentrated in a part of the body. For example, in a **bone scan**, a measured dose of a radioactive isotope is given to the patient. The injected isotope is carried by the blood stream into the bones. Then a radioactive isotope detector, the **scanner**, records on film the position of the isotope by means of its emissions. The picture, however, is less discrete than that produced in X-radiography. What is formed is really a pattern of the deposits of radioactive isotope. A single scan may produce three or four projections which might include an anterior view, posterior view, lateral view, or one of the more complex positions.

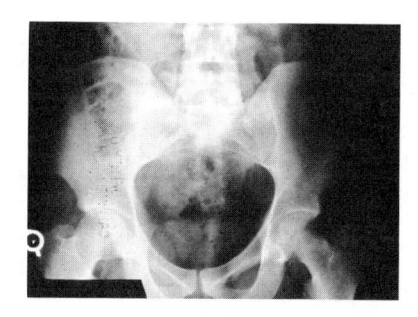

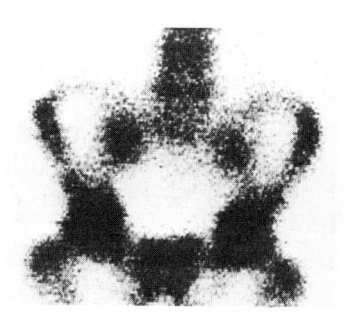

Figure 19-13: X-ray of pelvis. Picture produced by scanner is less discrete.

Many new whole body scanners are currently in use, such as the **scintiscanner**, which picks up and records the **scintillation** (emission of sparks) from the gamma rays emitted by the concentration of radioactive isotopes in the tissues. The subsequent images produced are called a **scintiscan**. Each such new piece of equipment and imaging technique adds to the diagnostic tools available for health care.

CASE STUDY

Joshua Scott, 22, tall and excessively thin, was admitted to the medical unit of Fayetteville General Hospital. A thyroid mass was easily palpable and he complained of excessive fatigue and weight loss. He said he felt as if "his motor was running overtime." He had a productive cough and had experienced one episode of hemoptysis. A heavy smoker, he had ignored the cough but the bloody sputum had frightened him. In addition, he had severe headaches which were becoming progressively frequent and worse. He had a high pressure sales job in a large industry.

The official admitting diagnosis was hyperthyroidism, R/O malignant thyroid with possible metastasis. The physician ordered the following series of diagnostic tests in hopes of establishing a definitive diagnosis:

1. Routine C.B.C. and urinalysis
2. Chest roentgenograms A-P, lateral, and oblique views
3. Radiographic skull series
4. Prepare for thyroid scan with radioactive iodine on Friday
5. Prepare for bronchoscopy and bronchogram on Wednesday
6. Brain scan for Monday A.M.

Please schedule with radiology and nuclear medicine.

When the nurse explained the schedule of tests that were to be performed, the patient became quite agitated and alarmed. He said he didn't understand the words she was using and besides, he was afraid he would become sterile if any radioactive substances were used on him.

She quietly and slowly defined roentgenography in simple everyday terms. She went on to explain that the bronchogram is also radiography but that a contrast media is used to enhance the radiogram formed on the radiographic film.

She further described the thyroid and brain scan as requiring no special preparation. She said that

Figure 19-14: Joshua Scott was admitted with a diagnosis of Hyperthyroidism.

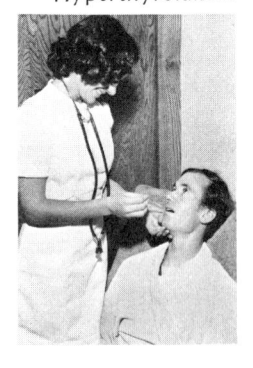

many patients relaxed enough during the procedures to doze off, since there is no discomfort. The nurse was also able to assure him that both tests had been performed on millions of patients in relative safety. She admitted that massive doses of radiation could make a man temporarily sterile, but emphasized that the amount of radiation used for medical diagnosis is so minimal that there is no danger to the gonads.

Throughout the following two weeks, Joshua submitted to the various radiologic tests that had been ordered for him. He cooperated in every way with the radiologic and nuclear medicine technicians. When all the test results were completed, Joshua's attending physician and the house intern had a conference with the chief radiologist.

The radiology report confirmed the presence of a lesion in the thyroid gland. Only biopsy could confirm the diagnosis. The situation was explained to the patient and he agreed to surgery, so he was scheduled for a thyroid biopsy and possible thyroidectomy. The biopsy revealed adenocarcinoma of the thyroid with some metastasis and a partial thyroidectomy was performed.

As a follow-up to the surgery, radiotherapy was planned. Six months later, Joshua is still receiving radiotherapy. He has not experienced any depilation but the skin on his neck has desquamated to some extent. His prognosis, once guarded, is much improved.

SUMMARY

Radiation science applied to the diagnosis and treatment of disease is improving the prognosis for many patients. Highly trained technicians utilize radiologic technique in the care of patients. From the early day of Roentgen's work to the vastly complicated electronic techniques of today, the controlled scientific concepts of radiation science have proved beneficial to mankind.

PRACTICE & REVIEW

Explain and define the new special terms you have been using. Remember, you learned how to pronounce them at the beginning of this chapter.

1. radioactive _____
2. roentgenography _____
3. radiolucent _____

4. radiopaque _____
5. irradiation _____
6. craniocaudad _____
7. fluoroscopy _____
8. pneumoencephalography _____
9. tomography _____
10. scintiscanner _____

Now, double-check the meaning of the terms above by studying the brief definitions given in the Glossary-Index at the back of this book.

Test yourself quickly before going on to learn other medical and professional terms. Use these short review exercises to practice for your new work in health services. Your teacher will also help by recommending various other Study Activities.

A. Read the terms below and then write a synonym for each in the space provided:

1. roentgenogram _____
2. roentgenography _____
3. roentgen rays _____
4. exposure _____
5. view _____

B. Match the word at the right with one of the ten definitions below:

____ 1. Word used to mean hidden image	a. gamma rays
____ 2. Another name for roentgenogram	b. Fe
____ 3. Electromagnetic radiations	c. electrons
____ 4. Primary chemical substances	d. pass box
____ 5. The symbol for the element Iron	e. latent
____ 6. Negative particles that are part of an atom	f. scout
	g. elements
____ 7. Term used to describe the release of radiation	h. cassette
	i. I
____ 8. Lightproof film holder	j. emission
____ 9. Name given to film transfer box	k. radiogram
____ 10. Name given to a preliminary film	

After studying Chapter 20

Communication with Medical Records

You should be able to:

* Pronounce and define each of its new medical words and phrases and use the new technical jargon.

* Identify eight record forms used by health personnel.

* Describe a "daily care plan."

PRONOUNCE THESE EIGHT NEW WORDS WITH YOUR TEACHER: MEDICAL WORDS

cardex (kar-deks)
chart (chärt)
clinical (klin′ikl)
parentally (pah-ren′tah-le)
diarrhea (di″ah-re′ah)
guerney (gr-nĭ)
litter
discogenic (dis″ko-jen′ĭk)

Record keeping is an important responsibility of all health workers. Some records, such as notes taken during a report, are unofficial. Other records are "official." These official records are compiled as the patient's chart. Official records are kept about the patient in the physician's office, in referral clinics, and in the hospital.

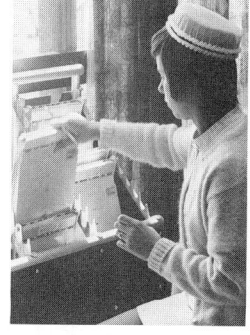

Figure 20-1: Official records are compiled as the patient's chart.

UNOFFICIAL RECORDS

Unofficial records of the patient and his care include the notes made by the health worker during the report period or conference. These are frequently just notations in a small notebook and are meant only for the writer. They may also be made on a patient's daily care plan.

Daily care plans are printed check lists. They facilitate the planning of patient care because the worker can simply check or circle the parts which apply to each patient. The daily care plans or notebooks are usually carried by the worker as she/he goes about caring for assigned patients. Having a summary at hand saves the worker the effort of constantly returning to the

Figure 20-2: Patient care sheet used during report.

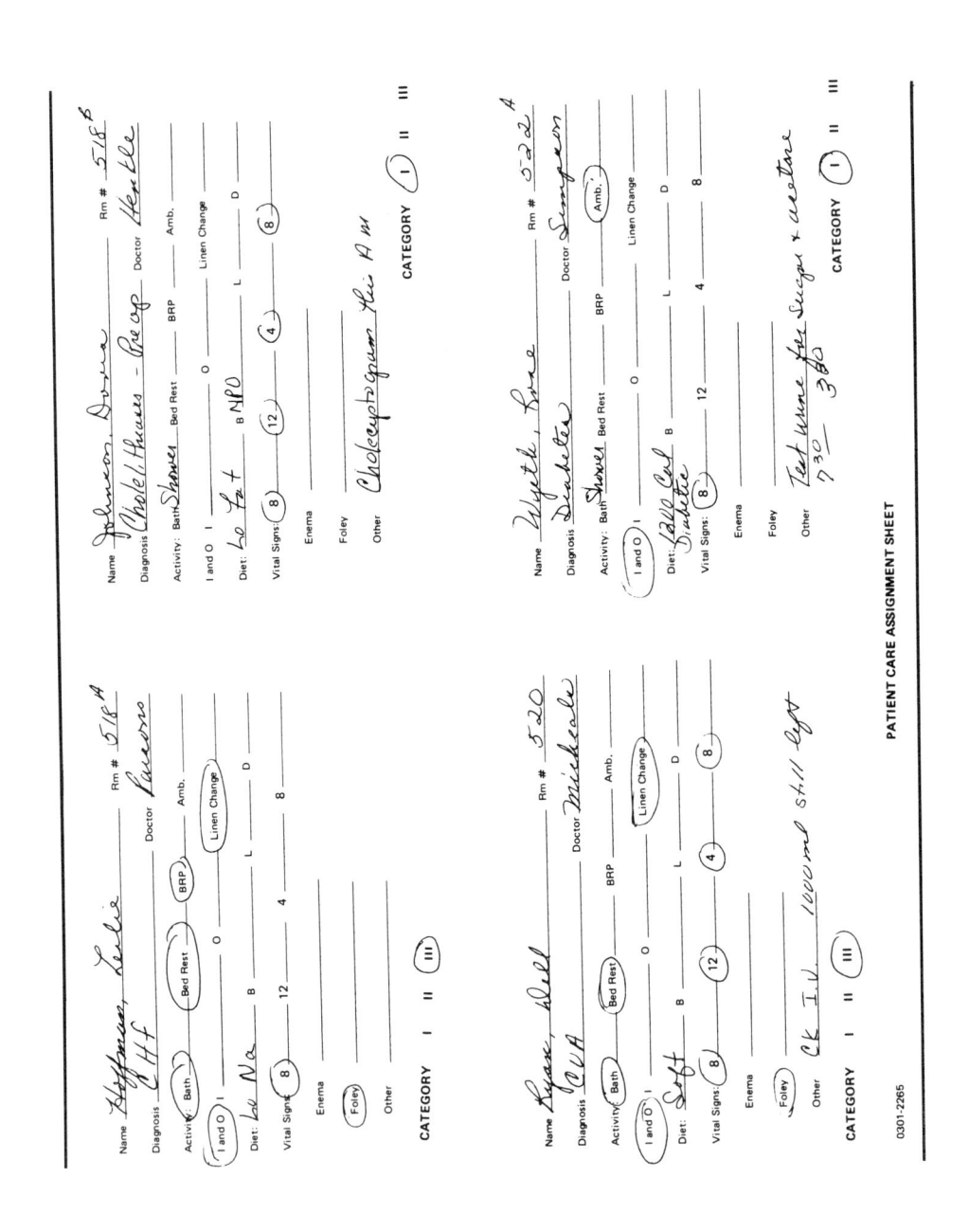

316 COMMUNICATION WITH MEDICAL RECORDS

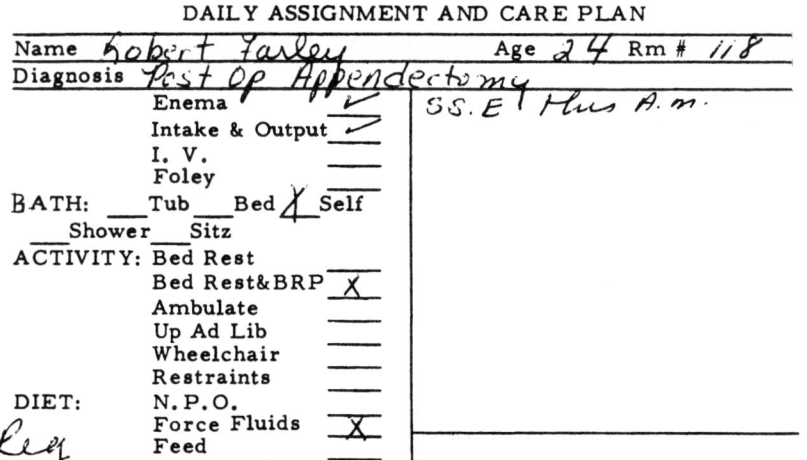

DAILY ASSIGNMENT AND CARE PLAN	
Name Robert Farley Age 24 Rm # 118	
Diagnosis Post Op Appendectomy	
Enema ✓	SS.E Plus A.m.
Intake & Output ✓	
I.V.	
Foley	
BATH: ___Tub ___Bed X Self	
___Shower ___Sitz	
ACTIVITY: Bed Rest ___	
Bed Rest & BRP X	
Ambulate ___	
Up Ad Lib ___	
Wheelchair ___	
Restraints ___	
DIET: N.P.O. ___	
Reg Force Fluids X	
Nurse Feed ___	

Figure 20-3: Daily Assignment and Care Plan is used to summarize patient information.

nurse's station to look at the official orders to confirm his activities.

All such records must be carefully handled so that information about a patient doesn't fall into improper hands. Any additional notations made on the care plans during the day are later transferred to the official record.

The patient report is given to the oncoming shift from another unofficial record called the **cardex**. The cardex sheets are kept in a binder called the cardex or cardex backing. The information written or typed on the cardex is taken from the official record, the Doctor's Order Sheet. The physician writes specific orders regarding the patient's care and therapy. These orders are transferred to the cardex, usually by a ward clerk or by the nurse in charge.

Other special information about the patient is added to the cardex after a nursing assessment has been made. A **nursing assessment** is a plan for specific nursing care and approaches based on nursing expertise and on observations of the patient's sociological, psychological and general physical needs.

The unofficial daily care records are destroyed before the worker leaves the hospital after each tour of duty. The cardex sheets, which are changed daily according to the patient's need, are destroyed when the patient is discharged. Frequently these sheets accompany the official record if a patient is transferred to a new location. In any event, despite their unofficial status all records or notations are private patient information and that information must be protected.

Figure 20-4: (left) The Cardex.

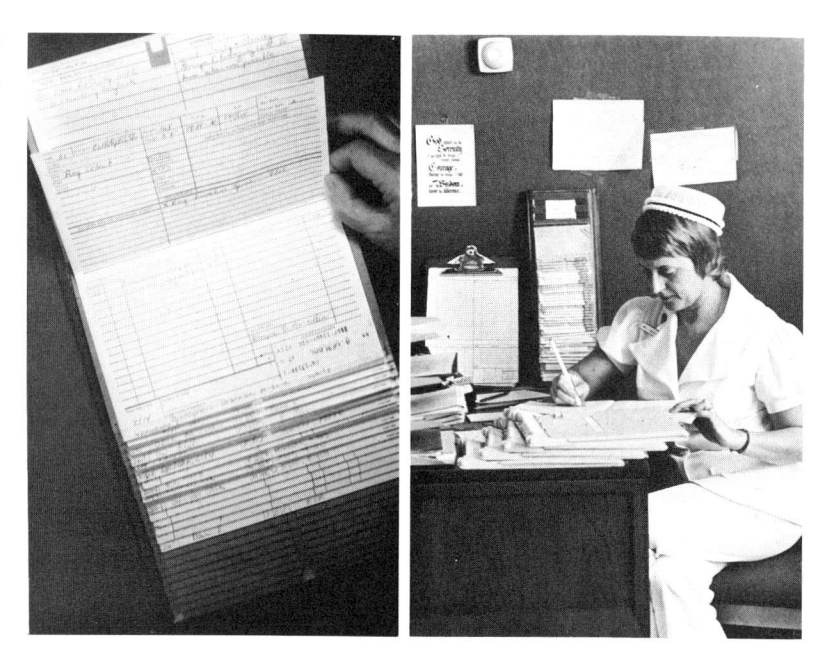

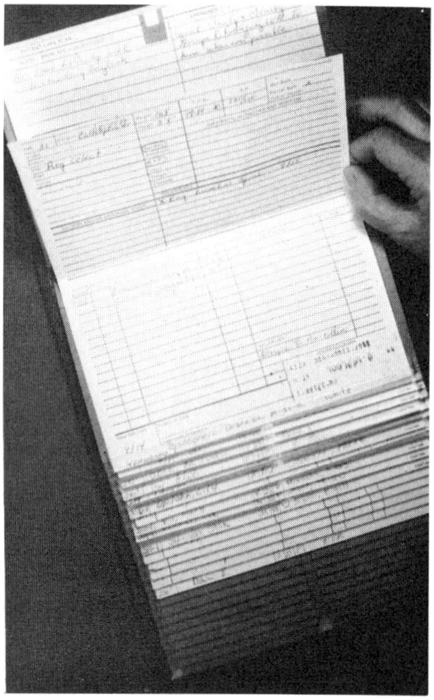

Figure 20-5: (right) The nurse reviews the physician's orders and makes a nursing assessment.

OFFICIAL RECORDS

Official records are legal records whose contents are governed by law; they are considered privileged and confidential. But to be effective as a team, every member of the team must know what the diagnosis, prognosis, and progress are for the patient, and the ultimate goal desired from the therapy. So all health workers should have access to the information contained on the official record either directly from the recorded sheets or through the cardex and reports.

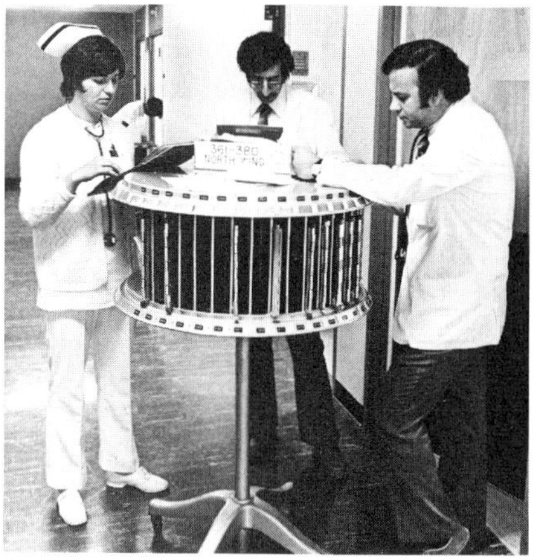

Figure 20-6: The physician, nurse and intern all use and contribute to the official records.

*318 COMMUNICATION WITH MEDICAL RECORDS

The Chart

The official record is called the patient's **chart**. The chart is made up of a variety of forms, each designed to record some special type of information. Most hospitals or agencies use standard patient forms, although some health agencies devise their own forms to cover their particular need.

The term "chart" is an English term which has been adopted by medicine. Like many English words, "chart" may be used as either a noun, an adjective, or a verb. For example, the nurse on duty may chart the fluid intake on the patient's chart. The various chart forms are bound together in a **chart book** and stored in a chart **rack** or **caddy** so as to make them accessible to all personnel. In some facilities, only professional personnel make notations on the patient's chart; in others, any person giving care is responsible for recording that information.

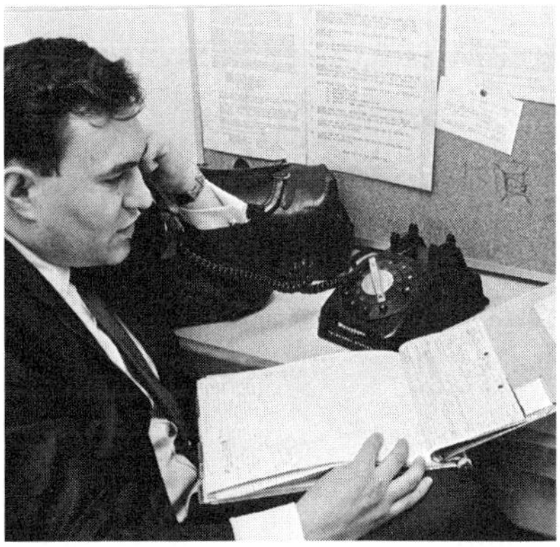

Figure 20-7: (left) The physician dictates his findings into the dictaphone. The report will be typed, signed and added to the chart in his hand.

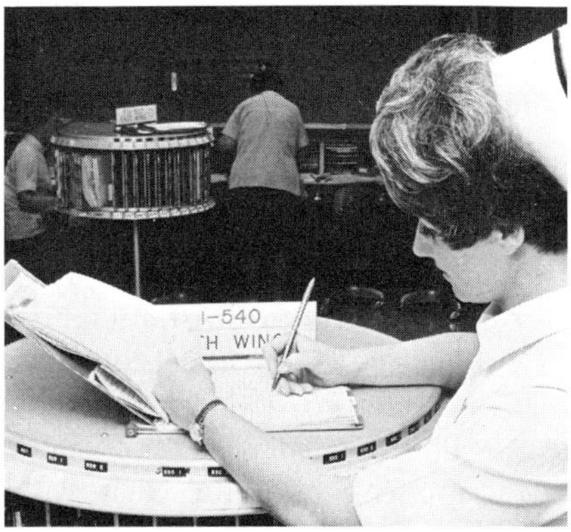

Figure 20-8: (right) The registered nurse is charting a medication she has just given on the patient's chart.

In a hospital, notations or notes are the summaries made of information pertinent to each patient. They are usually charted as phrases rather than as full sentences to conserve space. Each **entry** (notation) is made in a manner prescribed by the general rules of medical charting. Since everything on the chart is about the patient, neither the word patient nor the patient's name is included in each entry. For example, a patient who has had a regular House Diet ordered but who eats poorly because of nausea, would have the incident recorded in this manner—"Reg. Diet, poorly taken, C/O nausea." Each entry must be signed or initialed by the responsible person and no blank lines must be left.

Every sheet of the chart must be identified with the patient's name, hospital number, date of admission, and name of the physician. A stamped and printed card similar in appearance to a commercial charge plate is made at admission time

Figure 20-9: The Addressograph is used to imprint the patient's name and other identifying information on every sheet of the chart.

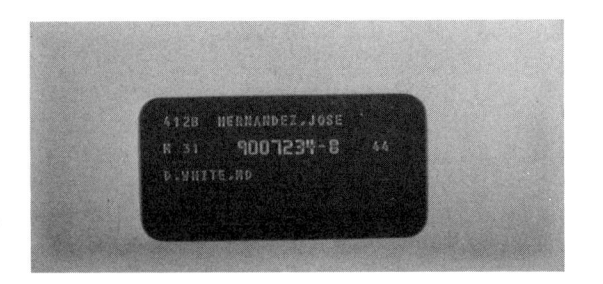

for use with each patient. It carries the patient's name and address and other data and is made like an Addressograph plate. This plate is used to imprint the identification on each of the patient records. If an Addressograph plate is not used in a given hospital, each sheet must be properly identified in handwriting. In this way, mistakes are avoided.

The chart is made up of several basic forms which include the **admission** or front sheet, the Doctor's Orders, the Physical and History form, the Nurse's Notes, and the Graphic chart (**clinical** sheet).

The **front sheet** is filled in by the admitting officer on admission of the patient. It provides personal and general background information, financial data, and the admission diagnosis. This particular sheet is completed and signed by the physician upon discharge.

The **Doctor's Order sheet** is used by the physician to describe the care he wishes the patient to have. Usually the physician writes the orders himself, dates and signs them. Sometimes, however, the physician relates his directions to a nurse who writes them on the form. The nurse then writes out the physician's name and initials it, thus indicating that the orders were given orally (by voice). For example, "V.O. Dr. Frankcus BA . . . ."

The physical, history and progress forms are also completed by the physician. The **physical and history** form is a combined summary of the physician's examination of the patient and the history of the patient's medical problems.

The **nurses notes** and the **graphic sheet** as well as many of the supplemental form sheets are completed by the nursing staff. The Nurses Notes record the care the patient receives and includes pertinent observations by the staff on the patient and his condition. The **Graphic Sheet** includes information which may also appear on the Nurses Notes in a graphic or abbreviated form. Vital signs, records of total fluid intake or output are frequently listed on this sheet.

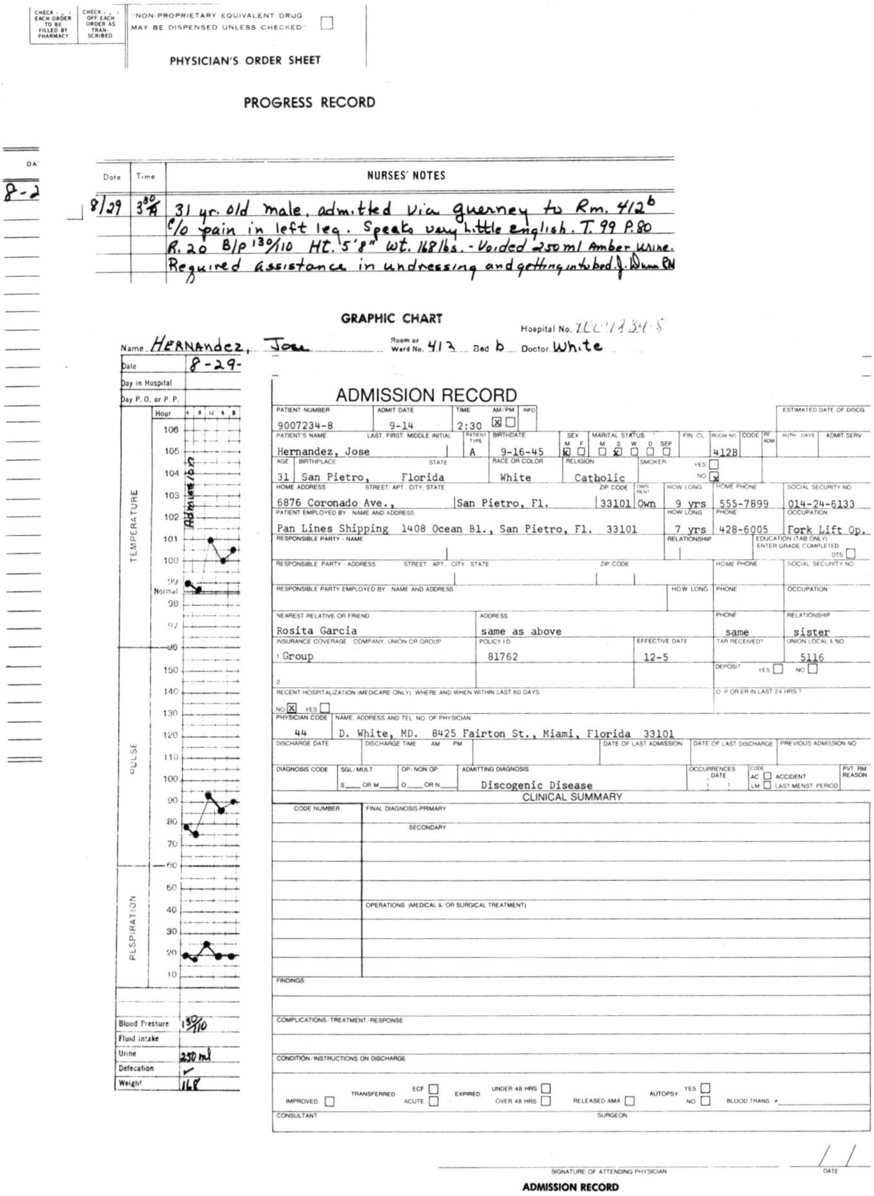

CHECK EACH ORDER TO BE FILLED BY PHARMACY | CHECK OFF EACH ORDER AS TRANSCRIBED | "NON-PROPRIETARY EQUIVALENT DRUG MAY BE DISPENSED UNLESS CHECKED" ☐

PHYSICIAN'S ORDER SHEET

PROGRESS RECORD

NURSES' NOTES

Date	Time	
8/29	3³⁰P	31 yr. old male, admitted via guerney to Rm. 412b c/o pain in left leg. Speaks very little english. T. 99 P. 80 R. 20 B/P 130/10 Ht. 5'8" wt. 168 lbs. - Voided 250 ml Amber urine. Required assistance in undressing and getting into bed. J. Dunn RN

GRAPHIC CHART

Name Hernandez, Jose Room or Ward No. 412 Bed b Doctor White Hospital No. 9007234-8

Date 8-29-

Day in Hospital

Day P. O. or P. P.

Hour

Temperature: 106, 105, 104, 103, 102, 101, 100, 99 Normal, 98, 97, 96 (Admitted)

Pulse: 150, 140, 130, 120, 110, 100, 90, 80, 70, 60

Respiration: 50, 40, 30, 20, 10

Blood Pressure 130/10

Fluid Intake

Urine 250 ml

Defecation ✓

Weight 168

ADMISSION RECORD

PATIENT NUMBER	ADMIT DATE	TIME	AM/PM
9007234-8	9-14	2:30	☒ AM ☐ PM

PATIENT'S NAME (LAST, FIRST, MIDDLE INITIAL)	PATIENT TYPE	BIRTHDATE	SEX	MARITAL STATUS	ROOM NO
Hernandez, Jose	A	9-16-45	M ☒	S ☒	412B

AGE	BIRTHPLACE	STATE	RACE OR COLOR	RELIGION	SMOKER
31	San Pietro,	Florida	White	Catholic	NO ☒

HOME ADDRESS	CITY, STATE	ZIP CODE	OWN/RENT	HOW LONG	HOME PHONE	SOCIAL SECURITY NO
6876 Coronado Ave.,	San Pietro, Fl.	33101	Own	9 yrs	555-7899	014-24-6133

PATIENT EMPLOYED BY - NAME AND ADDRESS	HOW LONG	PHONE	OCCUPATION
Pan Lines Shipping 1408 Ocean Bl., San Pietro, Fl. 33101	7 yrs	428-6005	Fork Lift Op.

RESPONSIBLE PARTY - NAME | RELATIONSHIP | EDUCATION (TAB ONLY) ENTER GRADE COMPLETED

RESPONSIBLE PARTY - ADDRESS | ZIP CODE | HOME PHONE | SOCIAL SECURITY NO

RESPONSIBLE PARTY EMPLOYED BY - NAME AND ADDRESS | HOW LONG | PHONE | OCCUPATION

NEAREST RELATIVE OR FRIEND	ADDRESS	PHONE	RELATIONSHIP
Rosita Garcia	same as above	same	sister

INSURANCE COVERAGE - COMPANY, UNION OR GROUP	POLICY I.D.	EFFECTIVE DATE	UNION LOCAL & NO
1 Group	81762	12-5	5116

RECENT HOSPITALIZATION (MEDICARE ONLY) WHERE AND WHEN WITHIN LAST 60 DAYS — NO ☒ YES ☐

PHYSICIAN CODE	NAME, ADDRESS AND TEL. NO. OF PHYSICIAN
44	D. White, MD. 8425 Fairton St., Miami, Florida 33101

DISCHARGE DATE | DISCHARGE TIME | DATE OF LAST ADMISSION | DATE OF LAST DISCHARGE | PREVIOUS ADMISSION NO

DIAGNOSIS CODE	ADMITTING DIAGNOSIS
	Discogenic Disease

CLINICAL SUMMARY

CODE NUMBER | FINAL DIAGNOSIS PRIMARY | SECONDARY

OPERATIONS (MEDICAL &/OR SURGICAL TREATMENT)

FINDINGS

COMPLICATIONS/TREATMENT/RESPONSE

CONDITION/INSTRUCTIONS ON DISCHARGE

IMPROVED ☐ TRANSFERRED ECF ☐ ACUTE ☐ EXPIRED UNDER 48 HRS ☐ OVER 48 HRS ☐ RELEASED AMA ☐ AUTOPSY YES ☐ NO ☐ BLOOD TRANS. #

CONSULTANT | SURGEON

SIGNATURE OF ATTENDING PHYSICIAN | DATE

ADMISSION RECORD

Figure 20-10: Basic forms found on the patient's chart.

Other special forms are added to the chart as the need arises. For example, a **Diabetic Form** would be made out for the patient with diabetes. Significant information recorded on this form will include the results of urine testing and insulin administration. Similarly, the patient with a cranial injury has a **Neurological Record** known as a "head sheet" included on his

Figure 20-11: Supplementary forms that are added to the basic chart forms as needed.

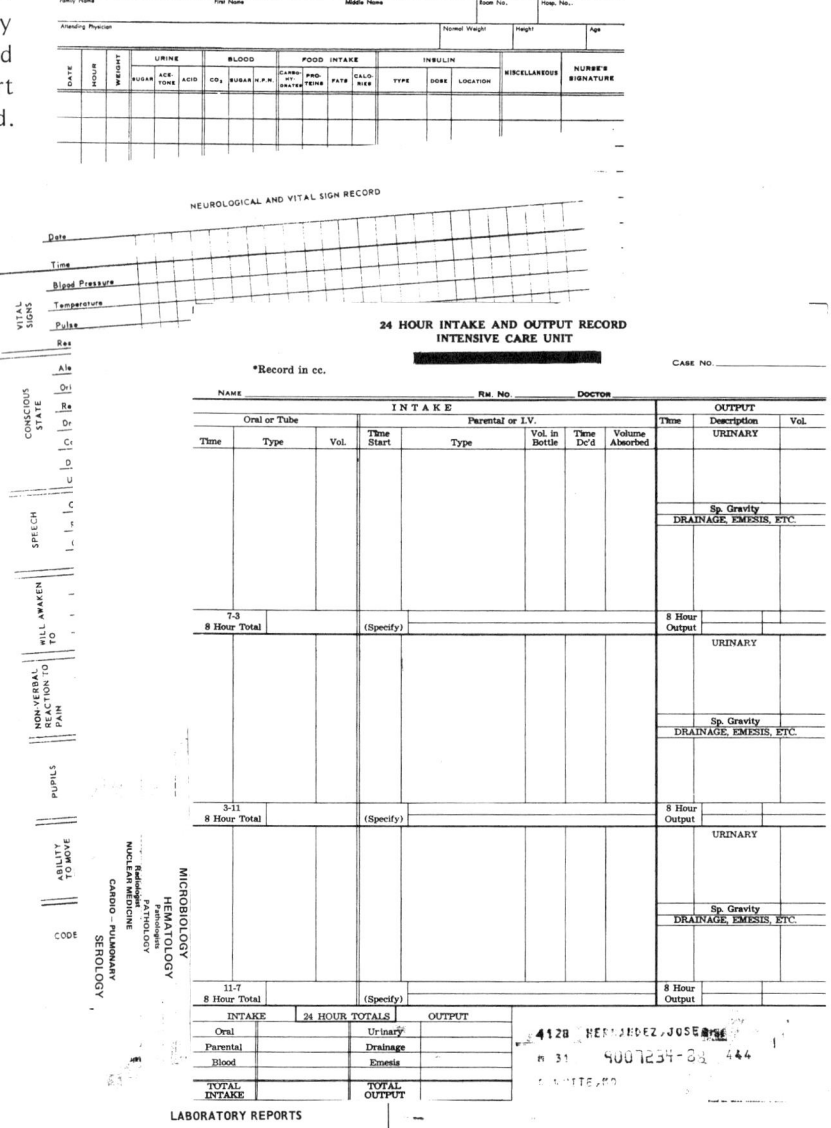

chart. The head sheet provides information at a glance about the patient's neurological status.

An **Intake and Output Record Sheet** summarizes total amounts of fluid taken into the body orally, **parentally** (entering through a route other than by mouth to the alimentary canal), and through other routes such as a naso-gastric tube or

*322 COMMUNICATION WITH MEDICAL RECORDS

gastrostomy (opening into the stomach) tube. The Intake and Output sheet also summarizes the total fluids lost from the body through emesis, urine, **diarrhea** (watery stools), and other forms of drainage such as nasogastric tubes. Copies of laboratory reports are attached to the **laboratory report** sheet, with the latest report on top.

When a patient enters the hospital for care, he/she voluntarily entrusts his well-being to many strangers. So there must be some sort of positive assurance that these people recognize the patient as himself and that only the specific care ordered by his doctors will be administered to him.

PATIENT IDENTIFICATION

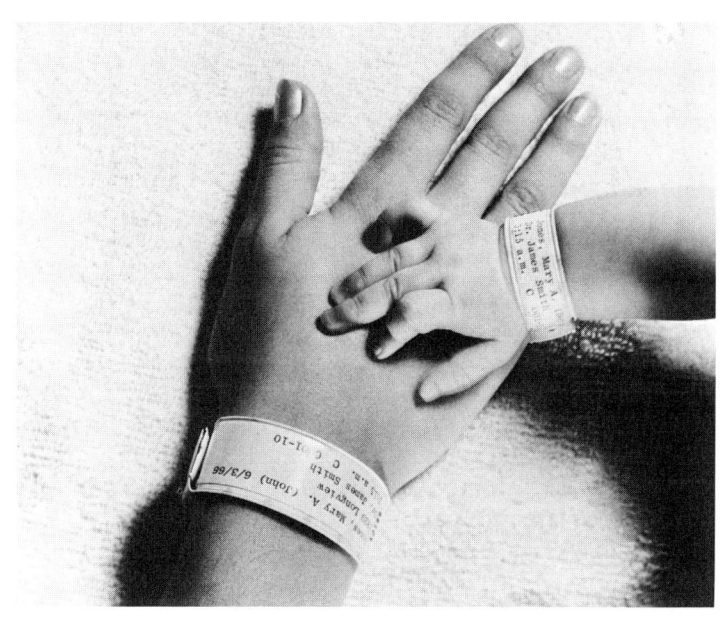

Figure 20-12: "Matching identification bracelets" *(courtesy of Sherwood Medical Industries).*

One method of assuring the proper identity of the patient in a large hospital is to stamp every patient record sheet with that person's addressograph plate. Another way to prevent accidents because of mistaken identity is to tag the patient himself. So plastic covered arm bands (**identification bands**) are placed on the patient's wrist during the admission procedure. They are not and must not be removed until after the patient is discharged and leaves the hospital. In addition to calling the patient by name, the health worker must always be sure to look at his arm band before administering any medication or carrying out any procedure. In obstetrics, at delivery, matching identification bands are placed on both mother and baby before the

Figure 20-13: "Footprints for identification of newborn" *(courtesy of American Hospital Supply Corporation).*

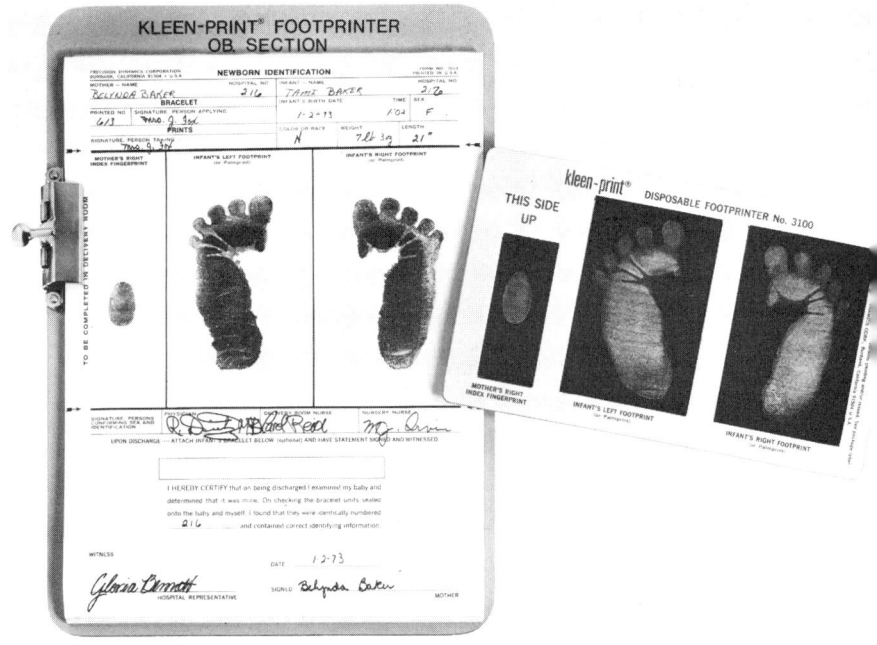

neonate is moved out of the delivery room. In addition, the baby's footprint and mother's thumb print are placed side by side on the birth record.

If a test or examination is ordered, it is important that every relevant specimen be properly identified with the patient's name, number, doctor, date, and time and be accompanied by the appropriate requisition form.

Medication Records

As orders for medications are taken from the physician's order sheet and transferred to the cardex, the pharmacy is notified and a medicine card is prepared for each drug to be given. Medicine cards are usually color coded for specific time intervals such as T.I.D., Q.I.D., B.I.D., H.S., Stat and A.C. or P.C. Each medicine card also states the name of the patient and room location, the medication, dosage, and method of administration. This card accompanies the medication to the patient's bedside. There it is compared to the identifying arm band before the medication is administered. As soon as the medication or treatment has been given, the fact is and must be recorded on the appropriate record form and signed by the responsible person.

Special Orders

Special signs are placed on the chart or at the bedside to alert all personnel to special orders. For example, identical alerting strips will be placed at the bedside and on the front of

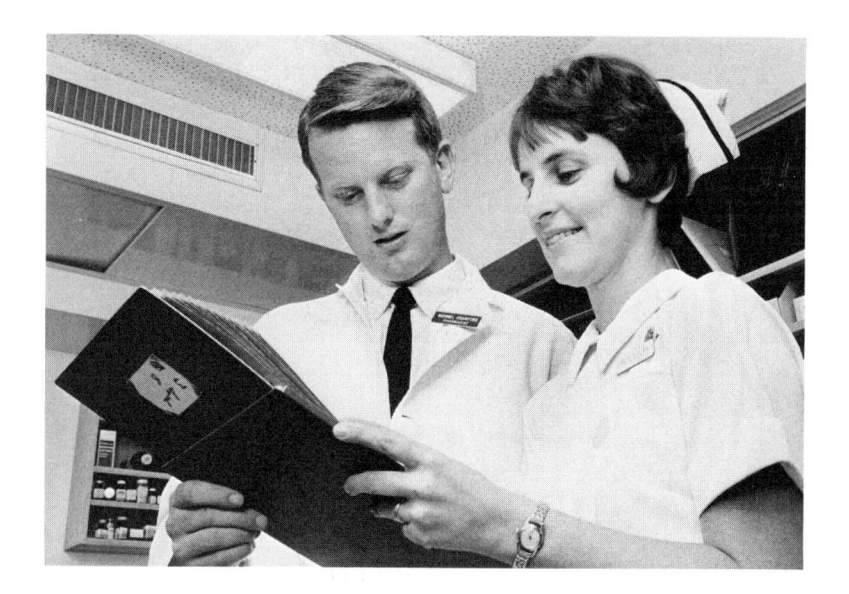

Figure 20-14: The pharmacy is notified as each new medication is added to the cardex from the doctor's order sheet.

Name	Scott, E.
Room Number	111 d
Doctor	Toyota
Med	ASA grs X
	Prn for Headache

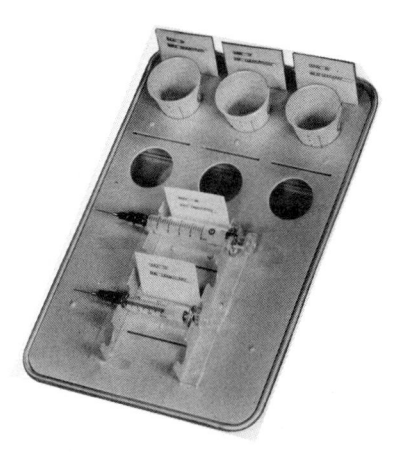

Figure 20-15: "Medication cards must be checked against wrist bands for proper identification" *(courtesy of American Hospital Supply Corporation).*

the chartback of a patient whose intake and output needs have to be measured.

Hospitals are usually large, busy places, with patients moving from area to area throughout the day to receive different therapies. At times a single patient may be moved from his originally assigned bed to three or four different locations in a single 24-hour period.

For example, Mike Dooley, a 42 year-old engineer with a diagnosis of cholecystitis, was assigned to Room 217 bed B. One morning at 7:45 a.m., the porter from radiology came to the unit for Mr. Dooley and transported him by wheelchair to

Figure 20-16: Signs on charts or over the patient's bed alert personnel to important orders *(courtesy of American Hospital Supply Corporation)*

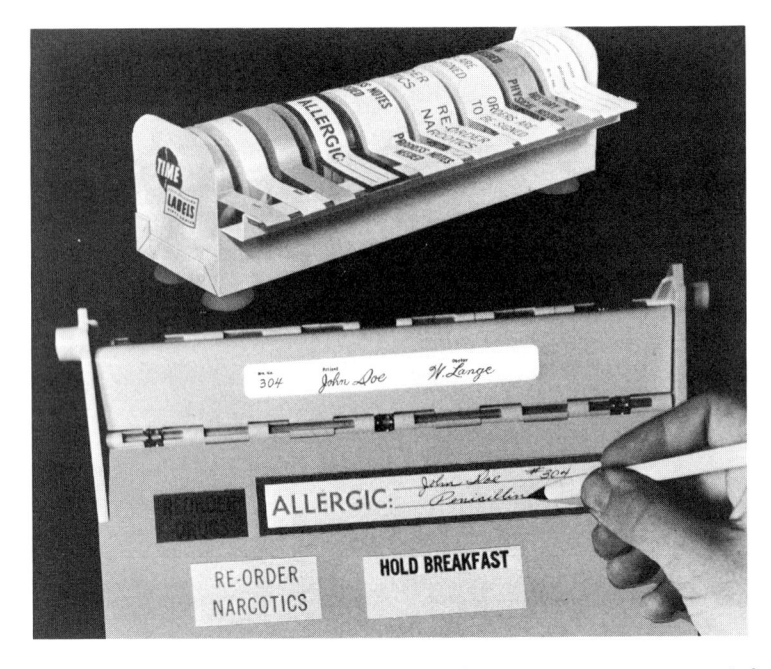

Figure 20-17: The patient location board keeps all personnel aware of the patient's location at all times.

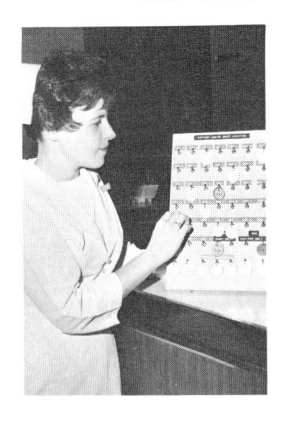

the radiology department for a cholecystogram. Returned from radiology, the patient was back in bed 217B for only about one hour when the nursing assistant escorted him to the floor treatment room so his physician and the consulting surgeon could examine him.

After that examination, Mr. Dooley was returned to his bed. But almost immediately, preparations were begun for his impending surgery. Within two hours, he was moved to the operating room for a cholecystectomy and choledochostomy. His post-operative diagnosis was cholecystitis with choledocholithiasis. He spent the night in the post-operative recovery room. It wasn't until about 9 a.m. of the next day that the patient was returned to the bed of his original admission on the second floor.

During that time, three separate work staffs assumed responsibility for the care of the patients on the second floor. In addition, during this same period personnel from the radiology staff, the O.R. staff, and the recovery staff all shared in the responsibility for this one particular patient, Mr. Dooley.

One way that the care given Mr. Dooley by all those health workers was coordinated was by means of the chart which moved from location to location with him. The floor staff also keep each other informed about the status of each patient through reports and by means of some form of patient location board.

* 326 COMMUNICATION WITH MEDICAL RECORDS

A patient location board has a space labelled with the room number opposite each patient's name. As a patient is moved from one location to another, a new location marker is affixed to the board so that all staff members are informed of the patient's whereabouts.

Patient Location Board

Patients are usually politely discouraged from bringing valuable personal property to hospitals, but if for some reason such property is brought it can be placed in a marked "property envelope" and stored in the hospital safe. Such envelopes are not ordinarily returned to the patient until he/she is discharged.

Personal Property Safeguards

The official records on the chart are not destroyed when the patient no longer needs care and is discharged. They are routinely stored in the hospital records system. Many huge hospitals commit the records to a microfilm retrieval system so they are ready for review if they are ever needed again. In any event, all hospital records are stored safely in some systematic manner for a considerable time. Record keeping is an important responsibility of the medical assistant as well as a responsibility of the hospital staff.

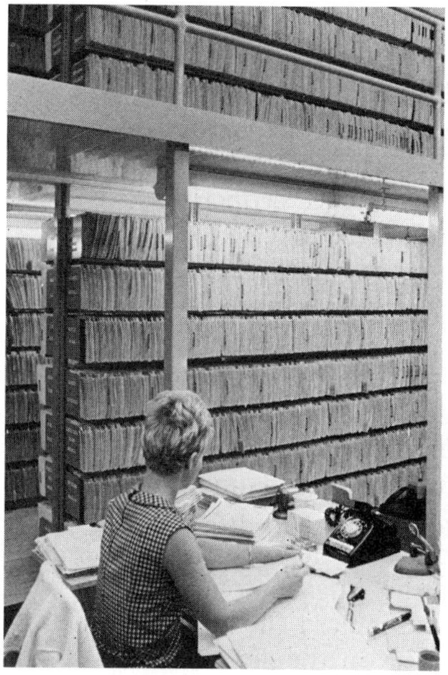

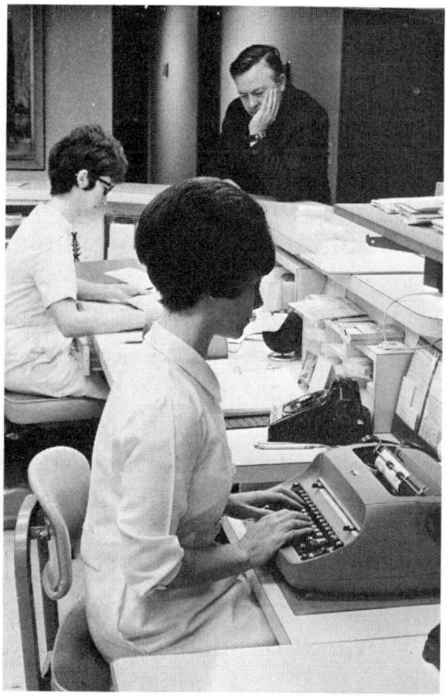

RECORD STORAGE

Figure 20-18: (left) Patient charts are never destroyed but must be safely stored for easy retrieval.

Figure 20-19: (right) The Medical Assistant keeps records for the physician *(courtesy of American Association of Medical Assistants, Inc.).*

The records maintained in the physician's office are similar in nature to those maintained in the hospital. Recall that on the first visit, the patient fills out or helps fill out a general form

Physician's Office Records

RECORD STORAGE 327 *

that provides information that is used to begin the patient file. This **case history file** is the physician's permanent official record and is maintained on each patient. If the office visit is due to an occupationally related injury, a report may also have to be filed with one or more governmental agency.

Most of the other forms found in the doctor's office are one or the other of three types: summaries of the physician's findings as they relate to the physical examination, history, and current patient complaints; laboratory reports; and business forms such as insurance forms and **statements** (billings). The physician is ultimately responsible for the information on the patient record but the office assistant aids the physician in the compilation of the records and assures their accessibility by accurate filing. The medical assistant also makes appointments for the physician and keeps records of them so that adequate time is allowed for each visit.

Whether it is done in the hospital or in the office, the keeping of accurate, confidential records is not only an ethical responsibility for all health personnel, but in many instances a legal one as well. Just as in the hospital, the medical records in the physician's office are confidential and nothing of their nature must be revealed.

CASE STUDY

José Hernandez, a 31 year-old dock worker was loading a ship with a forklift on the harbor night shift. One of the crates was wedged tightly and he was unable to position the forklift properly, so he jumped down from the machine to take a closer look. Landing heavily on one foot, he lost his balance and toppled over in a heap. When he attempted to get up he experienced severe pain in his left leg and had to be assisted. His foreman then had him taken home with instructions to see a doctor in the morning.

The next day, Mr. Hernandez made an appointment to see his physician. He arrived on time and answered the questions on the patient form for the case history file. He needed some help from his sister who interpreted much of the English for him. The doctor's medical assistant completed the information requested under the headings on the general history and occupational injury forms and then helped record the physician's findings on the physical evaluation form.

* 328 *COMMUNICATION WITH MEDICAL RECORDS*

Convinced that there was the possibility of **discogenic** (intervertebral disc involvement) **disease**, Dr. White sent Mr. Hernandez to City Hospital for admission to the orthopedic service on the fourth floor. Misunderstanding the physician, the patient waited until early the next morning to go to the hospital. But the night admissions officer was still on duty and completed a Front Sheet and attached a regular identifying band to Mr. Hernandez's wrist. Noting the severity of the patient's pain, the admissions officer asked the porter to transport him on a **guerney** (stretcher or **litter**) to his room.

In the room the nurse helped Mr. Hernandez into bed, took his vital signs, and then left to complete his chart. She charted his vital signs and output on the graphic chart and completed the nurse's notes, summarizing her observations during the admission. She added a progress record and a physician's order sheet to the front sheet, making sure they were all properly identified with the patient's name, hospital number, physician and date by stamping each sheet with the patient's Addressograph plate.

She placed the sheets together in a chart back and put the chart into the chart caddy so that it would be accessible to the staff. A cardex form was started and placed in the cardex to be finished as soon as the physician completed the physician's order sheet. She then located the patient on the location board so that the entire staff would be alert to his presence in Rm. (room) 412B.

SUMMARY

Records are summaries of the patient's condition and his response to treatment. Some are permanent and legal and must be completed and maintained according to accepted procedure. Using appropriate forms, many members of the health team contribute their observations to the final official record.

Non-official records are made for the immediate professional use of personnel while they are giving care. These records are not part of a patient's official record and must be destroyed when they are no longer being used. All patient information must be held in confidence.

PRACTICE &   *Explain and define the new special terms you have been using. Remember,*
REVIEW   *you learned how to pronounce them at the beginning of this chapter.*

1. cardex _____
2. chart _____
3. clinical _____
4. parentally _____
5. diarrhea _____
6. guerney _____
7. litter _____
8. discogenic _____

Now, double-check the meaning of the terms above by studying the brief definitions given in the Glossary-Index at the back of this text.

Test yourself quickly before going on to learn other medical and professional terms. Use these short review exercises to practice for your new work in health services. Your teacher will also help by recommending various other Study Activities.

A. Write a brief explanation underneath each of these signs that are used in patient care:

1. I & O

2. Caution: O_2 in use

3. N.P.O.

B. Circle the number of the terms below which designate official records:

1. Physical and History
2. Nursing assessment plan
3. Cardex
4. Assignment sheet
5. Intake and output
6. Progress notes
7. Physician's orders
8. Nurse's notes
9. Laboratory reports
10. Daily care plan

C. Complete these ten statements with the best word or words from the list below:

entry   intake/output   Addressograph   skull sheet
caddy   legal   doctors   neurological record
nurse's notes clinical   aide   chart

1. The patient's record is an official or _____ record.
2. The official patient's record is called his _____ .
3. A notation made on a patient's official record is called an _____ .
4. Many hospitals identify each sheet of the official record by using an _____ similar to a charge plate.
5. Charts are kept in a chart _____ or rack for easy accessibility.
6. Another name for the graphic chart is the _____ record.
7. Instructions of the patient's therapy are written on the _____ order sheet.
8. The nurse records her observations on the _____ .
9. Another name for the "head sheet" is the _____ record.
10. The _____ record summarizes the total amount of fluids taken in and lost from the body.

D. Answer each of the following with a brief phrase or term:

1. What technique was used to keep track of Mr. Dooley as he moved from department to department? _____
2. How must official records be cared for? _____
3. Who, besides the doctor, has responsibility for record keeping in the physician's office? _____
4. What is the patient's hospital record called? _____
5. What other record does the office assistant keep? _____

E. Reread the case history and underline any medical words or forms which have been introduced in this chapter:

patient form   occupational injury form
physical evaluation form   general history
identifying band   front sheet
chart   charted
graphic chart   nurse's notes
progress record   Addressograph
physician's order sheet   chart back
cardex   location board

RECORD STORAGE 331 *

Symbols

$\bar{\bar{aa}}$	equal part of each	$\bar{\bar{ss}}$	one half
$\bar{q}\ 4°$	every 4 hours	℥	ounces
′	feet	+	positive charge
♀	female	$\bar{p}$	p.m. or afternoon
f ℥	fluidram	℈	scruple
f ℥	fluiounce	℞	take
″	inches	$\bar{c}$	with
$\bar{A}$	morning or a.m.	$\bar{s}$	without
−	negative charge		

Glossary

The definition for the words in this Glossary are written in the context of their use in this book.

Medical phrases and jargon have not been pronounced. Jargon as applied in *Foundation of Medical Communication* means "technical or specialized language characteristic of the medical health workers."

The source for the pronounciation of words is the *Encyclopedia and Dictionary of Medicine and Nursing* by Miller and Keane, published by W. B. Saunders Company.

a, an (a, an) without, not, deficient, 59
ab (ab) away from, 59
abate (ah-bat') diminish, 126
abd.—abdomen or abdominal, 87
abdomen (ab-do'men) area of trunk between the thorax and pelvis, 81
abduction (ab-duk'shun) movement of a part away from midline,
A.B.G.—arterial blood gas, 288
abnormalities (ab"nor-mal'ĭ-ties) defects, 12
abortion (ah-bor'shun) pregnancy lost before the end of the third month, 134
abrasion (ah-bra'zhun) a rubbed or scraped area, 153
a.c.—before meals, 88
accelerator nerve (ak-sel'er-a"tor) (nerv) nerve which carries impulses to increase heart rate, 202
accomodate (ah-kom"o-dat) to dilate pupils of the eyes, 309
accreditation—approval, 22
acetone—solvent for cleansing skin before injections, 220
acid intoxication—acidosis or acid state, 259
acidosis (as"ĭ-do'sĭs) an acid state, 220
acoustic (ah-koos'tĭk) pertaining to hearing, 229
acquired—obtained, 106
acromegaly (ak"ro-meg"ah-le) condition due to hypersecretion of STH after maturity, 219

ACTH—adrenocorticotropic hormone, 216
active (ak'tĭ-v) used with case means current; used with immunity means antibodies self-produced, 106
ad (ad) to, toward, increase, 53
addressograph—a printed plate similar to a charge plate used to identify patient records, 320
adduction (ah-duk'shun) movement of a part toward the midline, 183
aden (ad-en) gland, 53
adenoidectomy (ad"ĕ-noĭ-dek'to-me) surgical removal of adenoids, 164
adenoids (ad'ĕ-noids) pharyngeal tonsils which are masses of lymphoid tissues, 164
adenohypophysis (ad"ĕ-no-hi-pof'ĭ-sĭs) anterior or glandular lobe of pituitary gland, 2q2, 213
ADH—antidiuretic hormone, 214, 264
adherent—attached, 166
adipose (ad'ĭ-poz) fatty tissue; a form of connective tissue, 140
adjuvants (ad'joo-vants) assistants, 284, 289
ADL—activites of daily living, 238
ad lib—as desired, 87
adrenal glands (ah-dre'nal) endocrine glands located above the kidneys in the rentroperitenial space, 214
adrenalin (ah-dren'ah-lĭn) hormone produced by adrenal medulla, 216

333 *

adrenocorticotropic hormone (ah-dre"no-kor"ti-ko-trop'ĭk) an anterior pituitary hormone which influences the activity of the adrenal cortex, 216, 217

aeration (a"er-a'shun) exchange of carbon dioxide for oxygen, 292

aerosols (a'er-o-sol'z) fine mists of medicine, 287

afferent (af'er-ent) another name for sensory fibers, 227

afferent vessel (af'er-ent) terminal branch of the renal artery leading into the glomerulus), 106

agglutinins (ah-gloo'tĭ-nĭns) antibodies which cause the antigen to clump together, 106

agranulocytes (a-gran'u-lo-sits") cells without stainable particles in the cytoplasm, 196

airway (ar'wa) passageway for air, 290

albuminuria (al-bu"mĭ-nu're-ah) presence of albumin in the urine, 257, 259

alcoholism (al'ko-hol"izm) habitual and excessive drunkeness, 9

algia (al'je-ah) pain, 61

alignment—position, 187

alimentary tract (al"ĭ-men'tar-e trakt) gastrointestinal tract, 242

alkalosis (al"kah-lo'sĭs) excess alkalinity, 257, 259

alleles (ah-lel's) two genes controlling a given characteristic, 130, 132

allergens (al'er-jens) foreign substances which produce hypersensitivity, 154

allergies (al'er-jes) hypersensitivity, 154

alopecia (al"o-pe'she-ah) loss of hair, 146, 149

alpha and beta cells—masses of endocrine tissue located in the pancreas, also called Islets of Langerhans, 214

alpha particles (al'fa par'tĭ-kls) particulates of radiation, 300

alveolus (al-ve'o-lus) pertaining to the jaw bones; a socket in which a tooth sits; terminal parts of respiratory system, 161, 244

ambient (am'bĭ-ent) atmospheric or room air, 284

ambulatory (am'bu-lah-tor"e) up, walking, or mobile, 116

amenorrhea (a-men"o-re'ah) absence of menses, 271

amino acid (am'ĭ-no) simplest form of proteins, 243

ammonia (ah-mo'ne-ah) a metabolic waste product, 259

amnesic (am-ne'zĭk) no memory of events, 239

amniocentesis (am"ne-sen-te'sĭs) technique for withdrawing a small amount of amniotic fluid for examination, 13

amniotic sac (am"ne-ot'ĭk sak) membrane containing the fetus and its surrounding fluid, 134

amphiarthrotic (am'fe-ar-thrak'tik) slightly moveable joints, 174

amt.—amount, 88

amylase (am'ĭ-las) enzymes which acts upon starches, 249

anabolism (ah-nab'o-lizm) formation of complex substance from simple ones, 243

anal sphincter (a'nal sfingk'ter) circular muscle guarding anal exit, 249

analgesic (an"al-je'sĭks) pain relieving, 126

anaphylactic shock (an"ah-fi-lak'tĭk shok) severe allergic reaction which may be fatal, 293

anastomose (ah-nas"to-mo'sd) communication tube between organs, 209

anatomy (ah-nat'o-me) study of structure, 124

ancillary (ancillary) auxilliary or assisting, 1, 14, 24

anemia (ah-ne'me-ah) too few erythrocytes or too little hemoglobin, 132, 196

anesthesia (an"es-the'ze-ah) technique used to reduce sensations or feelings, 21, 234

anesthesiologist (an"es-the"ze-ol'o-jĭst) physician who administers anesthesia, 20-21

aneurysms (an'u-rĭzm) weakened blood vessels, 271, 280

angina pectoris (an-je'nah pek"to-rĭs) temporary cardiac ischemia, 208

ano (an-o) pertaining to anus, opening of lower bowel, 57

* 334 GLOSSARY

anorexia (an″o-rek′se-ah) lack of appetite, 69, 78

anosmia (an-oz′me-ah) loss of smell, 163

anoxia (an-ok′se-ah) no oxygen, 160

ANS—autonomic nervous system, 228

antagonists (an-tag′o-nĭsts) muscles which oppose the action of other muscles, 184

ante (an′te) before, 53

anteflexion (an″te-flex′shun) pronounced anterior flexion of the uterus, 273

anterior (an-ter′e-or) front or ventral, 81

anterior fontanel (an-ter′er-or fon″tah-nel) unossified area between frontal and parietal bones, 180

anti (an′tĭ) against, 64

antibiotics (an″tĭ-bi-ot″ĭkz) chemical compounds used to control some infectious microbes, 99

antibodies (an′tĭ-bod″es) protective substances which form in response to the presence of an antigen, 105

antidiuretic (an″tĭ-di″u-re-tĭk) hormone which inhibits urine production, 214, 217

antigen (an′tĭ-jen) a substance which engers the production of antibodies, 96, 105

antipyretics (an″tĭ-pi-ret″ĭkz) drugs to reduce fever, 113, 126

antiseptic (an″tĭ-sep′tĭk) anti-infectious agent used on living tissue. 109

antitoxins (an″tĭ-tok′sins) antibodies which neutralize the toxin, 106

anuria (an-nu′re-ah) no urine, 265

anus (a′nus) terminal opening, 246

aorta (a-or′tah) an artery; It is the largest vessel in the body and it arises out of the left ventricle, 200

A-P (anterior-posterior) x-ray beam directed from front to back, 307

A & P—procedure to correct systocele, called anterior colporrhaphy, 277

apex (a′peks) a pointed portion of an organ, 166

aphasia (ah-fa′ze-ah) inability to communicate, 117, 238

aphonia (a-fo′ne-ah) loss of voice, 169

aphrasia (ah-fra′ze-ah) inability to make speech, 117

apnea (ap′ne-ah) respiratory pattern wherein respirations cease, 168

apoplexy (ap′o-plek″se) common name for cerebral vascular accident or stroke, 238

appendages (ah-pen′dĭ-jes) arms and legs; accessory structure, such as nails and glands, 81, 146

appendectomy (ap″en-dek′to-me) removal of the appendix, 126

appendicitis (ah-pen″dĭ-si′tĭs) inflammation of the appendix, 105

appendicular (ap″en-dĭk′u-lar) referring appendages, 175

appendix (ah-pen′dĭks) small finger-like pouch extending out of the cecum, 250

apprehensive (ap″re-hen′sĭv) fearfully anxious, 238

arachnoid mater (ah-rak′noid) cob web mother, the middle layer of the meniges, 130, 140

areola (ah-re′o-la) pigmented area around the nipple, 150

arrhythmias (ah-rign′me-ahs) irregularity in rhythm, 193, 203

arterial blood gas analyzer—machine which determines the level of gases in arterial blood, 288

arteries (ar′ter-ez) blood vessels which carry blood away from the heart, 200, 203

arterio (ar-te″re-o′) relating to a blood vessel, 59

arteriogram (ar-te″re-o-gram″) artery X-ray, 209, 239

arterioles (ar-te′re-ols) small arteries, 203

articular cartilage (ar-tik′-u-lar) hyaline cartilage found at the ends of bones which articulate in synodial joints, 181

articulate (ar-tik′-u-lat) meet, 181

artificial (ar″ti-fish′al) when used with immunity, means coming in contact with the antigen or antibody through an artificial means such as injection, 106

arth (ar'th) joint, 57, 184
arthralgia (ar-thral'je-ah) pain in a joint, 184
arthrectomy (ar-threk'to-me) excision of a joint, 184
arthritis (ar-thri'tis) inflammation of a joint, 184
arthrocele (ar'thro-sel) joint swelling, 184
arthrochalasis (ar"thro-kal'ah-sĭs) abnormal relaxation of a joint, 174, 184
arthroclasia (ar"thro-kla'ze-ah) joint manipulation, 184
arthrodesis (ar"thro-de'sis) surgical fusion of a joint, 184
arthrodynia (ar"thro-din'e-ah) pain in a joint, 184
arthroempyesis (ar"thro-em"pi-e'sis) suppuration in a joint, 184
arthrogram (ar-thro'-gram) film obtained in arthrography, 309
arthrography (ar-throg'rah-fe) a joint radiogram after instillation of contrast media, 309
arthrophyte (ar'thro-fit) abnormal growth in a joint cavity, 184
arthrotomy (ar-throt'o-me) incision of a joint, 184
ascending sensory tract—bundles of axon carrying afferent messages to higher centers, 232
asepsis (asep'sis) without infection, 96
A.S.H.D.—arteriosclerotic heart disease, 75
asis (ah-sis) state, condition, 56
asphyxia (as-fik'se-ah) death due to cessation of ventilation, 284, 297
aspirating (as"pi-ra-tĭng) withdrawing fluid, 294
assimilated (ah-sĭm-ĕ-la-ted) absorbed into the body, 242
asthma (as'mah) allergic condition associated with breathing, 155
atelectasis (at"i-lak'tah-sĭs) collapse of all or part of a lung, 160, 169, 170, 293
atomizer (at'om-iz"er) mechanism for converting medication into a fine spray, 290
atoms (at'oms) tiny particles of which elements are composed, 301

atresia (ah-tre'ze-ah) congenital absence of a body opening, 125
atresia (ah-tre'ze-ah) lack of development, 113, 125, 262
at risk—more apt to develop an abnormal condition, 12
atrophy (at'ro-fe) decrease in size and function, 125
atrophy (at'ro-fe) wasting, 190
atrium (a'tre-um) upper heart chamber, 198
atrioventricular valves (a"tre-o-ven-trik'u-lar) refers to tricuspid valves, 200
atrioventricular mass or node (a"tre-o-van-trik' u-lar mass) special node tissue found in right atrium close to interventricular septum, part of conduction system, 201
attending physician—doctor in charge of a particular case, 19
audio (aw-de-o) hearing, 64
auditory meatus (aw'dĭ-to"re me-a'tus) external ear canal, 148
auscultate (aw'skul-tat) examination by listening, 69, 78
autoclave (aw'to-klav) a machine used for sterialization by steam, 108
autonomic (aw"to-nom'ĭk) involuntary nervous system composed of visceral, efferent fibers, 228
autotrophs (aw'to-trof) organisms that live on inorganic matter, 100
A.V. node—atrioventricular node, 201
axial (ak'si-al) pertaining to skeleton; includes cranium, vertebrae, ribs, and sternum, 175
axilla (ak-sĭl'ah) armpit area, 307
axillary (ak'sĭ'ler"e) pertaining to the arm pit, 151, 206, 307
axon (ak'son) extension of neuron which conducts the nerve impulse away from the cell body, 225

bacillus (bah-sĭl'us) rod shaped bacterium, 99
bactericidal (bak-tēr"ĭ-si'dal) lethal for bacteria, 104

bacteriology (bak-te′re-ol′o-je) study of bacteria, 30
barium swallow—gastrointestinal series, 28
Bartholins glands (bar′to-lins) two small glands found on either side of the sublingual orifice, 276
basal matabolic rate—rate at which oxygen is consumed, 219
base—alkaline, 166, 258
basic four—refers to different food groups from which a balanced diet is made, 243
benign (be-nin′) not malignant, 124
beta particles (ba′tah) particles of radiation, 300
bi, bin (bi) prefix meaning two, 53
biceps brachii (bī′seps bra′ke-ī) muscle of anterior upper arm, 185
bicuspid (bikus′pĭd) pertaining to the two-flapped valve between left atrium and ventricle, 199
bifurcates (bi-fur′kāt) divides into two, 165
B.I.D.—twice a day, 88
bile (bil) hapatic secretion from mulsified fats, 249
biliary apparatus (bil′e-a′′re ap′′ah-ra′tus) refers to the system of ducts which convey bile, 251
biopsy (bi′op-se) examination of living tissue from the body, 84
blast (blast) suffix meaning bud, sprout, 52

blood gas barrier—thin tissue between the alveolus and blood, 161
blood pressure—pressure of blood exerted against the vascular walls, 203
BMR—basal matabolic rate, 219
bolus (bo′lus) soft mass which is ready to be swallowed, 246
botulism (bot′u-lizm) a serious form of food poisoning, 100
bowel (bow-el) intestine, 253
Bowman's capsule (Bomanz kap′sul) tubule surrounding the golmerulus part of the nephron, 263

B/P or B.P.—blood pressure, 75
bpm—beats per minute, 202
brachial (bra′ke-al) pertaining to or near upper arm, 206
brachium (bra′ke-um) the arm, 83
bradycardia (brad′′e-kar′de-ah) slow heart rate, 203
brain (bran) complex mass of nervous tissue found in the cranial cavity, 232
brain scan (bran skan) a technique for recording radioactive deposits in the brain, 312
breech (brēch) presentation of buttocks or feet at delivery, 137
bronchiectasis (brong′′ke-ĕk′tah-sĭs) abnormal permanent dialation of branchii, 293
bronchogram (brong′ko-gram) an x-ray of the bronchii, 309
bronchoscopy (brong′kos-ko-pe) a visual examination of the bronchii, 295
bronzing—a yellowish browning of the skin, 154
buccal cavity (buk′al kav-e-te) mouth, 242
Bulbourethral glands (Bul′bo-u-re′thral) cowpers glands, 279
bundle of His (bun′dl) interventricularbundle of special neuromuscular fibers; part of conduction system, 201
bypass—a surgical procedure which alters a normal route, 209

C.—centigrade scale, 150
Ca—calcium, 217
Ca^{++} (kal′se-um) calcium ion, 258
calcemia (kal-se′me-ah) excessive calcium ions in the blood, 260
calcium (kal′se-um) an element, 217
calciuria (kal′′se-u′re-ah) excessive calcium in urine, 260
calibrations (kal′′ĭ-bra′shuns) gradations, 150
calices (kal′ĭ-ses) cup like structure such as found in the kidney to collect urine, 263
calculi (kal-ku-li) stones or concretions, 261
cancellous (kan-sel′us) spongy bone, 178

cap.—capsule, 88
capillaries (kap′ĭ-ler″ez) semipermeable membranes for the interchange of substances between blood and body tissue, 203
capsules (kap′sūls) extra covering found on some microbes, 102, 203
carbohydrates (kar″bo-hi′drātes) sugars, 125
carbon monoxide (kar-bon mon-ok′sid) a gas which forms a permanent bond with hemoglobin, 293
cardi (kar′de) prefix meaning heart, 59, 207
cardiac arrest (kar′de-ak ah-rest′) heart stoppage, 44, 207
cardiac cateterization (kar′de-ak kath″e-ter-ĭ-za′shun) passage of a small tube through a vein into the heart, 209
cardiac cycle (kar′de-ak si-kl) the alternate rhythmic contraction and relaxation of the atrium and ventricles, 201
cardiac sphincter (kar′de-ak sfingk′ter) cureular muscle which surrounds the esphogus at its lower end, 246
cardialgia (kar″de-al′je-ah) heart pain, 207
cardiodynia (car″de-o-din′e-ah) pain the the heart region, 207
cardiogenic (kar″de-o-jen′ĭk) pertaining to the heart, 207
cardiograph (kar′de-o-graf″) instrument for recording heart movements, 207
cardiologist (kar″de-ol′o-jĭst) physician who treats heart conditions, 20, 207
cardiomegaly (kar″de-o-meg′ah-le) hypertrophy of the heart, 193, 207
cardiopathy (kar″de-o-pah-the) morbid heart condition, 207
cardiorrhexis (kar″de-o-tok′sĭs) rupture of the heart, 207
cardiotoxic (kar″de-o-tok′sĭk) poisonous to the heart, 207
cardiovascular system (kar″de-o-vas′ku-lar sĭs′těm) system of heart, blood vessels, and blood, 193
caries (ka′re-ēz) cavities, 246
carpal (kar′pal) pertaining to the wrist, 177

cartilage (kar′tĭ-lĭj) flexible connective tissue, 162
cartilaginous formation (kar″tĭ-laj′ĭ-nus fōr-ma′shun) method of bone formation, 179
case history file—physician's permanent official office record of each patient, 320
cassette (kah-set) a light-proof film holder, 306
cast (kast) rigid covering, 188
casts (kastz) sediments in the urine, 259
catabolism (kah-tab′o-lĭzm) process by which complex processes are converted to simple ones, 243
catheter (kath′ĕ-ter) tube, 266
cauda equina (kaw′da e-kwĭn′ah) mass of spinal nerves found in the vertebral canal extending below the cord, 232
CBC—complete blood count, 75
c.c.—cubic centimeter, 90
C.C.—current complaint, 76, 77
cecum (se′kum) beginning section of the colon, 250
cele (sēl) hernia, 51, 55
cell membrane (sel mem′brān) cell wall, 130
cellular respiration (sel′u-lar res″pĭ-ra′shun) process by which nutrients and oxygen are combined to form energy, water, and carbon dioxide, 160
centers—same as nuclei centers, masses of grey matter located in brain responsible for contributing a specific body function, 233
centesĭs (sen-te′sis) prefix meaning puncture, perforate, 64
centi (sen′tĭ) prefix meaning 1/100 of a unit of measurement, 69, 90
centĭgrāde scale (sen′ti-grad) scale for temperature measurement, 150
central neurons (sen′tral nu′ron) pertaining to neurons, are of internucial neurons which are found in the central nervous system, 227
central canal—small hole extending the length of the cord in the center of grey matter, 232
central nervous system (sen′tral ner′vs sĭs-tem) the brain and spinal cord, 227

central venous pressure—pressure exerted by the blood in the major veins, 203
cephal (sef'ah-l) prefix meaning head, 51, 61
cephalic presentation (sĕ-fal'ĭk prez"en-ta'shun) head first presentation at delivery, 137
cephalo-pelvis (sef"ah-lo pel'vĭk) head-pelvis relationship, 137
cerebrospinal bluid (ser"ē-bro-spi'nal floo'ĭd) thin watery fluid located in subarachnoid space, 140
cerebellum (ser"ĕ-bĕl-um) second largest portion of the brain, 233
cerebral palsy (ser'ĕ-bral pawl'ze) a group of disorders due to damage of cerebral motor areas, 236
cerebrum (ser'ĕ-brum) main portion of the brain, 224, 234
cerumen (se-roo'men) waxy substance secreted by ceruminous glands, 148
ceruminous glands (see-roo'men-us) secrete cerumen or waxy material, 148
cervical (ser'vĭ-kal) pertaining to the neck, 82
cervix (ser'vĭks) portion of uterus which protrudes into the vagina, 273
cesarean section (sĕ-sa're-an) hysterotomy to deliver the baby, 130, 137
chancre (shang'ker) primary lesion of first stage of syphilis, 271
chemotherapy (ke"mo-ther"ah-pe) treatment of disease by chemical agents, 102
chest physical therapy—techniques used to loosen pumonary secretions, 287
cheynes stokes (chān stoks) respiratory pattern of periodic deep shythmatic respirations following by shallow respirations or apnea, 168
C.H.F.—congestive heart failure, 75
chlorine (klo'ren) an element, 258
choana (ko-a'nah) nasal cavity, 160, 162
chole (ko'le) prefix meaning bile, 55, 252
cholecystectomy (ko"le-sĭs-tek'to-me) excision of the gall bladder, 127, 252
cholecystitis (ko"le-sĭs-ti'tis) inflammation of the gall bladder, 252
cholecystogram (ko"le-sĭs'to-gram) X-ray record of gall bladder function, 242, 252
cholecystography (ko"le-sis-tog'rah-fe) a diagnostic technique employing X-ray films, 252, 253, 309
choledochal (kol'e-kok"al) pertaining to the common bile duct, 252
choledochitis (kol"e-do-ki'tĭs) inflammation of the common bile ducts, 252
choledocho (ko-led'o-ko) prefix for common bile duct, 252
choledochoduodenostomy (ko-led"ŏ-do-du"o-dĕ-nos'to-me) anastomosis of the common bile duct to the duodenum, 252
choledocholithiasis (ko-led"o-ko-lĭ-thi'ah-sĭs) gall stones in common bile duct, 242, 253
choledocholithotomy (ko-led"opko-li-thot'o-me) incision of the common bile duct to remove stones, 252
choledocholithotripsy (ko-led"o-ki-lith'o-trip"se) crushing of a gall stone in the common duct, 254
choledochotomy (ko"led-o-kot'o-me) incision of the common duct, 252
cholelithiasis (ko"le-lĭ-thi'ah-sĭs) the presence of gallstones, 253
cholemesis (ko-lem'e-sĭs) vomiting of bile, 252
cholepathia (ko"le-path'e-ah) disease of the gall bladder, 252
cholerrhagia (ko"le-ra'je-ah) excessive bile flow, 252
chondr (kon"dr) prefix meaning cartilage, 52
chondrocytes (kon'dro-sits) cartilage cells, 179
chronic (korn'ĭk) long, continued illness, 105
chronic bronchitis (kron'ĭk brong-ki'tĭs) long term inflammation of bronchii, 169, 170
chyme (kim) liquid into which bolus of food is converted, 246, 250
cilia (sil'e-ah) hair-like projections that permit mobility in some microbes, 102, 104
Circle of Willis (ser'kl of wĭl-lĭs) system of vessels which supply, and are located at the base of, the brain, 205
circumcision (ser"kum-sĭzh'un) surgical removal of excess foreskin, 278

Cl (klo′rēn) chlorine, 258

clavicle (klav′ĭ-kl) collar bone, 166, 175

clear liquid diet—diet which supplies chiefly water and carbohydrates, 244

climacteric (kli-mak′ter-ĭk) menopause, 275

clinical sheet (klin′ĭ-kl) records information in an abbreviated form and graphs the vital signs, 315

clitoris (klit′o-rĭs) small cylindrical mass of erotic tissue, part of the external female reproductive organs, 277

chlorine (klo′ren) an element, 258

closed reduction—realignment of a fracture by manipulation, 188

clostridium tetani (klo-strid′e-um tet″ah-nĭ) microbe which causes the disease tetanus, 102

CNS—central nervous system, 227

c/o—complaining of, 77

C.O.—coronary occulsion, 75

coccus (kok′us) round bacterium, 99

code blue—special signal to alert personnel of a cardiac arrest, 44

code gray—signal that a security officer is needed, 44

code red—same as Doctor red, 44

code 66—same as code blue, 44

code 99—same as code blue, 44

coli(ko′li) prefix meaning colon, 250

colic (kol′ĭk) pertaining to the colon, 250

colitus (ko-li′tĭs) inflammation of the colon, 250

collecting tubules (ko-lect′ing tu′tulz) microscopic tubules draining urine through renal medulla, 263

colo (ko′lo) prefix meaning colon, 250

colocentesis (ko″lo-sen-te′sĭs) surgical puncture of the colon, 250

coloclysis (ko-lok′lĭ-sĭs) irrigation of the colon, 250

colon (ko-lon) large intestine, 250

colonitis (ko″lon-i′tĭs) inflammation of the colon, 250

colono (kol″o-no) prefix meaning colon, 250

colonopathy (ko″lon-op′ah-the) disease of the colon, 242, 250

colony (kol′o-ne) mass of microbes developed from one single organism, 103

colp or colpo (kolp) (kol′po) prefix meaning pertaining to vagina, 276

colpectomy (kol-pek′to-me) removal of vagina, 276

colporrhaphy (kol-por′ah-fe) repair of vaginal wall, 271, 276

columnar (ko′um-nar) pertaining to the mucous-producing epithelial cells which are column shaped, 163

CO_2—abbreviation for carbon dioxide, 288

comatose (ko′mah-tos) in coma, 238

commensalism (kŏ-men′sal-ĭzm) symbolic relationship wherein one organism derives benefit from the other but causes no harm, 96, 100

comminuted fracture (kom″i-nu-ted) the bone is broken or crushed into small pieces, 187

common bile duct—tube formed from cystic and hapatic duct carrying bile into small intestine, 249

communicable (kŏ-mu′nĭ-kah-bl) easily passed from person to person, 98

compact bone—hard bone, 178

compacted fracture—bone fragments firmly driven into each other, 187

complemental volume (kom′plĕ-men-tal) a- of air that can be drawn into lungs above tidal volume, 167

compliance (kom-pli′ans) elasticity, 276, 284, 285

compounds (kom′pownds) chemical combinations, 161

compression fracture (kom-pre-shun) bone fragments are pressed together, 187

concentrated urine (kon″sen-tra′ted) containing less water, 260

concretions (kon-kre′shuns) stones, 251

condyle (kon′dil) a rounded projection on a bone, 178

congenital (kon-jen′ĭ-tal) present at birth, 125

conjunctiva (kon″junk-ti′vah) delicate membrane which covers the eyes and lines the lids, 104
conjunctivitis (kon-junk″tĭ-vi′tĭs) inflammation of conjunctiva, 146
connecting (kon-nek′tĭng) central neuron, 227
connective tissue (kō-nek′tiv tĭ-sh′u) a group of tissues which connect other tissues of the body, 140
constipation (kon″stĭ-pa′shun) difficulty defecating, 254
constitutional (kon″stĭ-tu-shun-al) systemic or general body, 153
contamination (kon′tam′″ĭ-na′shun) soiling by contact with microbes, 96
continuum (kon′tin-u-um) continuous from, 14,
contract—to shorten, 149
contractures (kon-trak′tūrs) abnormal shortenings, 146, 157
contrast media—radiopaque materials used in radioscopy, 304
contusion (kon-too′zhun) bruise, 153
convalescent (kon″vah-les′ent) a person recovering, 7
convalescent hospital—another name for nursing homes, 10
convoluted tubules (kon″vol′ted) part of the nephron, 263
convolutions (kon″vol-lu′shuns) folds of cerebral cortex. 234
convulsions (kun-vul′shuns) involuntary muscle spasms, 236
C.O.P.D.—chronic obstructive pulmonary disease, 170, 171
copious (ko′pi-us) excessive amounts, 160, 171
copulation (kop″u-la′shun) sexual intercourse, 276
corium (ko′re-um) true skin or dermies, 147
coronal (kor′o-nal) imaginary line which divides the body into anterior and posterior parts, 81
coronal (ko-ro′nal) line of union between frontal and parateal bones, 178

coronary circulation (kor′o-na″re ser-ku-la′shun) vessels carrying blood to the heart, 205
coronary sinus (kor′o-na″re si′nus) vein which returns blood from myocardium to right atrium, 205
cor pulmonale (kor pul-mon-al-ĭ) heart disease developed secondarily to pulmonary disease, 286
corpus luteum (kor′pus loo′te-em) yellow body of tissue which forms after ovulation from the Graafian follicle, 275
cortex (kor′teks) outer portion of organ or structure, 216
corticotropin releasing factor (kor″ti-ko-tro′pin) hormone produced by the hypothalamus which stimulates release from the anterior pituitary, 216
cortisone (kor′ti-zone) hormone produced by adrenal cortex, 216
coryza (kor-ri′zah) a nasal discharge, 153
cost (cos″t) previs meaning rib, 52
Cowpers glands (kow-pĕrz) secrete part of the seminal fluid, 279
CPPB—Continuous Positive Pressure Breathing, 294
crani (kra′ne) skull, 61
cranial (kra′ne-al) pertaining to the head, 81
cranial nerves (kra′ne-al) pertaining to cranial nerves which are attached to the brain, 229
craniocaudad (kra′ne-o-kaw′dad) from head to tail, 300, 307
cranium (kra′ne-um) skull, 175
creatinine (kre-at′ĭ-nin) a metabolic caste product, 259
crest—bone marking meaning prominent ridge or border, 178
CRF—corticotropin releasing factor, 216
crust (krust) scab, 153
cryptorchidism (krip-tor′ki-dĭsm) undescended testes, 279
C.S.—central supply or central service, 73
culture (kul-tūr) growth of microorganisms; sample of infectious materials, 102

GLOSSARY 341 *

cupping (kup-ing) a technique of chest tapping to loosen secretions, 292
cutaneous (ku-ta'ne-us) pertaining to the skin, 152
C.V.A.—cerebrovascular accident, 75
C.V.P.—central venous pressure, 203
cyanosis (si"ah-no'sis) a bluish discoloration of the skin, 154
cyclopropane (si"klo-pro'pan) a medical gas, 289
cyst (sist) prefix meaning bladder, 55
cystic duct (sis'tik) passage way for bile out of gall bladder, 249
cystitis (sis-ti'tis) inflammation of urinary bladder, 266
cystocele (sis'to-sel) weakening of the anterior vaginal wall, 277
cystoscopy (sis-tos'ko-pe) procedure for looking into the bladder, 126, 261, 267
cyte (sit) suffix meaning cell, 51, 52
cytology (si-tol'o-je) study of cells, 30, 130
cytolysins (si-tol'i-sins) antibodies which dissolve the antigen cells, 106
cytoplasm (si'to-plazm) cell material outside the nucleus, 130

dc.—decimeter, 90
d.C.—discontinue, 88
D.C.U.—definitive care unit, an intermediate care service for patients, 73
deci (des'i) prefix meaning 1/10 of a unit of measurement, 69, 90
deciduous (de-sid'u-us) baby teeth, 245
decubitus (de-cu'bi-tus) an ulceration due to pressure, 153
defecated (def"e-cate-ed) eliminated, 250
deglutition (deg"loo-tish'un) swallowing, 229, 246
dehydrate (de"hi-dra'te) excessive water loss, 260
delivery room (de-liv'er-e) area of the hospital where babies are born, 27
dentes (den-tez) teeth, 244

denti (den-ti) prefix meaning tooth, 55
dentitions (den-tish'uns) sets of teeth, 245
dentures (den-turs) artificial teeth, 246
deoxygenated (de-ok"si-jen-na'ted) oxygen loss, 199
depilation (dep'i-la-shun) hair loss, 310
derma (der'mah) prefix meaning skin, 55
dermatitides (der"mah-tit'i-dez) inflammatory conditions of the skin considered collectively, 155
dermatitis (der"mah-ti'tis) skin inflammation, 105, 155
dermatologist (der"mah-tol'o-jist) physician who treats skin conditions, 20
dermatology (der"mah-tol'o-je) study of the skin, 146
dermis (der'mis) corium or true skin, 147
dermotropic (der"mo-trop'ik) affecting the skin, 98
descending motor tract—bundles of axons carrying efferent messages from higher centers, 232
desquamation (des"kwah-ma'shun) tissue shedding, 310
diabetes insipidus (di"ah-be'tez in-sip'i-dus) condition due to hyposecretion of ADH, 219
diabetic coma (di"ah-bet'ik koma) a state of acidosis due to diabetes mellitus, 220
dialysis (di-al'i-sis) movement through a semipermeable membrane, 194, 264
diaphragm (di'ah-fram) dome shaped cavity which separates the thoracic and abdominal cavity, 130, 139
diaphysis (di-af'i-sis) shaft of bone, 180
diarrhea (di"ah-re'ah) watery stool, 315, 323
diarthrotic (di"ar-thrak'tik) freely moveable joints, 181
diastole (di-as'to-le) period of dilation of the heart, especially of the ventricles, 202
diastolic (di"as'to-lik) pertaining to diastole, 203
diencephalon (di"en-sef'ah-lon) portion of brain composed of thalamus and hypothalamus, 233

diffusion (di-fu'zhun) movement of a gas across a membrane due to a greater concentration of blood on one side, 161

diplo (dip"lo) prefix meaning double or twofold, 101

diplococus pneumonia (dip"lo-kok'us nu"mo-ne-ah) bacterium which causes pneumonia and other infections, 103

diploe (dip'lo-e) cancellus bone of the skill, 179

diplopia (di-plo'pe-ah) double vision, 224

disaccharide (di-sak'ah-ride) double sugar, 243

disarticulated (dis-ar-tik'u-la"ted) separated, 175

discogenic disease (dis"ko-jen'ik) intervertebral disc involvement, 315, 329

discrete (dis-kret) clear cut, 304

disoriented (dis-o"re-en-ted) unable to recognize time, place, or person, 122

dissociate (dis-so"se-at) come apart, 257

distal (dis'tal) furthest away from point of attachment, 81

distention (dis-ten'shun) stretching,

diuresis (di"u-re'sis) increased secretion of urine,

dl.—deciliter, 90

dm.—decimeter, 90

DOA—dead on arrival, 209

Doctor Red—signal that there is a fire, 44

dominant (dom-i-nant) when used with genes means only one gene needed for expression, 133

dorsal (dor'sal) posterior or back, 81

dorsum (dor'sum) back, 81

dosimeter (do-sime'ter) an instrument to record radiation exposure, 306

ductless (dukt-les) without ducts, referring to glands of internal secretion, 148

ducts (dukts) tubes, 147

ductus deferens (duk' def'er-enz) vas deferens, 279

duodenum (du"o-de'num) first 10 inches of intestinal tract, 248

dura mater (du'rah ma'ter) tough mother, outer layer of meninges, 140

D/W—dextrose and water, 87

dwarfism (dwar'fizm) a condition of childhood due to hyposecretion of STH, 218

Dx.—diagnosis, 77

dys (dis) prefix meaning painful, abnormal, 53

dysarthria (dis-ar'thre-ah) slurred speech, 237

dysarthrosis (dis-ar-thro'sis) deformity of a joint, 113, 126

dyscrasias (dis-kra'ze-ahs) abnormalities, 196

dysmenorrhea (dis"men-o-re'ah) painful menstruation, 124

dyspareunia (dis"pah-ru'ne-ah) painful copulation, 276

dyspepsia (dis-pep'se-ah) indigestion, 242, 253

dysphagia (dis-fa'je-ah) difficulty swallowing, 284, 295

dysphonia (dis-fo'ne-ah) difficulty speaking, 160, 165

dyspnea (disp-ne'ah) respiratory pattern of difficult, painful respirations, 168

dystocia (dis-to'se-ah) difficult birth, 137

ecchymosis (ek"i-mo'sis) a flattened, black and blue spot due to bleeding into tissues, 146, 153

E.C.D.—exploration of the common duct,

ECG—electrocardiogram, 71

ectomy (ek'tom-me) suffix meaning excision, removal, 56

ectopic (ek-top'ik) pregnancy outside the uterus, 137

eczema (ek'ze-mah) a skin rash that itches, oozes, blisters and scales, 155

edema (e-de'mah) excess fluid in interstitial space, 194

edematous (e-dem'a-tus) swollen, 163

EEG—electroencephalogram, 71

effector (e-fek'tor) muscle or gland that responds to nervous stimulation, 227

efferent (ef'er-ent) neuron transmitting messages from the central nervous to an effector, 227

GLOSSARY 343 *

efferent blood vessel—drains blood from the glomerulus, 263

efferent or tubular capillary bed—a system of capillaries which surround tube system of the nephron, 263

ejaculation (e-jak″u-la′shun) passage of semen through the tube system during intercourse, 279

ejaculatory duct (e-jak″u-la-tori̅) formed from seminal vessels and vas deferans and carries sperm, 279

elastic connective tissue—stretchable connective tissue, 140

electrolytes (e-lek′tro-lites) salts, 157

electromagnetic radiations—pure energy with no mass or substance, 310

electrons (e-lek′trons) negatively charged atomic particles found outside the nucleus, 301

electroscope (e-lek′tro-skop) exposure meter that records level of radiation, 306

element (el′e-ment) a primary chemical substance, 301

emaciated (e-ma′se-a-ted) appearing wasted, 257, 266

embolus (em′bo-lus) moving clot, 205

embryo (em′bre-o) term applied to the baby during the first trimester, 134

emesis (em′ĕ-sis) vomiting, 57

emet (e-met′) prefix meaning vomiting, 57

EMG—electromyogram, 75

empyema (em″pi-e′mah) pyothorax, 169, 170

emphysema (em″fi-se′mah) pathologic accumulation of air in tissues, 160, 169, 170, 171

E.M.T.—Emergency Medical Technician, 72

encephal (en-sef′ahl) prefix meaning brain, 61

encephalalgia (en″sef-ah-lal′je-ah) pain in the head, 235

encephalatrophy (en″sef-ah-lat′ro-fe) atrophy of brain tissue, 235

encephalitis (en″sef-ah-li′tis) inflammation of the brain, 235

encephaloecele (en-sef″ah-lo-se̅l) protrusion of brain through an opening in the skull, 235

encephalogram (en-sef′ah-lo-gram″) x-ray picture of the brain, 235

encephaloid (en-sef′ah-loid) resembling brain tissue, 235

encephaloma (en-sef″ah-lo′mah) a brain tumor, 235

encephalopyosis (en-sef″ah-lo-pi-o′sĭs) brain abscess, 235

encephalorrhagia (en-sef″ah-lo-ra′je-ah) brain hemorrhage, 235

encephalosclerosis (en-sef″ah-lo-sklĕ-ro′sĭs) hardening of the brain tissue, 224, 235

endemic (ĕn-dĕm′ik) small number of cases always present in the community, 99

endo (ĕn′do) prefix meaning within, 59

endocrine (ĕn′do-krĭn) internally secreting gland, 148

endocrine glands (ĕn′do-krĭn) glands of internal secretion, also called ductless glands, 148, 212

endocrinologist (ĕn″do-kri-nol′o-jist) physician who treats endocrine conditions, 20

endometrium (ĕn″do-me′tre-um) vascular lining of uterus, 273

endosteum (ĕn-dos′te-um) bone lining, 180

endothelium (ĕn″do-the′le-um) smooth epithelial cells which line heart and blood vessels, 198

endotracheal (ĕn″do-tr′ke-al) within the trachea, 289

enema (ĕn′ĕ-mah) introduction of fluid into the rectum, 253

enterectomy (ĕn″tĕr-ĕk′to-me) excision of a portion of the intestine, 249

enteritis (ĕn″tĕ-ri′tis) inflammation of intestines, 249

entero (ĕn′tĕr-o) prefix meaning intestine, 57, 249

enterocentesis (ĕn″tĕr-osĕn-te′sĭs) puncture of intestines to withdraw gas or a fluid, 246, 249

enterocinesia (ĕn″tĕr-osi-ne″se-ah) peristalsis, 242

enterodynia (ĕn″ter-odin′e-ah) pain in the intestines, 249

enterogenous (ĕn″tĕr-o-j-ĕ-nus) arising within the intestines, 249

* 344 GLOSSARY

enterotropic (ĕn″tĕr-otrop′ĭk) affecting the intestinal tract, 98

enzymes (ĕn″zĭms) chemicals which initiate or alter a chemical reaction, 103

eosinophils (e″o-sĭn′o-fĭls) leukocytes which take an eosin stain, 197

epi (ĕp′ĭ) prefix meaning above, upon, 52

epidermis (ĕp″ĭ-der′mĭs) outer layer of skin which is constantly being shed, 147

epididymides (ep″ĭ-dĭd′ĭ-mĭ-dĕs) the two 20 feet tubules which are coiled on top of the testes, 279, 280

epididymitis (ep″ĭ-dĭd″ĭ-mĭ′tĭs) inflammation of the epididymis, 271, 280

epilepsy (ĕpĭ-lep″se) a noninfectious disorder due to a cerebral lesion, 236

epiphyseal cartilage (epĭ-fĭz′ahl kar′tĭ-lĭj) area between diaphysis and epiphysis of children, the point at which growth in length of bone takes place, 180

epiphysis (ĕ-pĭf′ĭ-sĭs) end of bone, 174, 180

epistaxis (ĕp″ĭ-stak′sĭs) nose bleed, 163

epithelial (ĕp″ĭ-the″le-al) term applied to tissues characterized by cells packed together, 139

equilibrium (e″kwĭ-lĭb′re-um) sense of balance, 229

E.R.—emergency room, 73

erythema (er″ĭ-thema) redness of the skin, 146, 153, 155

erythro (ĕ-rĭth′ro) prefix meaning red, 52

erythropoietin (e-rĭth″ro-poĭ′tĭn) hormone believed to be produced by the renal cells, 265

Escherichia coli (ĕsh″ĕ-rĭk′e-ah ko″lĭ) a bacterium normally found in the intestinal tract, 96, 101

esophagus (ĕ-sof′ah-gus) a muscular cylinder extending from pharynx to stomach, 246

estrogen (ĕs′tro-jen) hormone produced by ovaries, 215

etiology (e″te-ol′o-je) cause, 22, 124

ethmoid (ĕth′moĭd) bone which helps form the internal skull, 163

ethmoidal (ĕth-moĭ′dăl) pertaining to the ethmoid, 163

eupnea (ūpne′ah) respiration of normal rate and rhythm, 168

eustachian (ū-sta′ke-an) refers to tubes which lead from nasal pharynx to middle ear, 164

ex (ĕks) prefix meaning out, 62

exacerbation (ĕg-zas″er-ba′shun) period of increased severity of symptoms, 113, 126

exanthema (ĕg″zan-the′mah) rash, 153

excoriation (ĕk″sho-re-a′shun) superficial loss of substance such as that produced by scratching, 146, 153

exocrine gland (ĕk′so-krĭn) gland which secretes externally; also called ducted gland, 148

exophalmic (ĕk″sof-thal′mĭk) eyes protruding out, 219

exopthalmic goiter (ek″sof-thal′mĭk goĭ′ter) condition due to hypersecretion of thyroxin, 219

expectorant (ĕk-spĕk′to-rant) medication to aid expectoration, 296

expectorated (ĕk-spĕk″to-ra-tĕd) expelled from airway, 291

expectoration (ĕk-spĕk′to-ra′shun) ejection of mucus from the lung, 171

expiration (ĕk″spĭ-ra′shun) exhalation,

extension—movement by which the two ends of any jointed part are drawn away from each other, 183

extensors (ek-sten′sors) muscles which bring about extension of a joint, 185

external respiration (ĕks″ter-năl rĕs″pĭ-ra′shun) changes of gases between alveolus and blood,

extracorporeal (ĕk″strah-kor-po′rĕ-al) outside the body, 193, 202

extremities (ĕk-strĕm′ĭ-tes) arms and legs, 175

extrinsic (ĕxtrĭn sĭk′) of external origin, 198

exudate (ĕks′u-dāt) fluid which accumulates as the result of inflammation, 105

F.—Fahrenheit scale for measuring temperature, 150

facet (fas′ĕt) small flat surface, 178

Fahrenheit scale (far'ĕn-hīt sk-āl) a temperature measurement scale, 150

Fallopian tube (făh-lo'pe-an tub) oviduct, 134, 273

fascia (făsh'e-ăh) connective tissues which hold internal structure together, 149

fasting blood sugar—test of glucose level after fasting, 221

Father O'Malley—same as code grey, 44

fat—essential nutrient, 243

fatty acids—break down of fat digestion, 243

FBS—fasting blood sugar, 221

Fe—symbol for iron, 301

feces (fe'sez) semi-solid waste eliminated from the body, 250

femoral (fem'o-ral) pertaining to the femur (e.g., artery, vein or nerve), 205

femur (fe'mur) thigh bone, 177

fertilization (fer"ti-li-za'shun) union of male and female gametes, 133

fertilized ovum (fer"ti-līz-d o'vum) original cell formed from union of sperm and ovum, 133

fetal (fe'tal) applies to the baby before birth, 12

fetus (fe'tus) name given to baby during second or third trimester, 135

F.F.—Force fluids, 87

F.H.—Family history, 77

fibrin (fi'brin) an insoluble protein formed by interaction of fibrinogen and thrombin, 196

fibrinogen (fi-brin'o-jen) a blood protein, part of the blood clotting mechanism, 196

fibrous connective tissue (fi'brus) firm connective tissue, 140

film badge—dosimeter, 306

filtrate (fil'trat) fluid which passes from the blood stream into Bowman's capsule and the convoluted tubules, 263

filtration (fil-tra'shun) movement of materials across a membrane due to weight column of fluid, 194

first degree burns—minimal burn damage to the epidermis, 155

fissure (fish'er) a narrow slit or cleft, 153

fissures (fish'ers) pertaining to cerebrum; deep grooves which divide cerebrum into lobes, 234

flaccid (flak'sid) soft, flabby muscle; lacking tone, 185, 224

flagella (flah-jel'a) whiplike appendages that permit mobility in some microbes, 102

flatulence (flat'u-lens) excessive gas, 253

flatus (fla'tus) excessive gas, 247

flexion (flek'shun) act of bending, or condition of being bent, 183

flexors (flek'sors) muscles which bring about flexion of a joint, 185

flow meter—an instrument for controlling the gas flow, 289

flourescence (floo"o-res'ens) shining with light from an outside source, 309

fluoroscopy (floo"or-os'ko-pe) special X-ray technique which examines the deep parts of the body, 300, 309

focus (fo'kus) center of infection, 164

follicular stimulating hormone (fol-ĭk-u-lar stim'u-lating hor'mon) pituitary hormone which stimulates maturation; an ovarian follicle, 213, 217

fomites (fo'mī-tezs) contaminated inanimate objects, 96, 108

fontanels (fon"tah-nel'z) areas of unossified skull of newborn baby, 180

foramen (fo-ra'men) bone marking, meaning large opening, 178

foramen ovale (fo-ra'men o-vale) opening in interatrial septum of fetal heart valves, 199

foreskin (for'skin) Prepuce—loose tissue covering the penis and clitoris, 278

fossa (fos'ah) basin-like depressions, 177

Fossa ovale (fos-ah o-vale) oval depression in interatrial septum, 199

Fowlers position—a sitting position, 78

fractures (frak'tūrs) breaks in the continuity of bones, 125, 187

frontal (frun'tal) pertaining to the forehead or frontal bone, 163

F.S.H.—follicular stimulating hormone, 213

functional (fungk'shun al) a disease with no discernable lesion, 124
fundus (fun'dus) rounded base of stomach, 273

gall (gawl) another name for bile, 251
gallbladder (gawl'blad-er) small sac found on the posterior inferior hepatic surface storing bile, 251
gametes (gam'ets) reproductive sex cells, 133
gamma globulin (gam'ah glob"u-lin) blood protein containing antibodies, 107
gamma rays—very short wave lengths with great penetrating power, 300
ganglion (gang'gle-on) collection of nerve cell bodies, 231
gastr (gas'tr) prefix meaning stomach, 57
gastralgia (gas-tral'je-ah) stomach pain, 247
gastrectomy (gas-trek'to-me) removal of the stomach, 127, 247
gastric (gas'trik) pertaining to or near the stomach, 206, 242, 247
gastritis (gas-tri'tis) inflamed stomach, 247
gastrology (gas-trol'o'je) study of the stomach, 247
gastroparalysis (gas"tro-pah-ral'i-sis) paralysis of the stomach, 247
gastrotomy (gas'tr ot'o-me) surgical opening into the stomach, 323
general paresis (jen'er-ahl pah-re'sis) degeneration of the brain, 280
genes (jēns) cell proteins which carry the characteristics from one generation to the next, 1, 13
genetic (jĕ-net'ik) relating to the genes; study of the genes, 13, 125
genitals (jen'i-tals) reproductive organs, 271
genotype (jē'no-tip) genetic makeup of an individual, 132
germinal layer (jer'mi-nal) reproductive layer, 147
gero—prefix meaning aged, 57
gestation (jes-ta-shun) the period of growth and development of the new individual in the uterus, 134
G.I.—gastrointestinal tract, 246
giantism (ji'an-tizm) a condition of childhood due to hypersecretion of STH, 218
gingivae (jin-ji'vah-e) gums, 244
gingivitis (jin"ji-vi'tis) inflammation of the gums, 244
glans (glanz) tip of penis, 278
glenoid fossa (gle'noid fos'ah) depression on temporal bone, 177
gliomas (gli-o-mahs) tumors of the neuroglia, 236
glomerulonephritis (glo-mer'u-lo-nĕ fri'tis) inflammation of glomeurli, 257, 266
glomerulus (glo-mer'u-lus) tuft of capillaries; part of the nephron, 263
gloss (glos') prefix meaning tongue, 57
glossopharyngeal (glos"o-fah-rin'je-al) pertaining to the muscles of the tongue and throat; name of cranial nerve nine, 229
glottis (glot'is) opening in center of vocal cords, 165
glucagon (gloo'kah-gon) hormone produced by pancreatic alpha cells, 217
glucose (gloo-kōs) a simple form of carbohydrate, 194
glucose tolerance (gloo'kōs tol'er-ans) a diagnostic test which tests the body's ability to respond to a glucose challenge, 221
gluteal (gloo'te-al) pertaining to the buttocks, 84
glycerol (glis'er-ol) the alcohol component of fats, 243
glycogen (gli'ko-jen) stored glucose, 217
glycosuria (gli"ko-su're-ah) sugar in the urine, 212, 220
gm.—gram, 90
golgi apparatus (gol'je ap"ah-ra'tus) cell organelle responsible for carbohydrate formation, 130
gonads (go'nads) name for ovaries and testes, 215

gonococcus (gon″o-kok′us) microbe which causes gonorrhea, 101
gonorrhea (gon″o-re′ah) infectious, highly communicable disease, 101
gr.—grain, 89
graafian follicle (graf′e-an fol′ĭ-kl) structure in which the ova matures in the ovary, 275
gram (gram) suffix—basic unit of dry weight in metrics; record, 64
granules (gran′ūls) particles, 196
granulocytes (gan′u-lo-sīts″) cells which have stainable particles in the cytoplasm, 193, 196
graphic charts—clinical sheets; records information in an abbreviated form and graphs the vital signs, 320
graphic sheet—records information in an abbreviated form and graphs the vital signs, 320
gravida (grav′ĭ-dah) number of pregnancies, 78, 136
gray matter—nervous tissue consisting mainly of nerve bodies, 232
greater omentum (o-men′tum) partition of peritoneum hanging like an apron over the intestines, 250
greenstick fracture (grēn-stik) bone only partly through the skin, 187
grs.—grains, 88
GTT—glucose tolerance test, 221
gtts.—drops, 89
guerney (gr-ni) stretcher or litter, 315, 329
gustation (gus-ta′shun) taste, 224
Gyne (jin″ĕ) gynecology, 73
gynecological (jin″ĕ-kol′o-je-kal) pertaining to female reproduction, 275
gynecologist (jin″ĕ kol′o-jist) physician specializing in conditions of the female reproductive tract, 20
gynecology (jin″ĕ kol′o-je) study of conditions of the female reproductive tract, 20
gyrus (ji′rus) rounded portion of the convolution, 234

H+—hydrogen ion, 77, 258
H.A.—Health Assistant, also known as a Nurse Aide or Orderly,
hay fever—an allergic condition associated with itching and running nose, 155
Hb—hemoglobin, 75
HCL—hydrochloric acid, 247
HCO_3—bicarbonate ion, 258
heart block (hart blok) condition which prevents the nodal tissue from carrying out its activity, 202
hebetic age (hĕ-bĕt′ĭk) pertaining to puberty, 275
helium (he′le-um) a medical gas, 289
hemacyte (he′mah-sit) a blood corpuscle, 179, 198
hemato (hem″ah-to′) prefix meaning blood, 198
hematology (he″mah-tol′o-je) study of blood, 30
hematopoiesis (hem″ah-to-poi-e′sis) blood producing, 174
hematuria (hem′ah-tu′re-ah) blood in the urine, 257, 267
hemi (hem′ĭ) prefix meaning half, 61
hemiplegia (hem″ĭ ple′je-ah) paralysis of one side of body, 234
hemisphere (hem′ĭ-sfer) half spheres pertaining to 1/2 of the cerebrum, 234
hemo (he′mo) prefix meaning blood, 52
hemodialysis (he″mo-di-al′ĭ-sis) blood dialysis, 257, 266
hemodialyzer (he″mo-di′ah-lizer) a machine which performs hemodyalysis, 268
hemoglobin (he″mo-glo′bin) a pigmented protein found in red blood cells, 161
hemolymph (he′mo-limf) blood and lymph, 198
hemolysis—rupturing of red blood cells, 198
hemoptysis (he-mop′tĭ″sĭs) spitting up blood, 284, 297
hemorrhage (hem′ŏ-rij) escape of blood, 196
hemorrhoids—varicose veins of the rectum, 253
hemotology (he″mo-tŏl′o-je) blood study, 198

Henle's loop (hen'lez) part of the nephron, 263
hepar (he'par) liver, 251
hepat (hep'aht) prefix meaning liver, 252
hepatalgia (hep"ah-tal'je-ah) pain in the liver, 242, 252
hepatectomy (hep"ah-tek'to-me) surgical removal of part of the liver, 252
hepatic (hĕ-pat'ik) pertaining to or near the liver, 206, 249
hepatic duct—passageway for bile out of the liver, 249
hepatitis (hep"ah-ti'tis) inflammation of the liver, 98, 252
hepatodynia (hep"ah-to-din'e-ah) pain in the liver, 252
hepatolith (hep'ah-to-lith") a gall stone in the liver, 252
hepatologist (hep'ah-tal-o-jist) a liver specialist, 252
hernia (her'ne-ah) protrusion of a part of an organ through an abnormal opening, 127
herniation (her"ne-a'shun) protrusion, 127
herniorrhaphy (her"ne-or'ah-fe) surgical repair of a hernia, 113, 127
herpes zoster (her'pez zos"ter) viral infection attached to the dorsal root ganglion, 236
heterotroph (het'er-o-trōf") organism that lives on organic matter, 100
heterozygous (het"er-o-zi'gus) a person with two unlike genes with same characteristics, 130, 132
histoplasmosis (his"to-plaz-mo'sis) lung infection caused by a mold, 293
hg—mercury, 203
hilum (hi'lum) indentation for blood vessels and nerves, 165
histamine (his'tah-min) a chemical released in the body during an allergic reaction, 154
histology (his-tol'o-je) study of tissues, 139
homeostasis (ho"me-o-sta'sis) constancy, 287
homozygous (ho"mo-zi'gus) a person having like genes for the same characteristics, 132

horizontal recumbent—supine position; lying down, 78
hormone (hōr'mon) secretion of endocrine glands; substance produced by the endocrine glands, 150, 212
House Diet—another name for regular diet, 244
H.S. or h.s.—Hour of Sleep; bedtime, 88
H.V.D.—hypertensive vascular disease, 75
hyaline cartilage (hi'ah-lin) smooth connective tissue, 181
Hymen (Hi'men) thin membrane found at external vaginal os, 276
hydro (hi-dro') prefix meaning water, 62
hydrocephalus (hi"dro-sef'ah-lus) a condition due to accumulation of cerebral spinal fluid in the ventricles, 231
hydrochloric acid (hi"dro-klor'ik) an acid produced by cells lining the stomach, 247
hydrogen ion (hi'dro-jen i'on) a positively charged particle whose presence makes a solution acid, 258
hydronephrosis (hi"dro-nĕ fro'sis) distention of renal pelvis and tubules with urine, 266
hydrothorax (hi"dro-tho'raks) an accumulation of fluid in the chest, 297
hydroxyl ion (hi-drok'sil i'on) a negatively charged particle whose presence makes a solution alkaline, 258
hyper (hi'per) above, excess of, 59
hyperacidity (hi"per-ah-sid'i-te) excessive production of hydrochloric acid, 247
hyperbaric (hi"per-bar'ik) under greater than atmospheric pressure, 296
hypercapnia (hi"per-kap'ne-ah) accumulation of CO_2 in the blood, 288
hypercarbia (hi"per-kar'be-ah) accumulation of CO_2 in the blood, 284, 288
hyperglycemia (hi"per-gli-se'me-ah) excess blood sugar, 218, 221
hyperkalemia (hi"per-kah-le'me-ah) excess potassium ions in the blood stream, 257, 259
hypernatremia (hi"per-na-tre'em-ah) excess of sodium ions in the blood stream, 257, 259

hyperpnea (hi″perp-ne′ah) respiration pattern of increased rate and depth, 160, 168

hypersecretion (hi″per-se-kre′shun) oversecretion, 217

hypertension (hi″per-ten′shun) high blood pressure, 114

hyperthermia (hi″per-ther′me-ah) greatly increased temperature, 150

hyperventilation (hi″per-ven″ti-la′shun) overventilation, 288

hypo (hi′po) prefix meaning under, deficiency of, 59

hypocapnia (hi″po-kap′ne-ah) lack of CO_2 in the blood,

hypocarbia (hi″po-kar′be-ah) lack of CO_2 in the blood,

hypoglycemia (hi″po-gli-se′me-ah) deficient blood sugar, 212

hypokalemia (hi″po-kah-le′me-ah) too few potassium ions in the blood stream, 259

hyponatremia (hi″po-na-tre′me-ah) too few sodium ions in the blood stream, 259

hypophysis (hi-pof′i-sis) another name for the pituitary gland, 213

hyposecretion (hi″po-se-kre′shun) under secretion, 218

hypospadias (hi″po-spa′de-as) abnormal urethral opening on or under surface of penis or perineum, 262

hypotension (hi″po-ten′shun) low blood pressure, 203

hypothalamus (hi″po-thal′ah-mus) portion of the brain stem found inferior to the thalamus; lower part of diencephalon, functions as reflex center of visceral activities, 214, 233

hypothermia—greatly reduced temperature, 150

hypoventilation (hi″po-ven″ti-la′shun) underventilation, 288

hypoxemia (hi″pok-se′me-ah) insufficient oxygen in the blood, 196

hypoxia (hi-pok′se-ah) diminished levels of oxygen, 125, 152, 160

hyster (his′ter) Prefix meaning uterus, 53

hysterectomy (his″ter-eck′to-me) surgical removal of the uterus, 276

hysterodynia (his″ter-o-din′e-ah) pain in the uterus, 276

hysterology (his″te-rol′o-je) study of the uterus, 276

hysterometer (his″te-rom′e-ter) instrument for measuring the uterus, 276

hysteropathy (his″te-rop′ah-the) disease of the uterus, 271, 276

hysteropexy (his′ter-o-pek″se) uterine suspension to repair a prolapse, 273

hysterotomy (his″te-rot′o-me) surgical opening into the uterus,

I.C.C.—Intensive Coronary (or Cardiac) Care Unit, 73

ICSH—Interstitial Cell Stimulatine Hormone, 217

ileocecal valve (il″e-o-se′kal) oneway valve preventing movement of materials back from the colon to the small intestine, 248

ileum (il′e-um) final portion of small intestine, 175, 248

iliac (il′e-ak) pertaining to or near ilium, 205

im, in (im, in) prefix meaning into, in, not, 57

Impotence (im′po-tns) inability to perform sexually, 279

infarction (in-fark′shun) death of tissues, 193, 198

inferior (in-fer′e-or) below another part, 81

inferior vena cava (in-fer′e-or ve′nah ka-vah) vein bringing blood from lower extremities, 199

infiltrated (in-fil′trate-ed) invaded, 296

infra (in′frah) prefix meaning below, 61

infused (in-fu′zd) introduced into vein by gravity, 266

inguinal (ing′gwi-nal) pertaining to the groin,

inhalation therapist—respiratory care therapist, 287

inorganic (in″or-gan′ik) matter which has never had life, 100

insertion (in-ser′shun) distal point of attachment of skeletal muscle, 185

insomnia (in-som′ne-ah) sleeplessness, 78

inspiration (in″spĭ-ra′shun) inhalation,
insufflate (in″su-fla′t) blow up or into, 296
insulin (in′su-lin) hormone produced by the pancreatic beta cells, 217, 221
integument (in-teg′u-ment) skin, 146
integumentary system (in″teg″u-men′tar″e sis′tem) system of the body consisting of the skin and its appendages, 146
intensifying screens (in″ten′si-fi-ing) found in the cassette used to supplement x-ray energy of production of energy, 302
inter (in′ter) prefix meaning between, 64
interatrial (in′ter-atra-al) between the atria, 199
intercellular (in″ter-sel′u-lar) between the cells, 130, 138
intercostal (in″ter-kos′tal) between the ribs, 206
intern (in′tern) person who has completed his basic medical school education and is gaining experience in a clinical area, 22
internal respiration (in′ter-nal res″pĭ-ra′shun) exchange of gas between blood and tissue cells, 161
internuncial (in″ter-nun′shal) central neuron, 227
interstitial (in″ter-stich′al) intercellular; tissue fluid, 130, 138, 194
Interstitial Cell Stimulating Hormone (in″ter-stish′al) stimulates the testes to produce sperm, 217
interventricular (in″ter-ven-trik′u-lar) between the ventricles, 198
Interventricular Bundles (in″ter-ven-trik′u-lar) The Bundle of His which is part of the conduction system of the heart, 201
intra (in′trah) prefix meaning within, 52
intracellular (in″trah-sel′u-lar) found within the cell, 194
intracorporeal (in″tra-kor-po′re-al) inside the body, 202
intralaryngeal (in″tr-lar-ing′eal) within the larynx, 160, 165
intrapleural cavity (in″trah-ploo′ral kav-e-tee) potential space between the two layers of pluera, 166

intrapulmonic space (in″trah-pul-mon′ĭk) within the lung, 166
intravascular (in″trah-vas′ku-lar) within the vessels, 194
intubation (in″tu-ba′shun) passing a tube, 289
involuntary muscle—a type of muscle forming the walls of organs, also known as visceral or smooth muscle, 142
involuntary nervous system (in-vol′en-tar″e) another name for autonomic nervous system, 230
I. & O.—intake and output, 87
ionize (i′on-iz) dissociate in solution, 257
ions (i′ons) electrically charged particles, 257
I.P.P.B.—intermittent positive pressure breathing, 171, 291
iron (i′ern) an element, 301
irradiate (i-ra-de-at) to subject to radiation, 300, 305
ischemia (is-ke′me-ah) diminished blood flow to an area; forming the inferior-posterior pelvis, 113, 125, 198
isotopes (i′so-tops) radioactive elements of unusual weight, 301
itis (i′tis) suffix meaning inflammation, 56, 169
I.V.—intravenous, 87
I.V.C.—inferior vena cava, 199

jaundice (jawn′dis) a yellowish coloration of the skin, 154, 251
jejunum (je-joo′num) middle portion of small intestine, approximately 3-4 feet, 248
joints—point of articulation between bones, 181

K⁺ (po-tas′e-um) potassium ion, 258
keloid (ke′loid) a tumor-like growth of scar tissue, 153
ketonuria (ke″to-nu′re-ah) presence of ketone bodies in the urine, 259
ketosis (ke″to′sis) another name for acidosis or diabetic coma, 212, 220
kidneys (kid′nes) two organs which produce urine, 260

kilo (kil'o) prefix meaning 1000 x the unit of measurement, 69, 90

kyphosis (ki-fo'sis) hunchback or pronounced thorax curve, 189

labia majora (la'be-ah ma'jor-ah) two large, hair-covered, lip-like structures; part of the vulva, 277

labia minora (la'be-ah min'or-ah) two hairless lips found beneath the labia majora, 277

laboratory monitors—monitors radiation build-up, 306

laceration (las"ĕ-ra'shun) cut or break in skin, 146, 153

lactase (lak'tās) intestinal enzymes acting to convert lactose to monosaccharides, 248

lactation (lak-ta'shun) process of secreting milk, 150

lactiferous (lak-tif'er-us) milk-conveying, 150

lactogenic hormone (lak"to-jen'ik) prolactin, stimulates lactation or milk production, 217

lactose (lak'tos) a disaccharide, 248

laparo (lap'ah-ro) loin, flank, 55

laparotomy—surgical incision through the flank, 84

laryngeal adenocarcinoma (lah-rin'je-al ah"dĕ-no-kar"si-no'mah) a malignant tumor of larynx, 293

laryngectomy (lar"in-jek'to-me) removal of larynx, 293

laryngopharynx (lah-ring"go-far'ingks) portion of pharynx which leads into the larynx and esophagus, 164

laryngoscopy (lar"ing-gos'ko-pe) visualization of the larynx, 295

larynx (lar'ingks) voice box, 164

lateral (lat'er-al) part away from midline; X-ray beam directed from the side, 81

lesions (le'zhuns) pathologic tissue change, 124

lesser omentum (o"men'tum) partition of peritoneum between stomach, duodenum, and liver, 250

lethargic (leth"ar'jik) drowsy and functionally slow, 219

leuk (lu'k) white, 51

leukocytosis (lu"ko-si-to'sis) increased numbers of white blood cells, 105

L.H.—luteinizing hormone, 217, 273

Licensed Practical Nurse—Licensed Vocational Nurse, 24

Licensed Vocational Nurse—a person educated in nursing techniques who has been licensed by the state to carry out those functions under professional supervision, 23

ligaments (lig'ah-ments) tough fibrous connective tissue bands holding bones together, 182

lipase (li'pas) enzyme which breaks down fat, 249

liter, litre, or L—basic unit of liquid volume in metric system, 69, 90

lith (lĭth) stone, 56

lithotomy position—patient on back with legs flexed and separated, 78

liver (liv-er) largest organ of the body; functions include blood filtration, bile secretion, and glycogen storage, 251

LLQ—left lower quadrant, 81

lobes (lōbs) division of an organ, 165, 166

Lo Na—Low sodium, 87

longitudinal fissure (lon"ji tu'di-nal fish'er) deep cleft or groove dividing the cerebrum into right and left hemispheres, 234

long term facilities (nursing homes, rest homes, convalescent hospitals) provide patient care for patients with disabilities that exist for a long period of time, 10

lordosis (lor-do'sis) swayback or pronounced lumbar curve, 189

L.P.N.—Licensed practical nurse, 24, 72

L.R.S.—lower respiratory system, 162

lumbar (lum'bar) pertaining to the loins, 206

lumbar puncture (lum-bar pung-tūr) technique for withdrawing cerebrospinal fluid from the vertebrae, 239

lumen (lu'men) tube, cavity, 248

LUQ—left upper quadrant, 81

luteinizing hormone (lu'te-in"ĭ-zing) hormone produced by the anterior pituitary gland which promotes ovulation, 217, 273

* 352 GLOSSARY

L.V.N.—licensed vocational nurse, 24, 72
L & W—living and well, 77
lymph (limf) fluid found in lymphatic vessels, 194
lymphadenitis (lim-fad″ĕ ni′tis) inflammation of lymph nodes, 193
lymphatic capillaries (lim-fat′ĭk kap′ĭ-ler″es) small vessels which drain tissue fluids into lymph vessels, 203
lymph nodes (limf nōds) small masses of lymphoid tissues, 195
lymphocyte (lim′fo-sīt) a granular phagocytic leukocyte, 195, 197
lysis (lī′sis) breaking up, dissolving, 56

M.A.—medical assistant, 72, 79
macule (mak′ūl) colored, nonelevated spot, 153
malaise (mal-āz′) a general feeling of ill health, 146
malignant (mah-lig′nant) life-threatening, 124
malnutrition (mal″nu-trish′un) poor nutrition, 125
malpractice (mal-prak′tis) a neglect of professional duty or skill that results in injury, 121
maltase (mawl′tas) an intestinal enzyme which converts maltose to monosaccharides, 248
maltose (mawl′tos) disaccharide, 243
mamma (mă′ma) milk-secreting gland, 150
mammary glands (mam′ar-e) breasts, 150
mammography (mah-mog′rah-fe) a radiologic technique used to visualize breast abnormalities, 152
mammoplasia (mam″o-pla′ze-ah) breast development, 150
mandible (man′dĭ-bl) lower jaw bone, 177
mandibular fossa (man″dĭb′u-lar fos′ah) depression of temporal bone, 177
marrow (mar′o) soft bone tissue, 196
mast (mast) breast, 57
mastication (mas″tĭ-ka′shun) chewing, 224
mastoid process (mas′toid) projection of temporal bone, 185

maxilla (mak-sil′ah) cheek bone, 163
maxillae (mak-sil′e) cheek bones, 163
maxillary (mak′sil-eri) pertaining to the maxilla, 163, 229
maxillary nerve (mak′sil-ar-e) branch of the trigeminal nerve, 229
meatus (me-a′tus) an opening or passage, 178
media (me′de-ah) special substance used to grow microbes, 102
medial (me′de-al) part close to midline, 81
mediastinum (me″de-ah-sti′num) space between the pleural cavities posterior to the pericardial space, 139
medical (med′i-kl) pertaining to nonsurgical treatment of condition, 25
mediolateral (med″i-o-lat′er-al) X-ray view with beam directed from midline to side, 307
Med/Surg—abbreviation for medical and surgical, 73
medulla (mĕ-dul′ah) middle portion of an organ, 166, 216
medulla oblongata (me-dul′ah ob-loon-ga′ta) lowest part of brain stem, frequently referred to as "medulla," 233
medullary canal (mĕ-dul′ari) center cavity of long bone, 180
megakaryocyte (meg″ah-kar′e-o sit″) large cell from which thrombocytes are derived, 193
melanin (mel′ah-nan) dark pigment, 147
membranes (mem′brāns) thin sheet of tissue which covers a surface, lines a cavity, or divides a space or organ, 134, 139
membranous formation (mem′brah-nus) refers to one method of bone formation, 179
menarche (me-nar′ke) first menstrual cycle, 271
meninges (mĕ-nin′jez) three-layered serous membrane lining dorsal cavity, 130, 140
meningococcus (mĕ-ning″go-kok′us) diplococcus which causes meningitis and other infections, 150
menorrhagia (men″o-ra′je-ah) excessive menstrual flow, 275
menses (men′sēz) menstruation, 212, 215, 275

GLOSSARY 353 *

menstrual cycle (men'stroo-al si-kl) length of time between menses, 272

mental retardation—lack of mental development, 133

mesentery (mes'en-ter"e) extension of peritoneum binding most of the intestines to posterior abdominal wall, 250

mesophilic (mez'o-fīl-ik) organisms which grow best at middle temperature, 108

metabolism (mĕ-tab'o-lizm) the utilization of nutrients by the body, 125, 243

metastasis (mĕ-tas'tah'sis) spread of tumor cells away from original site, 124, 151

meter (m) basic unit of length in metric system, 90

metra, metro (me'trah, me'tro) uterus, 53

metrectomy (me"trek'to-me) surgical removal of the uterus, 276

metritis (me-trī'tis) inflammation of the uterus, 276

metrodynia (me"tro-din'e-ah) Pain in the uterus, 276

metropathy (me-trop'ah-the) uterine disease, 276

metrorrhagia (me"tro-ra'je-ah) irregular menstrual flow, 275

metrorrhea (me"tro-re'ah) an abnormal uterine discharge, 276

mg—milligram, 88

M.H.—marital history, 77

micro (mi'kro) small, 64

microbes (mi'krōbs) microorganisms, 96

microbiology (mi"kro-bi-ol'o-je) study of microorganisms, 96

microns (mi'krons) a unit of measurement—.001 mm, 100

micturating (mik'tu-ra-ting) the act of emptying the bladder, 260

mid brain—portion of brain stem superior to pons, 233

midsagittal (mid-saj'i-tal) midline which divides the body into right and left halves, 81

milli (mil'e) prefix meaning 1/1000 of a unit measurement, 69, 90

m—minim or meter, 89

/min—per minute, 87

minimal air (min'i-mal air) volume of air that cannot be forced out of lungs, 168

miscarriage (mis"k-ar'ij) pregnancy lost after first trimester, 134

mitochondrion (mi-to-kon'drion) a cellular organelle which produces energy for the cell, 130

mitosis (mi-to'sis) cell multiplication or division, 133

mitral (mi-tral') another name for bicuspid valve, 199

mixed infection—an infection caused by more than one organism, 101

mixed nerves—contain somatic and visceral afferent and efferent fibers, 230

ml.—milliliter, 88

m—mix, 88

M.S.D.W.—married, single, divorced, widowed, 77

monocytes (mon'o-sits) a granular leukocyte, 197

monosaccharide (mono"sak'ah-ride) simple sugar, 243

mons pubis (mons pu'bis) fat-covered pad over pubic bone of female, 271

mons veneris (mons ven'er-is) mons pubis, 277

morbid (mor-bid) disease, 150

morbidity (mor'bid'i-te) number of cases, 96

moribund (mor'i-bund) dying, 209, 267

mortality (mor-tal'i-te) number of deaths, 99

motor (mo'tor) refers to activity or neurons which transmit a message from the central nervous system to an effector, 227

M.S.—multiple sclerosis, 76

mucolytic (mu"ko-lit'ik) 291

mucosa (mu-ko'sah) mucous membrane lining, 248

mucous membrane (mu'kus mem'brān) secrete mucus, 139

mucus (mu'kus) secretion of mucous membranes; thick sticky fluid, 104

Muscular Dystrophy (mus'ku-lar dis'tro-fe) a condition in which there is a loss of muscular protein resulting in muscular atrophy, 190

mutualism (mu'tu-al-izm") symbiotic relationship wherein each organism derives benefit, 100

my (mi) muscle, 59

myasthenia gravis (mi"as-the'ne-ah gra-vis) chronic disease characterized by muscle weakness, 190

myc (mi'k) prefix meaning fungus, 64

Mycobacterium tuberculosis (mi"ko-bak'te"re-um tu-ber'ku-lo'sis) microorganism known as tubercal bacillus that causes tuberculosis, 103, 170

mycology (mi-kol'o-je) study of yeasts and molds, 97

myelin sheath (mi'e-lin she'th) fatty insulation found around axons and dendrites, 226

myelo (mi'e-lo) prefix meaning spinal cord, 236

myelodiastasis (mi"e-lo-di-as'tah-sis) disintegration of the spinal cord, 224, 236

myelogenous (mi"e-loj'e-nus) referring to bone marrow, 174, 179

myelography (mi"e-log'rah-fe) radiogram of spinal cord following injection of contrast media, 309

myelogram (mi'e-lo-gram") radiogram obtained during myelography, 309

myelomalacia (mi"e-lo-mah-la'she-ah) abnormal softening of the spinal cord, 236

myelon (mi'e-lon) spinal cord, 236

myeloplegia (mi"e-lo-ple'je-ah) paralysis caused by a lesion of the spinal cord, 236

myelosclerosis (mi"e-lo-skle-ro'sis) hardening of the spinal cord, 174

myo (mi'o) prefix meaning muscle, 185

myocardium (mi"o-kar'de-um) muscular wall of the heart, 198

myology (mi-ol'o je) study of muscles, 186

myomalacia (mi"o-mah-la'she-ah) softening of muscles, 186

myometrium (mi"o-me'tre-um) muscular uterine wall, 273

myopathy (mi-op'ah-the) diseases of muscles, 186

myosclerosis (mi"o-skle-ro'sis) hardening of a muscle, 186

myospasm (mi'o-spazm) involuntary muscular contraction, 186

N.A.—nursing assistant, 72

Na$^+$—sodium ion, 258

NaCl—symbol for sodium chloride, 198

nares (na'res) opening into the nasal cavities, 162

nasolacrimal ducts (na"zo-lak'ri-mal) ducts which drain tears into nasal cavities, 162

nasopharynx (na"zo-far'ingks) upper throat, 164

naturally acquired active immunity—self-produced resistance developed without unusual means to an antigen, 106

NCU—Neurovascular Care Unit, 238

nebulizer (neb'u-liz"er) mechanism for converting medication into fine spray, 284, 290

necrotic (ne-krah-tik) pertains to cells which have died, 125

Neisseria gonorrhea (ni-se're-ah gon"o-re'ah) organism which causes gonorrhea, 103

neo (ne'o) new, 53

neonatal (ne"o na'tal) new born, 14

neoplasms (ne'o-plazm) new growths, 124

neph (nef) kidney, 62

nephrectomy (ne-frek'to-me) removal of a kidney, 265

nephritis (ne'fri'tis) inflammation of the kidney, 265

nephro—prefix meaning kidney, 265

nephrogram (nef'ro-gram) X-ray of the kidney, 265

nephrolith (nef'ro-lith) kidney stone, 265

nephron (nef'ron) microscopic kidney units which produce the urine, 262

nephropathy (ne-frop'ah-the) kidney pathology, 265

nephropexy (nef'ro-pek"se) surgical fixation of nephroptosis, 265

nephroptosis (nef"rop-to'sis) displacement of kidney, 257, 262

GLOSSARY 355 *

nerve (nerv) a bundle of axons and dendrites, 224

nerve impulse—an electrical wave which transmits a message, 140

nervous tissue (ner′vus ti sh′u) highly specialized tissue capable of conducting a nerve impulse, 140

neurilemma (nu″ri-lem′ah) membrane covering the myelon of the peripheral nerve fibers, 226

neuritis (nu-ri′tis) inflammation of a nerve, 235

neuro (nu′ro) nerve; abbreviation for neurology, 61, 73

neurofibroma (nu″ro-fi-bro′mah) tumor of nervous tissue caused by excessive growth of binding connective tissue, 235

neuroglia (nu-rog′le-ah) supporting tissue of the nervous system, 224

neurohypophysis (nu″ro-hi-pof″i-sis) posterior or nervous lobe of pituitary gland, 213

neurological record (nu-ro-log′i-kal) also known as head sheet or head chart used to record neurological observations, 321

neurologist (nu-rol′o-jist) physician who treats conditions of the nervous system, 20, 235

neuroma (nu-ro′mah) nervous tissue tumor, 224, 235

neuromuscular (nu″ro-mus′ku-lar) pertaining to nerves and muscles, 235

neuromuscular junction (nu″ro-mus′ku-lar jungk′shun) point of contact between nerve and skeletal muscles, 235

neuron (nu′ron) nerve cell, 224

neuroparalysis (nu″ro-pah-ral′i-sis) loss of function due to nerve damage, 235

neuropathy (nu-rop′ah-the) any disease of the nerve, 235

neurosclerosis (nu″ro-skle-ro′sis) abnormal hardening of nerve tissue, 235

neurotomy (nu-rot′o-me) surgical dissection of a nerve, 235

neurotransmitter (nu-ro′trans-miter) chemical which carries stimulus across the synapse, 226

neurotropic (nu″ro-trop′ik) affecting the nerves, 98

neutrons (nu′trons) particles with no electrical charges which are found in the nucleus of atoms, 301

neutrophils (nu′tro-fils) leukocytes which take a neutral stain, 197

nipple (nip′l) the area of the breast through which the milk flows, 150

neisseria meningitidis (ni-se′re-ah men″in-ji′ti-dis) bacterium which causes meningitis, 103

nitrogen (ni′tro-jen) a gas, 285

nitrous oxide (ni′trus ok′sid) a medical gas, 289

nodal tissue (no-dal tish′u) special neuromuscular tissue found in the heart, 201

noct—in the night, 88

non rep—do not repeat, 88

non vegetative (non vej′ĕ-ta″tiv) non-active or non-producing forms of microbes, 102

N.P.O.—nothing by mouth, 88

norm—a fixed standard, 166

normal flora (nor′mal flo′rah) refers to the microbe population found in various body areas, 100

nosocomial infection (nos″o-ko′me-al) hospital acquired infection, 110

N.S.—normal saline or salt solution, 171

nuclei (nu′kle-i′) centers—masses of grey matter located in brain responsible for controlling a specific body function, 233

nucleus—center of the atom containing neutrons and protons, 301

nullipara (nu-lip′ah-rah) no living child, 136

nurse practioners (ners prak-tish′on-urs) specially trained nurses who practice nursing independently, 4

nutrients (nu′tre-ents) foods which supply essential substances; essential elements for growth and repair, 125, 245

nutritional disease—disease resulting from the lack of or the inability to utilize nutrients, 125

O_2—symbol for a molecule of oxygen, 160
O.B.—obstetrics, 73
obligate intracellular parasites (ob'li-gāt in″trah-sel'u-lar par'ah-sits) microbes that must live within a living cell, 97
oblique (o-blēk) X-ray beam directed at an angle, 307
obstetrician (ob″stĕ-trish'an) one who practices obstetrics, 20
obstetrics (ob″stĕt'rics) care of the female during pregnancy, labor, and puerperium, 1, 2, 20
occlude (o-klood') block, 205
oculomotor (ok″u-lo-mo'tor) pertaining to eye movement, cranial nerve three, 229
official patient records—records which are governed by law, 318
OH⁻—hydroxyl ion, 258
olfactory (ol-fak'to-re) pertaining to the sense of smell, cranial nerve one, 163, 229
oliguria (ol″i-gu're-ah) scant urine, 265
ology (ol'o-je) suffix meaning study of, 64
oma (o'mah) suffix meaning tumor, 54
O.O.B.—out of bed, 87
open reduction—surgical procedure to realign a fracture, 188
opthalmic nerve (of-thal'mik) name of a branch of the trigeminal, 229
opportunists—microbes that cause disease only under special conditions, 101
opsonins (op-so'nins) antibodies which make antigens sticky, 106
opthalm (of-thal'm) prefix meaning eye, 51, 61
opthalmologist (of″thal-mol'o-jist) physician who treats eye conditions, 20
opthalmoscope (of-thal'mo-skop) instrument to view the eye,
optic (op'tik) pertaining to nerve eight, cranial nerve two, 79
O.R.—operating room, 28, 73
orchitis (or-ki'tis) inflammation of the testes, 280
orderly (or'der-le) name given to a male health assistant, 23

organelles (or'gah-nel's) organ-like structure of the cell, 130
organic (or-gan'ik) matter that is living or has had life, 100
organic disease (or-gan'ik) a disease in which a lesion is present, 124
organs (or'ganz) tissues grouped together for a specific function, 142
orifice (or'i-fis) opening, 104
origin (or'i-gin) proximal point of attachment to skeletal muscle, 185
oropharynx (o″ro-far'ingks) portion of pharynx which communicates with the mouth, 164
orrhaphy (or'ah-fe) suffix meaning repair of, 127
orthopedics (or″tho-pe'diks) pertaining to bone, 1, 2
orthopedist (or-tho-pe'dist) physician who treats conditions of the musculoskeletal system, 22
orthopnea (or″thop-ne'ah) ability to breathe in an upright position only, 168
os—opening, 273
ossa coxae (os'sa kok'si) pelvic girdle, 175
osis (o'sis) process, condition, 59
osmosis (oz-mo'sis) water-drawing power, 194
oss or osteo (os, os'te-o) bone, 52
osseous (os'e-us) bone tissue; a form of connective tissue, 140
ossification (os″i-fi-ka-shun) conversion into bone, 179
ossified (os″i fid) converted to bone, 179
ostalgia (os-tal'je-ah) pain in the bone, 180
ostectomy (os-tek'to-me) excision of a bone, 180
osteectopia (os″te-ek-to'pe-ah) displacement of a bone, 180
osteitis (os'te-i'tis) bone inflammation, 180
ostempyesis (ost″em-pi-e'sis) suppuration within a bone, 180
osteoarthritis (os″te-ar-thri'tis) inflammation of bones and joints, 180, 190
osteoclasis (os″te-ok'lah-sis) surgical fracture of a bone, 180

osteocytes (os'te-o-sīts") bone cells, 179

osteodynia (os"te-o-din'e-ah) pain in the bone, 175, 180

osteoma (os"te-o'mah) bone tumor,

osteomalacia (os"te-o-mah-la'she-ah) softening of a bone, 180

osteometry (os"te-om'ĕ-tre) measurement of a bone, 180

osteomyelitis (os"te-o-mi"ĕ-li'tis) pyogenic bone infection, 180

osteopathology (os"te-o-pah-thol'o-je) disease of the bone, 180

osteoporosis (os"te-o-po-ro'sis) metabolic bone disease, 180

osteotome (os'te-o-tom) a bone-cutting knife, 180

osteotomy (os"te-ot'o-me) surgical cutting of a bone, 180

ostomy (os'to-me) to create an opening, 63

ot (o't) ear, 60

O.T.—occupational therapist, 238

otologist (o-tol"o-jist) physician who treats ear conditions, 20

otomy (ot'o-me) suffix meaning cutting into, 56

otoscope (o'to-skōp) instrument to view the ear, 79

ova (o'vah) egg; female gamete, 272

ovarian (o-va're-an) pertaining to or near ovary, 206

ovaries (o'var-ez) endocrine glands located in female pelvis; female gonads, 214, 272

oviduct (o'vi-dukt) Fallopian Tube, 134, 273

ovulate (o"vu-lat) extrude an ova, 272

ovulation (o"vu-la'shun) process of extruding an ova from the ovary, 275

ovum (o'vm) female gamete, 272

oxia (ok'se-ah) pertaining to oxygen, 59

oxygen—an odorless, colorless gas essential for life, 195

oxygenated (ok'si-jĕ-na"ted) loaded with oxygen, 199

oxyhemoglobin (ox"si-he"mo-glo'bin) combination of oxygen and hemoglobin in which oxygen is transported, 161

oz.—ounce, 88

P—phosphorus, 217

P.—pulse, 77

P–A posterior-anterior, X-ray beam directed from back to front, 297

pacemaker (pas'mak-er) another name for S.A. node, 202

palate (pal'at) structure which separates the nasal cavity from oral cavity, 162

palatine tonsils (pal'ah-tin ton'sils) masses of lymphoid tissues found in posterior oral cavities, 164

pallor (pal'or) an absence of color, 154

palpate (pal'pat) examine by feeling, 78

pan (pan) prefix meaning all, 57

pancreatic duct (pan"kre-at'ik) an exocrine duct carrying digestive enzymes into small intestine, 249

pancreas (pan'kre-as) one of the abdominal viscera which has both endocrine and exercrine functions, 212, 216

pandemic (pan-dem'ik) widely spread epidemic, 99

papule (pap'ul) a small rounded elevation, 153

para (par'ah) prefix meaning around, near; number of pregnancies carried to age of viability, 53, 78

paralysis (pah-ral'i-sis) loss of motor function, 234

paramedics (par"ah-med'ĭks) Emergency Medical Technicians, 6

parameters (pah-ram'ĕ-ters) boundaries, 121

paraparesis (par"ah-pah-re'sis) partial paralysis of the legs, 234

paraplegia (par"ah-ple'je-ah) paralysis of lower part of body or legs, 234

parasite (par'ah-sit) heterotrophs which live on living matter, 100

parasitism (par'ah-si"tizm) symbiotic relationship in which one organism derives benefit at the others' expense, 100

parasitology (par"ah-si-tol'o-je) study of parasites, 30

parasympathetic (para"sim"pah-thet'ĭk) refers to one division of the autonomic nervous system, 228 parathyroid hormone—hormone produced by parathyroid glands, 217

parathyroid gland (par"ah-thi'roid) endocrine glands located embedded in posterior thyroid gland, 214

paraenchyma (pah-reng'kĭ-mah) essential organ parts, 160, 165

parentally—entering the body other than via the alimentary canal, 322

paresis (pah-re'sis) suffix meaning paralysis, 51, 61, 234

parietal (pah-rĭ'ĕ'tal) pertaining to the wall; referring to a membrane layer which lines a cavity, 140

parotiditis (pah-rot"i-di'tĭs) mumps, 99

parturient—giving birth, 136

pass box—transfer box, 303

passive—used with immunity—means antibodies are developed outside the person's own body, 106

pasteurization (pas"tur-i-za'shun) technique used to destroy pathogens with heat, 109

patella (pah-tel'ah) knee cap, 177

pathogenic (path"o-jĕ'nik) disease producing, 97

patholgoist (pah-thol'o-jist) studies and describes the disease process, 19

pathology (pah-thol'o-je) study of the disease process, 124

pathy (path'e) suffix meaning abnormality or disease, 54

p.c.—after meals, 88

pediatric (pe'de-at'rik) pertaining to children, 25

pediatrician (pe"de-ah-trish'an) physician who cares for infants and children, 19, 25

Peds—pediatrics, 69, 73

pelvic cavity (pel'vik kav'ĭ-te) that portion of peritoneal cavity surrounded by pelvic bones, 139

pelvic girdle (pel'vik) os coxae or fusing of the ilial, ischial, and pubic bones, 175

penis (pe'nĭs) male organ of copulation, 278

pepsin (pep'sĭn) a gastric enzyme which begins digestion, 249

peptidase (pep'tĭ-das) enzyme which converts proteins to amino acids, 249

per—through, 88

percussion hammer (per-kush'un) tapping, 79

peri (per'e) prefix meaning around, 52, 75

pericardium (per"i-kar'de-um) membrane around the heart, 139

perfusion (per-fu'zhun) blood flow, 205, 284

perikaryon (per-i-kăr'ĭ-ŏn) nerve cell body, 225

perineum (per"i-ne'um) area between anus and scrotum of male or anus and vagina of female, 262, 277

peridontal (per"e-o-don'tal) around a tooth, 244

periosteum (per"e-os'te-um) around the bone, 180

perirenal (per"i-re'anl) around kidney, 260

peristalsis (per"i-stal'sis) rhythmic or smooth muscle contractions, 246

peritoneal cavity (per"i-to-ne'al kav'ĭ-te) that portion of abdominal cavity surrounded by peritoneum, 139

peritonitis (per"i-to-ni'tĭs) inflammation of the peritonium, 250

peritoneum (per"i-to-ne'um) a serous membrane surrounding the peritoneal cavity, 139

petrie dish (pi-tri dish) flat plates used to cultivate microbes, 102

pH—acid base level, 258

P.H.—past history, 77

phagocytes (fag'o-sits) cells cepable of phagocytosis, 105

phagocytosis (fag"o-si-to'sis) ingestion of foreign particles by phagocytes, 104, 105

pharmacist (far'mah-sist) a licensed person who dispenses drugs from prescriptions, 6

pharynx (far'ingks) throat, 164

phenotype (fe'no-tip) obvious physical characteristics of hereditary make-up, 132

phimosis (fe-mo'sĭs) condition wherein the foreskin cannot be retracted, 271, 278

P—phleb (fleb') prefix meaning vein, 51, 57

phlebitis (fle-bi'tis) inflammation of the veins, 193, 205

phlegm (flem) heavy mucus, 170

phobia (fo'be-ah) suffix meaning fear, 51

phonation (fo-na'shun) voice production, 165
phosphorus—an element, 217
physician of record—attending physician, 22
Physiology—study of function, 124
P.I.—present illness, 77
pia mater (piah ma'ter) soft mother; inner layer of meninges, 140
P.I.D.—pelvic inflammatory disease, 76, 280
pilomotor (pi"lo-mo'ter) related to muscles attached to the hairs, 149
pilose (pi'los) hairy, 149
pituitary gland (pi-tu'i-tăr"e) endocrine gland located in cranial cavity, 214
placenta (plah-sen'tah) afterbirth, 134
placenta previa (plah-sen'tah pre'vĕa) placenta implanted low in uterine wall, 137
plasm (plazm) suffix meaning substance, 54
plasma (plaz'mah) liquid portion of blood, 197
Plasmodium vivax (plaz-mo'de-um vi-vax) protozoa which causes malaria, 109
plasty (plas'te) suffix meaning surgical correction, 63
platelets (plat'lets) thrombocytes—rupture of these cell fragments begins the blood clotting process, 195
pleura—serous membrane that surrounds the lungs, 139
pleurisy (ploo'ri-se) inflammation of pleura, 169
plexus (plek'sus) network of nerve fibers, 232
pneum (nu'm) prefix meaning air, lung, 51, 64
pneumo (nu'mo) prefix meaning lung or gas, 64, 169
Pnumococcal pneumonia (nu"mo-kok'al nu-mo'ne-ah) inflammation of lung caused by pneumoccus microbe, 169, 170
pneumococcus (nu"mo-kok'us) diplococcus which causes pneumonia and other infections, 103, 150
pneumoencephalography (nu"mo-en-sefh"ah-log'rah-fe) radiogram of brain following injection of air, 239
pneumonectomy (nu"mo-nek'to-me) removal of a lung, 169

pneumonetry (nu-mon"ĕ-tri) measurement of inspired and expired air, 169
pneumonia (nu-mo'ne-ah) acute inflammation of the lung, 169
pneumonotomy (ne"mo-not'o-me) incision into the lungs, 169
pneumorrhagia (nu"mora'je-ah) hemorrhage from the lungs, 160, 169
pneumothorax (numo-tho'raks) air in the intrapleural space, 169
pneumotropic (nu"mo-trop'ik) having an affinity for the lungs, 98
PNS—peripheral nervous system, 228
poliomyelitis (po"le-o-mi"ĕ-li'tis) also called infantile paralysis, a viral infection which attacks motor cells of coordination, 99, 236
poly (pol'e) prefix meaning many, 59
polycythemia (pol"e-si-the'me-ah) excessive erythrocytes, 196
polydipsia (pol"e-dip'se-ah) excessive thirst, 212, 220
polymorphonuclear leukocytes (pol"e-mor"fo-nu'cle-ar) neutrophils named because of their many shaped nuclei, 197
polyphagia (pol"e-fa'je-ah) excessive hunger, 220
"polys" (pol'ez) abbreviation for polymorphonuclear luekocytes, 197
polysaccharide (poli-sak'ah-ride) complex saccharide, 243
polyuria (pol"e-u're-ah) excessive urine output, 220
pons varolii (ponz var-o'le) portion of brain stem between the medulla and mid-brain, 233
popliteal (pop"li-te'al) pertaining to the knee, 83
portal entry (por'tal) method of entering the body, 98
portal system (por'tal sis'tem) collection of vessels draining blood from digestive tract into the liver, 205
posterior (pos-ter'eor) back or dorsal, 81
posterior fontanel (pos-ter'e-or fon"tah-nel')

unossified area of skull between the parietal bones and occipital bone, 180
post mortem (post mor'tem) after death, 209
postpartum—after delivery, 14, 20
postprandial (post-pran'de-al) after meal, 242, 253
postural drainage (pos'tu-ral) a technique which puts the patient's head and thorax in a dependent position to promote gravity drainage of secretion, 291, 292
potassium (po-tas'e-um) an element, 258
pre (pre) prefix meaning before, 53
premature (pre"mah-tur') babies before term or low birth weight, 135
prenatal (pre-na'tal) before birth, 13
prenatal period (pre-na-tal per'i od) before birth, 138
prepping—preparing the skin before surgery, 70
prepuce (pre'pus) foreskin of clitoris or penis, 277
prime mover—major muscle responsible for an action, 185
primipara (pri-mip'ah-rah) women pregnant for the first time, 1, 12, 136
p.r.n.—whenever necessary, 87
process—bone marking meaning prominence, 178
procidentia (pro"si den'she-ah) uterine prolapse, 138, 273
procto (prok'to) prefix meaning rectum, 57
Proctologic position—position assumed by patient for a rectal examination, 78
progesterone—hormone produced by ovaries, 215
prognosis (prog-no'sis) probable outcome, 17
projection—angle at which X-ray is taken, 307
prolactin (pro-lak'tin) another name for lactogenic hormone, 217
prolapse (pro'laps) descending out of position, 273
prolapses (pro'lap-zes) drops down out of place, 273
pronation (pro-na'shun) radius rotated over ulna palm down, 183

proprioceptors (pro"pre-o-sep'tors) receptors found in muscles and tendons, 224, 226
proteases (pro'te-as-es) enzymes which break down proteins, 242, 249
protein (pro'te-in) an essential body nutrient, 243
prothrombin (pro-throm'bin) a blood protein, part of the blood clotting mechanism, 196
protons (pro'tons) positively charged particles found in nucleus of atoms, 301
prostate gland (pros'tat) gland of male reproductive system which surrounds the urethra. It secretes part of the seminal fluid, 279
prostatectomy (pros"tah-tek'to-me) removal of part of the prostate gland, 271, 279
prosthesis (pros'thĕ-sis) artificial part, 127
proximal (prok'si-mal) closest to a point of attachment, 81
pruritus (proo-ri'tus) itching, 154
pseudo (su'do) prefix meaning false, 51, 61
pseudopodia (su"od-po'de-ah) false feet, 96, 102
Psych (si-k) psychiatry, 73
psychiatrist (si-ki'ah-trist) physician who treats emotional illness, 17, 22
psycho (si'ko) prefix meaning mind, 51, 61
pt.—pint, 88
P.T.—Physical Therapist, 238
PTH—parathyroid hormone, 217
puberty (pu'ber-te) sexual maturity, 212
pubic (pu'bik) pertains to the pubic bone, 83
pubis (pu'bis) bones forming anterior pelvis, 175
pudendum (pu-den'dum) vulva, 277
pulmonary (pul'mo-ner"e) pertaining to the lung, 9
pulmonary artery (pul'mo-nor"e ar"ter-e) blood vessel which carries deoxygenated blood from right ventricle to the lungs, 200
pulmonary embolism (pul'mo-ner"e em'bo-lizm) clot in the lungs, 205
pulmonary tuberculosis (pul'mo-ner"e tuber'ku-lo'sis) infectious disease caused by a bacterium, 170

pulmonary veins (pul′mo-ner″e vans) return blood from lungs to left atrium, 199

pulse (puls) wave of pressure exerted against wall of arteries in response to ventricular systole, 202

pulse pressure (puls presh′ur) difference between systolic and diastolic pressure, 203

Purkinje fibers (pur-kin′jez) terminal fibers of conduction system imbedded in the myocardium, 201

pursed lip breathing—respiratory pattern to allow the patient to more completely empty his lungs on expiration, 292

pustule (pus′tul) small elevation filled with pus, 153

py (pi) prefix meaning pus, 62

pyelitis (pi″ĕ-li′tis) inflammation of the renal pelvis, 266

pyloric (pi-lor′ik) pertaining to or near pylorus, 247

pylorus (pi-lor′us) narrowed portion of stomach which connects to small intestine, 247

pyogenic (pi″o-jen′ik) pus producing, 105

pyorrhea (pi′o-re-ah) pus from alveolus, 245

pyosalpinx (pi″o-sal′pinks) pus in the Fallopian Tubes, 281

pyothorax (pi″o-tho′raks) pus in the intrapleural space, 170

Pyramids (per′ah-mids) macroscopic mounds of collecting tubule found in the medulla of the kidney, 263

pyre (pi′re) prefix meaning fever, 64

pyretic (pi-ret′ik) feverish, 150

pyretogenous (pi″rĕ-toj′ĕ-nus) fever producing, 146, 150

pyrexia (pi-rek′se-ah) elevation of temperature above normal, 105, 150

pyuria (pi-u′re-ah) pus in the urine, 259

q.d.—every day, 88
Q.I.D.—four times a day, 88
q.n.—every night, 88
q.o.d.—every other day, 88

q.s.—as much as required, 88
qt.—quart, 88
quadrant (kwod′rant) refers to the four imaginary sections of the surface of the abdomen, 81

R.—respiration, 75, 77
R—roentgen rays, 302
radi (ra′de) prefix meaning ray, 64
radiable (ra′de-ah-bl) capable of X-ray examination, 304
radial (ra′de-al) pertaining to or near radius, 205
radiant (ra′de-ant) spreading out, 300, 305
radical mastectomy (rad′i-kal mas-tek′to-me) surgical removal of entire breast, the underlying muscle, and lymph node, 150
radioactive cobalt—radioactive isotope of cobalt, 311
radioactive iodine—radioactive isotope of iodine, 311
radioactive phosphorus—radioactive isotope of phosphorus, 311
radiogram (ra′de-o-gram) X-ray picture, 302
radiography (ra″de-og′rah-fe) photography by X-ray, 302
radiologist (ra″de-ol′o-jist) a physician trained in radiologic technique, 18
radiology (ra″de-ol′o-je) study or science of radiation, 28
radiolucent (ra″de-o-lu′sent) permits passage of X-rays, 300, 302
radiopaque (ra″de-o-pah′k) impervious to radiation, non-penetrable, 300, 303
radioscopy (ra″de-os′ko-pe) examination of deep body structure by X-rays, 304
radiosensitive (ra″de-o-sen′si-tiv) effected by radiation, 310
radiotherapy (ra″de-o-ther′ah-pe) radiation used in treatment of disease, 40, 300, 301
radium (ra′de-um) a naturally occurring radioactive element, 300
rales (rahls) respiratory patterns with moist breathing sounds, 168

rarefied (rar'e-fid) areas of lessened density, 304

RBC—red blood cells, 75, 196, 198

R.C.T.—respiratory care therapist, 72

receptors (re-sep'tors) peripheral nerve endings responsive to stimuli, 226

recessive—when used with genes, not expressed, 133

Rectocele (rek'to-sel) a weakening of the posterior vaginal wall, 277

rectum (rek'tum) final 6-8 inches of alimentary tract, 249

recuperating (rĕ-kŭ'per-a-tĭng) recovering, 188

recuperative (re-ku'per-a-tive) recovery, 188

reduction—realignment of a fractured bone, 188

reflex—simplest nervous mechanism, 228

reflex arc (re'fleks) a sequence of events resulting in a reflex response, 228

Registered Nurse—a person educated in nursing techniques who is licensed by the State to practice nursing, 23, 172

regular diet—unrestricted hospital diet, 244

Rehab—rehabilitation, 73

remission (re-mish'un) period of decreased severity of symptoms, 126

ren (ren) prefix meaning kidney, 62

renal (re'nal) pertaining to or near the kidney, 206

renal colic (rĕ'nahl kol'ĭk) acute paroxysmal intermittent pain, 267

renal fascia (re'nal fash'e-ah) fibrous capsule surrounding the kidneys, 260

renal suppression (re'nahl su'pre-shun) kidney failure, 266

reni (ren'ĭ) prefix meaning kidney, 265

renin (re'nin) an enzyme secreted by the renal cells, 264

renipelvic (ren''ĭ pel'vĭk) pertaining to the renal pelvis, 265

renitis (ren'i-tis)inflammation of the kidney, 265

renography (re-nog'rah-fe) X-ray study of the kidney, 265

renopathy (re-nop'ah-the) any disease of the kidneys, 257, 265

respiration (res''pi-ra'shun) process of bringing oxygen into body and expelling carbon dioxide, 160

respiratory (re-spi'rah-to''re) airway of respiratory system, 160

reticular connective tissue (rĕ-tĭk'u-lar) delicate connective tissues, 140

retro (ret'ro) prefix meaning backward, 62

retroflexion (ret''ro-flek'shun) uterus bent backwards, 273

retrograde pyelogram (ret'ro-grad pi'ĕ-lo-gram'') nephrogram, 267

retroperitoneal space (ret''ro-per'ĭ-to-ne'al spas) area of the anterior cavity behind the peritoneum, 130, 139

retroversion (ret''ro-ver'zhun) entire uterus tipped backwards, 273

R.H.D.—rheumatic heart disease, 73

rheumatoid arthritis (roo'mah-toid) inflammation of synovial joints characterized by periods of remission and exacerbation, 189

rhinal (ri'nal) pertaining to the nose, 162

rhinorrhea (ri''no-re'ah) excess mucus discharge, 169

ribosomes (ri'bo-soms) cell organelle involved with protein synethesis, 131

ribs (ribs) flat bones forming part of the thorax, 175

RICU—Respiratory Intensive Care Unit, 294

right lymphatic duct—drains lymph from right side of the head, neck, right arm and shoulder, 206

RLQ—right lower quadrant, 81

R/O—rule out, 84, 86

roentgen rays (rent'gen ra-is) X-rays, 302

roentgenism—radiotherapy, 310

roentgenogram (rent'gen-o-gram) a radiogram, 303

roentgenography (rent''gĕ-nog'rah-fe) photography by X-ray, 300, 302

rrhea—suffix meaning flow, discharge, 51, 54

R.T.—radiologic technologist, 72

Rubella (roo-bel'ah) German measles, 99
Rubeola (roo-be'o-lah) 7 day measles, 99
rubor (roo'bor) a reddening of the skin, 151
RUQ—right upper quadrant, 81

saccharides (sak'ah-ridz) carohydrates, 242
sacrospinalis (sa"kro-spi'nal-is) muscle extending from sacrum to occiput, 185
sacrum (sa'krum) bone of the lower part of the vertebral column which articulates with oscoxae, 175
salpinges (sal-ping'jes) passageway for ova and sperm), 273
salpingitis (sal"pin-ji'tis) inflammation of the oviducts, 280
saliva (sah-li'vah) a thin watery liquid produced by salivary glands, 244
salivary glands (sal'i-ver-e) excretory glands that produce saliva, 244
saprophytes (sap'ro-fits) heterotrophs that live on dead matter, 96, 100
sacral (sa'kral) pertaining to the sacrum, 204
S.A. node—sinuatrial node, 201
scales—thin flakes of epithelial cells, 155
scanner—radioactive isotope detector, 311
scapulae (skap'u-le) shoulder blades, 175
scar—a strong fibrous connecting tissue, 157
sciatica (si-at'i-kah) inflammation of sciatic nerve, 224, 236
scintillation (sin'ti-la-shun) emission of charged particles, 311
scintiscan (sin'ti-skan) image produced by scintiscanner, 312
scintiscanner (sin'ti-skan-r) a special whole body scanner which picks up gamma radiation from radioactive isotopes, 311
scler (skler') prefix meaning hard, 59
scoliosis (sko"leo'sis) lateral curviture of the spine, 189
scope—suffix meaning examine, 64
scout film—preliminary, 304
scrotum (skro'tum) sac-like pouch that holds the male gonads, 278

sebaceous (se-ba'shus) glands found in skin which secrete an oily substance, 147
sebum (see'bum) oily secretion of sebaceous glands, 147
second degree burns—epidermis is destroyed and vesicates form, 155
second trimester—months four to six of pregnancy, 135
secondary syphilis—period of syphilitic disease when the organisms have invaded the organs of the body, 280
secundines (se'kun"dinz) amniotic sac or membranes which surround baby in utero, 136
select diet—another name for regular or house diet, 244
semen (se'men) composite fluid composed of sperm, mucus and other alkaline secretions, 278
semilunar (sem'i-lu-nar) half moon, 200
seminal fluid (sem'inahl) composite fluid of sperm, mucus and other alkaline secretion, 278
seminal vessicles (sem"i-nahl) Pouch-like sacs which are found on the posterior wall of the bladder. They secrete part of the seminal fluid, 279
seminiferous tubules (sem"i-nif'er-us) tubules which form the testes in which the sperm is formed, 279
semi-permeable—allowing selective passage, 194
sensitizing contact—the first contact with an allergen, 154
sensorium (sen-so're-um) area of brain which perceives sensations, 149
sensory (sen'so-re) pertaining to sensation, fibers which carry messages toward the central nervous system, 227
sensory perceptions (sen'so-re per-sep'shuns) awareness, 224
sepsis (sep'sis) infection, 96
septicemia (sep"ti-se'me-ah) bacteria reproducing in the blood stream, 105
septum (sep'tum) dividing portion, 162
serous fluid (se'rus floo'id) thin watery fluid produced by serous membrane, 139

shoulder girdle—includes scapulae and clavicles, 175
siblings (sĭb'lings) brothers and sisters, 77
Sig or S.—label, 88
simple mastectomy (sĭm-pl mas'tek'to-me) removal of breast tissue, 150
singultus (sing-ul'tus) hiccoughs or involuntary respirations due to spasms of diaphram, 168
sinoatrial mass or node (si'no-a'tre-al) special nodal tissue which acts as pacemaker for the heart, 201
sinus (si'nus) cavity, 178
Sippy diet (sip'e) frequent feeding of milk and cream gradually progressing to include eggs, 244
skeletal muscle—a type of muscle which serves in movement, also known as voluntary or striated, 174
skull—bones of cranium and face, 181
skull plate—X-ray of skull, 239
smooth muscle—a type of muscle forming the walls of organs, also known as visceral or involuntary muscle, 142
S.O.B.—shortness of breath, 77
sodium chloride (so'de-um klo'rid) salt, 197-198, 257
soma (so'mah) body, 227
somatic afferent fibers (so-mat'ik af'er-ent fibers) nerve fibers transmitting messages from body to central nervous system, 227
somatic efferent fibers—conduct messages from the central nervous system to skeletal muscles, 228
somatotrophic hormone (so"mah-to-tro'fik) an anterior pituitary hormone which stimulates growth, 217
somni (som'ni) suffix meaning sleep, 57
S.O.S.—if necessary, 88
spec. (spek') specimen, 87
specie (spes'i) particular type of microbe, 102
specimen (spes'i-men) sample of body tissues or fluids, 24
speculum (spek'u-lum) instrument to enlarge a body opening, 69, 79
sperm (sperm) male gamete, 133

spermatic cord (sper-mat'ik) vas deferous and blood vessels and nerves leading from scrotum into pelvis, 279
spermatogenesis (sper'mah-to-jen'e-sis) sperm production, 271
sphenoid (sfe'noid) bone which forms inferior and lateral sides of skull, 163
sphenoidal (sfe-noi'dal) pertains to the sphenoid bone, 163
sphgmomanometer (sfig'mo-mah-nom'e-ter) instrument to measure blood pressure, 69, 79, 193, 203
"spilled over"—excreted, 221
spine—backbone or vertebral column, 177
spirillum (spi-ril'um) spiral shaped bacterium, 100
spirometer (spi-rom'e-ter) volume measuring instrument, 160, 166
spirochete (spi'ro-ket) bacteria that are tightly controlled, 100
splenic (splen'ik) pertaining to or near the spleen, 206
spores (spors) resistent microbial forms, 102
sputum (spu'tum) mucus from the lungs, 171
squamosal suture (skwa'mos-ahl soo'cher) line of union between parietal and temporal bones, 178
squamous (skwa'mus) scale like, 147
S.S.E.—soapsuds enema, 87
stable (sta'bl) refers to an atom which does not easily go into combination with other atoms, 301
staphylo (staf'i-lo) prefix meaning clustered, 101
staphylococcus epidermis (staf'i-lo-kok'us ep"i-der-mi-dis) organism commonly found on the skin, 101
stat—at once, 88
sterile (ster'il) no living organisms present; unable to reproduce, 42
sterilized (ster'i-lized) condition of being sterile, 108
sternocleidomastoid (ster"no-kli"do-mas'toid) muscle located in the neck attached to the sternum of the temporal bone, 174, 185

sternum (ster'num) breast bone, 175
stertor (ster'tor) snoring type of respirations, 168
STH—somatotrophic hormone, 217
stimulus (stim'u-lus) something which excites the nerve causing it to transmit a nerve impulse, 226
stomach (stum'ak) a dilated portion of the G.I. tract, 246
strepto (strep'to) prefix meaning twisted, 101
Streptococcus hemolyticus (strep"to-kok'us he"mo-lit'ik-us) a very virulent microbe, 101
striated muscle (stri'a-ted) another name for voluntary or skeletal muscle, 142, 184
stricture (strik'tūr) narrowing of a tube or passageway, 262
stroke—cerebrovascular accident, damage to the blood vessels of the brain, 9
sub (sub) prefix meaning under, 61
subarachnoid space (sub-ah-rak'noid) space between arachnoid mater and pia mater filled with spinal fluid, 140
subdural (sub-du'ral) potential space between dura mater and arachnoid mater, 231
sucrase (soo'kras) intestinal enzyme acts to convert sucrose to monossachride, 248
sucrose (soo'kros) a disaccharide, 248
suctioning (suk'shun-ing) withdrawing fluid, 294
sudoriferous glands (soo"do-rif'er-us) sweat glands, 146, 147
sulcus (sul'kus) indentation between two gyri, 234
superior (soo-pēr'e-or) toward head end of the body, 81
superior vena cava (soo-pēr'e-or ve'nah ka-vah) vein which drains blood into right atrium from head, neck and extremities, 199
supination (soo"pi-na'shun) position with ulna and radius parallel, palm up, 183
supine (soo'pin) lying face upward, 78
supine mediolateral—patient in lying position, during a mediolateral X-ray exposure, 307
supplemental volume (su'ple-men-tal) amount of air that can be forced out of the lungs after a normal inspiration, 167
supra (soo'prah) prefix meaning above, 62
suprarenally (soo"prah-re'nah-li), above the kidney, 212
surgeon (ser"jen) a doctor who treats patients with conditions that respond best to operations with instruments, 2
surgery (se'jĕr-e) the branch of medicine that treats disease by operative procedures with instruments, 2, 20
sutures (soo'cherz) materials which hold incisions together until healing takes place; pertaining to bone marking, means bone union, particularly relating to the skull, 178, 188
S.V.C.—superior vena cava, 199
symbiosis (sim"bi-o'sis) refers to the relationship which exists between organisms, 100
symmetrical (sem"me'tri-kal) two sides the same, 232
sympathetic (sim"pah-thet'ik) refers to one division of the autonomic nervous system, 228
Syphilis (sif'i-lis) a serious venereal disease, 279
symphysis pubis (sim'fi-sis pu'bis) band of connective cartilage between two pubic bones, 175
synarthrotic (sin"ar-thrak'tic) immoveable joints, 181
synergistic (sin"er-jist'ik) enhancing the action of others, 174, 185
synapse (sin'aps) space between axon of one neuron and dendrites of others, 226
syncope (sing'ko-pe) faint, 238
synovial fluid (si-no've-al floo'id) lubricating liquid produced by synovial membrane of movable joint, 140
synovial joints (si-no've-al) diathrotic joints, 181
systole (sis'to-le) contraction of cardiac muscle, 202
systolic (sis'tal-ik) pertaining to systole, 203
synthesis (sin'thĕ-sis) production or formation, 131
synthesized (sin'thĕ-si'zd) produced, 213

T & A—tonsillectomy and adenoidectomy, 164
tab—tablet, 88
tabes dorsalis (ta′bez dor-sa′lis) progressive wasting of spinal cord, 280
tachy (tak-e) prefix meaning fast, 59
tachycardia (tak″e-kar′de-ah) rapid heart rate, 127, 202
tachypnea (tak″ip-ne′ah) respiratory pattern of rapid shallow respirations, 168
taking a plate—production of radiograms, 304
talipes (tal′i-pēz) clubfoot, 189
target organ—organ affected by a hormone, 213
Tbsp. or T.—tablespoon, 88
telencephalon (tel″en-sef′ah-lon) cerebrum, 233
teletherapy (tel″e-ther′ah-pe) radiation ionization toward a patient from a distance, 311
tendons (ten′dons) fibrous band of connective tissue which attaches skeletal muscle to bones, 174, 185
tertiary syphilis (ter′she′a-re sif′i lis) third stage of syphilis, 280
testes (tes′tez) endocrine glands located in male scrotal sac, 214, 215
testosterone (tes-tos′te-rōn) hormone produced by testes, 215
tetanus (tet′ah-nus) another name for the disease "lockjaw," 100
tetany (tet′ah-ne) severe prolonged muscle spasm, 188
thalamus (thal′ah-mus) superior portion of diencephalon, major relay center for sensory input, 233
therapeutic (ther″ah-pu′tik) effective in the treatment of disease, 17, 18
therapeutic regime—planned treatment program, 1, 2
thermography (ther-mog′rah-fe) technique used to identify actively growing tissues by the heat they produce, 152
third degree burns—epidermis and dermis are destroyed and underlying tissues may have irreversible damage, 155
third trimester—months seven to nine of pregnancy, 135

thoraco (tho-rah-ko) relating to chest or thorax, 64
thoracentesis (tho″rah-sen-te′sis) drainage of the chest, 170
thoracic (tho′ra sik) pertaining to the chest, 64, 189
thoracic duct (tho-ras′ik dukt) large lymphatic muscle which drains lymph from left side of body, right trunk, and legs, 206
thorax (tho′raks) chest, 64, 81
thrombin (throm′bin) substance forms from the interaction of thromboplastin and prothrombin, 196
thrombo (throm′bo) prefix meaning clot, 52
thromboplastin (throm″bo-plas′tin) located in thrombocytes, an element in the blood clotting mechanism, 196
thrombus (throm′bus) a clot, 196
thyroid cartilage (thi′roid kar′ti-lij) largest cartilage of larynx, 165
thyroid gland (thi-roid) endocrine gland located in the neck near the thyroid cartilage, 214
thyrotropic releasing factor (thi″ro-trop′ik) substance secreted by brain which stimulates release of TSH from anterior pituitary, 215
thyroxin (thi″rok′sin) hormone which is produced by thyroid gland, 219
tibial (ti′be-al) pertaining to or near tibia, 205
tic douloureux (tik doo-loo-roo′) a condition of unknown etiology effecting the trigeminal nerve, 229
T.I.D.—three times per day, 88
tidal volume (ti′dal) volume of air which flows in and out with each normal respiratory movement, 167
tissues (tish′uz) group of cells performing a similar function, 138
T.I.A.—transitory ischemic attack, 208
tomogram (to′mo-gram) film obtained during tomography, 309
tomography (to-mog′rah-fe) special radiographic technique providing images of the body sections, 300, 309
tonsillectomy (ton″si-lek′to-me) removal of tonsils, 164

GLOSSARY 367 *

tonus (to'nus) steady state of partial muscle contraction, 185
tox (toks) prefix meaning poison, 62
toxins (tok'sins) poisonous products, 103
toxoids (tok'soids) weakened toxins, 107
tract (trakt) passageway, 98
tracheobronchial tree (tra"ke-o-brong'ke-ahl) conduction passageway for air, 295
tracheostomy (tra"ke-ot'o-me) opening into the trachea, 289
tracheotomy (tra"ke-ot'o-me) surgical opening into the trachea, 127
traction (trak'shun) pulling apart, 188
transducers (trans-du-sers) organ in which nervous energy becomes chemical energy, 213
transverse (trans-vers') imaginary line which divides the body into superior and inferior parts, 81
traumas (traw'mahs) a wound or injury, 125
Trendelenberg position—patient tilted so head is lower than trunk, 78
Treponema pallidum (trep"o-ne'mah pal'i-dum) organism which causes syphilis, 103
TRF—thyrotropin releasing factor, 215
triceps brachii (tri'seps bra'ke-i) muscle of posterior upper arm, 185
tricuspid (tri-kus'pid) pertaining to the three-flapped valve between right atrium and ventricle, 199
trigeminal (tri-jem'i-nal) has three divisions, name of cranial nerve five, 229
trigone (tri'gon) triangular area in base of bladder formed by the two ureters entering and urethra leaving, 261
trochanter (tro-kan'ter) a broad, flat process on the femur, 177
trunk—body, 81
tsp.—teaspoon, 88
TSH—thyrotropic stimulating hormone produced by pituitary gland, 215, 217
tubercle (tu'ber-kl) nodule formed by the tubercle bacillus, 103
tubercle bacillus (tu'ber-kl bah-sil'us) microorganisms causing tuberculosis, 103

tuberosity (tu"be-ros'i-te) bone marking meaning large, rounded, irregular projection, 178
tumors (tu'mors) neoplasms or new growth, 124
tunica (tu'ni-kah) covering or coat, 203
tunica adventitia (tu'ni-kah ad'ven-ti'ah) outer layer of vascular wall, 204
tunica intima (tu'ni-kah in'te-mah) innermost wall of the vessel, 203
Tunica media (tu'ni-kah me-di-ah) muscular layer of vessel wall, 204
turgid (tur'jid) firm, 278

UA—urine analysis, 87
ulcer (ul'ser) open sore or crater, 153
umbilical cord (um-bil'i-kal kord) structure which attaches the fetus to the placenta, 134
umbilicus (um-bil'e-kus) navel, 69, 81
upper gastrointestinal series—radiographic examination of stomach and intestines; barium swallow, 28
urea (u-re'ah) a protein waste product, 16, 259
uremia (u-re'me-ah) condition which results from renal failure, 266
uremic frost (u-re'mik) accumulation of uric acid on the skin, forming a white powder, 266
urethra (u-re'thrah) mucus lined tube leading from the urocyst, 262
urethritis (u"re-thri'tis) inflammation of the urethra, 280
U.R.I.—upper respiratory infection, 76
uric acid (u'rik) a metabolic waste product, 259
urinalysis (u'ri-nal'i-sis) examination of urine, 113, 126, 259
urinary sphincter—a round muscle guarding the bladder exit, 261
urine (u'ri-n) a liquid waste produced by kidneys, 142
uro, uria (u'ro) (u'riah) relating to urine, 62
uro (u'ro) prefix meaning urine, 62
urocyst (u'ro-sist) urinary bladder, 260
urodynia (u"ro-din'e-ah) painful urination, 265

* 368 GLOSSARY

urologist (u-rol'o-jist) physician who treats problems of the urinary tract, 22, 265

uromancy (u'ro-man'se) prognosis based on urine examination, 257

U.R.S.—upper respiratory system, 162

urticaria (ur"ti-ka're-ah) reddened patches called "hives," 155

uterine fundus—upper rounded portion of uterus above the entrance of the fallopian tubes, 273

uterus (u'ter-us) womb, 134, 273

uvula (u'vi-lah) small tab of mucous membrane-covered muscle found between oral cavity and oral pharynx, 164

vaccines (vak'sēns) weakened antigens, 107

vaginitis (vaj"i-ni'tis) inflammation of the vagina,

vagus (va'gus) 10th cranial nerve which carries impulses to the viscera and slows heart rate, 280

valves (valvs) folds which temporarily close a passageway, 199

varicella (var"i-sel'ah) chickenpox, 99

variola (vah-ri'o-lah) smallpox, 99

vas (vas) prefix meaning vessel, 59

vascular (vas'ku-lar) with many blood vessels, 163

vasculature (vas'ku-lah-tūr") system of vessels, 193

vas deferens (vas def'er-enz) the tube which carries sperm from the epididymis into the pelvis, 278, 279

V.D.—venereal disease, 76

V.D.R.L.—Venereal Disease Research Laboratory, 75

vector (vek'tor) animal carrier of microbes, 109

vegetative nervous system (vej'ĕ-ta"tive)

veins (vāns) blood vessels which return blood to heart, 200

venereal disease (vĕ-nĕ're-al) communicable disease easily transmitted through direct sexual intercourse, 279

venipuncture (ven"i-pungk'tur) to puncture a vein, 205

ventilation (ven"ti-la'shun) process of supplying with fresh air, 171

ventilators—machines which assist in ventilation, 284, 288

ventral (ven'tral) front or anterior, 81

ventricles (ven'tri-kls) pertaining to the heart, lower chambers; pertaining to cerebral, cavities within the brain filled with spinal fluid, 198, 231

venules (ven'ūlz) small veins, 203

verbal apraxia (ver-bal ah-prak'se-ah) inability to make sounds, 238

vertebrae (ver'tĕ-bra) backbone, 175

vesicle (ves'ikl) blister, 153, 155

vestibule (ves'ti-bul) area of external female reproductive organs enclosed by the labia minora, 277

vibrissae (vi"bris'ē) short coarse hairs found in the external nares, 104

view—angle at which x-ray is taken, 307

view box—film illuminator, 248

villi (vil'i) finger-like projection, 248

viral neutralizing (vi'ral nu'tral-iz-ing) antibodies which inactivate viruses, 106

virulent (vir'u-lĕnt) strongly pathogenic; exceedingly harmful, 101

viscera (vis'er-ah) organs, 142

visceral (vis'ser-al) pertaining to the organs; referring to a membrane, means the layer next to the organs, 140, 142

visceral afferent fibers (vis'er-al af'er-ent fi'bers) fibers transmitting messages from organs to Central Nervous System, 227

visceral efferent fibers (vis'er-al ef'er-ent) conduct messages from the central nervous system to the cardiac muscle, smooth muscle and glands, 228

visceral receptors (vis'er-al re-sep'tors) receptors found in the organs, 226

viscerotropic (vis"ero-trop'ik) affecting the viscera, 98

vital signs (vi'tal) living signs such as tempera-

GLOSSARY 369 *

ture, pulse, respiration, and blood pressure, 21, 168
V.O.—verbal orders, 87, 199
vocal cords—folds of tissue found in larynx associated with voice production, 165
voiding (void-ing) the act of emptying the bladder, 260
volume ventilators—ventilator that delivers a specific amount of air to patient, 291
voluntary (vol'un-tār"e) name applied to skeletal muscles, 142, 184
v.s.—vital signs, 75, 77
vulva (vul'vah) external female genitalia, 271

WBC—white blood cell, 75, 198
weaned (wēnd) gradually removed from dependence, 295

wt.—weight, 77
wheals (hwēls) local areas of edema and itching, 155
white matter—composed mainly of myelinated axons, 232
wks.—weeks, 77
womb (wo͞om) uterus, 271

X-ray (ek's-rā) common jargon for radiogram; short, penetrating wave lengths, 300
X-ray department (ek's-rā) area of hospital where radiologic techniques are carried out, 28

zygote (zi'got) name given to the early stage of fetal development, 134